Medical Innovation and Bad Outcomes:

Legal, Social, and Ethical Responses

Medical Innovation and Bad Outcomes:

Legal, Social, and Ethical Responses

Edited by
Mark Siegler
and by
Stephen Toulmin
Franklin E. Zimring
Kenneth F. Schaffner

Published in cooperation with
The American Society of Law & Medicine and
The Center for Clinical Medical Ethics
University of Chicago

Health Administration Press
Ann Arbor, Michigan
1987

Library of Congress Cataloging-in-Publication Data

Medical innovation and bad outcomes.

   At head of title: Center for Clinical Medical Ethics at the Univer-
sity of Chicago.
   Papers presented at a conference at the University of Chicago in
May, 1985.
   Includes index.
   1. Products liability—Drugs—United States—Congresses. 2. Prod-
ucts liability—Medical instruments and apparatus—United States—
Congresses. 3. Medicine—Research—Law and legislation—United
States—Congresses. 4. Medical innovations—Social aspects—
United States—Congresses 5. Medical ethics—United States—
Congresses. I. Siegler, Mark, 1941- II. University of Chicago.
Center for Clinical Medical Ethics. [DNLM: 1. Ethics, Medical—
congresses. 2. Quality of Health Care—congresses. 3. Technology
Assessment, Biomedical—congresses. W 84.1 M4893 1985]
KF1297.D7M43   1987   346.7303'82   86-14863
ISBN 0-910701-15-6   347.306382

Health Administration Press
1021 East Huron Street
Ann Arbor, Michigan 48104-9990

To Anna

And it is only for their intentions that men can be held responsible. The ultimate effects of whatever they do are far beyond their control.

Joseph Conrad, *Chance*

Contents

Contributors

Kurt Baier, Ph.D.
Distinguished Service Professor
  of Philosophy
University of Pittsburgh

Baruch S. Blumberg, M.D., Ph.D.
Associate Director for Clinical
  Research
Fox Chase Cancer Center
University Professor of Medicine
  and Anthropology
University of Pennsylvania

Alexander Morgan Capron, LL.B.
Norman Topping Professor of Law,
  Medicine, and Public Policy
The Law Center
University of Southern California

Patricia M. Danzon, Ph.D.
Associate Professor of Health Care
  and Insurance
Wharton School
University of Pennsylvania

Richard A. Epstein, J.D.
James Parker Hall Professor
School of Law
University of Chicago

Charles M. Gray, Ph.D.
Professor
Department of History
University of Chicago

James M. Gustafson, B.D., Ph.D.
University Professor of Theological
  Ethics
University of Chicago

Paul Meier, Ph.D.
Ralph and Mary Otis Isham
  Distinguished Service Professor
Departments of Statistics and
  Pharmacological and
  Physiological Sciences
University of Chicago

Kenneth F. Schaffner, M.D., Ph.D.
Professor of History and
  Philosophy of Science
Adjunct Professor of Medicine
University of Pittsburgh

Mark Sheldon, Ph.D.
Associate Professor of Philosophy
Adjunct Associate Professor
  of Medicine
Indiana University, Gary

Mark Siegler, M.D.
Professor of Medicine
Director, Center for Clinical
   Medical Ethics
Pritzker School of Medicine
University of Chicago

Alvin R. Tarlov, M.D.
President
Henry J. Kaiser Family Foundation
Menlo Park, California

Stephen Toulmin, Ph.D.
Professor
Committee on Social Thought and
   Department of Philosophy
Associate Director, Center for
   Clinical Medical Ethics
University of Chicago

Alan J. Weisbard, J.D.
Assistant Professor of Law
Cardozo School of Law
Yeshiva University

Franklin E. Zimring, J.D.
Professor of Law
School of Law (Boalt Hall)
Director, Earl Warren Legal
   Institute
University of California, Berkeley

Preface

Technological innovations generate benefit and harm. New products and new technologies—in both medicine and industry—are developed in the hope that benefits will outweigh harm, but with an awareness that some harm is likely to occur *as a result of* the innovation. Often, the incidence of bad outcomes is very low (for example, in the case of the polio vaccine or commercial jet airplanes), but at times the incidence of bad outcomes is tragically high (for example, diethylstilbestrol, asbestos use, or the connection between tonsillar irradiation and thyroid cancer).

This volume of commissioned essays uses modern medicine as an instance of technological innovation to examine how our society should establish liability and compensation rules for individuals who experience bad outcomes that may have been caused by the use of a medical innovation. Recent Congressional sessions have weighed bills that address liability and compensation problems arising from injuries suffered in medical, industrial, and environmental settings. Considerable debate has been generated by recent legislative and judicial efforts to deal with, for example, asbestosis, Agent Orange, DES, and the Dalkon Shield.

The essays clarify the fundamental conceptual issues of causation, moral responsibility, and legal responsibility—issues that appear to underlie efforts to change our current public policy regarding liability and compensation or, for that matter, that would support the decision to live with the system we now have.

A recurring tension here, and in policy debates on these issues, relates to the following question: Should the "progressive" nature of American society in the 1980s (and of American medicine of the 1980s) encourage us to rethink our views of moral and legal responsibility? Should we move from the negative view of responsibility for a bad outcome to a more positive view of responsibility for improving the science and practice of medicine? Should this positive view of responsibility modify compensation approaches for those who suffer unanticipated (and non-negligent) medical maloccurrences?

The essays in section 1 describe the progressive forces in American society, in medicine, and in medical research that would argue for a new, positive view of responsibility. Section 2 explores the fundamental concepts of causation and moral and legal responsibility, while section 3 examines alternative legal perspectives for establishing liability. Section 4 concludes by drawing upon the conceptual and legal analyses in sections 2 and 3 to offer policy recommendations for compensating those injured as a result of innovative medical care. These essays aim to clarify the basic concepts that should be taken into account in searching for a just and efficient system for assessing liability and for providing compensation.

HISTORY OF THE PROJECT

This research project brought together individuals from many disciplines: medicine, law, economics, statistics, history, philosophy, and public policy. The interactions among participants were useful and productive, largely because the central issue—how to provide just and efficient compensation for those who suffer as a result of medical innovation—was important and of genuine concern to each scholar involved. This may be the all too obvious secret for good interdisciplinary collaboration: find a topic that has a legitimate and pressing interest for a number of thoughtful people who represent a number of fields.

The project began with informal discussions between Mark Siegler and Kenneth Schaffner. A preliminary proposal was submitted to the Ethics and Values in Science and Technology program of the National Science Foundation and National Endowment for the Humanities, and Arthur Norberg, then director of the EVIST program, encouraged further development of these ideas. Stephen Toulmin and Franklin Zimring were soon added to the project, and a formal proposal was resubmitted to the EVIST program. Rachelle Hollander, then director, provided rigorous and constructive criticism of our original proposal. In 1982, the final research project was organized with financial support from the EVIST program.

The initial research involved an interdisciplinary faculty seminar at the University of Chicago. It soon became clear that additional scholars should be added to the core group, and Kurt Baier, Baruch Blumberg, Alexander Capron, Patricia Danzon, and Alan Weisbard graciously agreed to join our efforts. The research project concluded with a public conference at the University of Chicago in May 1985. At that time, the participants in this project presented papers which were the results of several years of interdisciplinary discussion and research. Thus, this book should not be regarded as the proceedings of a conference, but as a collection of commissioned research papers prepared after an extended interdisciplinary effort.

Mark Siegler

Acknowledgments

Projects that are interdisciplinary in scope and involve participants from both sides of the continent generate many debts of gratitude. In contrast to other forms of indebtedness, a debt of gratitude is one which can never be fully discharged, and it is fitting that this is so. Such cherished debts bring to mind all those wonderful persons without whose help and support a project such as this would not have been possible.

I begin by thanking Rachelle Hollander, director of the EVIST program, for her intellectual guidance and nurturance of this research effort. By helping to clarify our original ideas, she helped shape a research agenda that combined clarification of fundamental legal and philosophical concepts with practical public policy concerns.

Many of my colleagues in the University of Chicago-Pritzker School of Medicine provided clinical expertise and served as participants in the research effort. Marc Silverstein, M.D., from the Section of General Internal Medicine, provided a scholarly analysis of the risks and benefits of the hepatitis B vaccine. Leslie DeGroot, M.D., Chief of the Section of Endocrinology at the University of Chicago, reviewed the complex association between tonsillar irradiation and thyroid cancer, a relationship he helped to clarify through meticulous clinical research. Arthur Herbst, M.D., Chairman of the Department of Obstetrics and Gynecology at the University of Chicago, originally described the association between diethylstilbestrol (DES) use in mothers and the development of clear cell carcinomas in DES daughters. He provided our research team with a careful analysis of the DES literature. During the early years of the project, Alan Donagan, Ph.D., was a valued contributor to discussions about the relationship of moral and legal responsibility.

Arthur Rubenstein, M.D., Chairman of the Department of Medicine and a member of the original research group, constantly provided intellectual support, particularly regarding innovations in the area of diabetes. Equally important, however, was his enthusiasm and support for an unusual type of interdisciplinary research effort that would not, I daresay, be encouraged in most leading university departments of medicine in this country.

The concluding public conference of the research group—"Response to Biomedical Innovation: A Legal, Ethical, and Political Analysis"—was held at the University of Chicago, May 16-18, 1985. The meeting would not have been possible without the help of Jonathan Kleinbard, Vice-President for University News and Community Affairs, and of his splendid team, particularly Sharon Rosen and Verna McQuown. Thanks also to Patricia Swanson, Assistant Director for Science Libraries, for providing conference facilities at the new John Crerar Library of the University of Chicago.

Mark Sheldon, Ph.D., Associate Professor of Philosophy at Indiana University Northwest and Adjunct Associate Professor of Medicine at the Indiana University School of Medicine, has been a valued colleague throughout this project. At various stages of the work, Mark served as research associate, conference facilitator, and editorial assistant. In each role, he contributed substantially both to the intellectual content of the work and to the efficiency with which it was completed.

The secretarial support I received throughout this project was magnificent. My sincere thanks go to Evelyn Clark for her assistance in launching the project. Terry Kirkpatrick joined me at the eleventh hour and somehow, miraculously, managed to put it all together in order to complete the book. She knows how much I appreciate her help. Allisyn Gras was a wonderful help, both in managing the conference and in preparing the manuscript. She realizes how much her effort and ebullient spirit are appreciated by all.

And finally, a few words about Patti Bieghler, who did most of the work in organizing the conference, harvesting the manuscripts, and bringing the project to its conclusion. She provided the administrative and emotional glue that held the effort together. She was as competent and successful on this project as she has been on all her other endeavors. I cannot thank her enough for her friendship, diligence, and support.

Alvin Tarlov, M.D., has always been a friend and mentor. His advice and guidance were as valuable as ever. He encouraged the project from its inception and kept me focused on the important policy questions for physicians and for the medical profession.

Financial support for this project was provided by a grant (OSS-8018097) from the EVIST program of the National Science Foundation and the National Endowment for the Humanities. Additional financial support was provided by the Henry J. Kaiser Family Foundation and by the Andrew W. Mellon Foundation. The views expressed are those of the editors and authors and do not necessarily reflect those of the National Science Foundation, the National Endowment for the Humanities, the Kaiser Foundation, or the Mellon Foundation.

Finally, a word of thanks to Dillan, Alison, Richard, and Jessica, and especially to dear Anna, without whose love and support this project would have been neither achievable nor, for that matter, worthwhile.

Mark Siegler

1

Paying the Price of Medical Progress: Causation, Responsibility, and Liability for Bad Outcomes after Innovative Medical Care

Mark Siegler and Mark Sheldon

When a previously untreatable disease is conquered, everyone—physicians, researchers, funding agencies, as well as the public—has a sense of triumph and a touch of justifiable pride. The development of renal dialysis permits more than 50,000 Americans to survive, who, in earlier times, would have died from kidney failure; liver transplantation provides hope to children born with congenital and previously fatal liver disease; new and effective cancer treatments frequently enable physicians to cure diseases, such as Hodgkin's disease, leukemias in children, and testicular cancer, all previously incurable; while the development of effective immunizations against polio, measles, rubella, and hepatitis B have benefited millions of persons. These examples of medical triumph reflect the beneficent goal of medicine: to "do good."

Invariably, however, each of these medical "miracles" brings with it a small number of "bad outcomes," and people suffer harm despite the most conscientious treatment. Every medical innovation has the potential to cause immediate side effects and future injuries that were not foreseeable when the innovation was introduced. This tragic potential for causing harm exists with every medical breakthrough and is recognized by scientists and clinicians as a necessary cost of medical progress.

Of course, the price of a bad outcome is exacted from the individual who suffers the untoward reaction, whereas the benefit of the breakthrough is available to society as a whole.

These observations suggest a range of questions:

1. Should American society continue to encourage further medical progress, or should it opt for a period of retrenchment during which conservative standards of care would prevail?

2. Are the risks associated with medical progress sufficient to outweigh the benefits?

3. For the minority who suffer a bad outcome after receiving innovative medical treatment, who can be said to have "caused" their injury? Who is responsible? Who is liable?

4. Finally, who, if anyone, should compensate those who are injured, and according to what standards?

The general problem addressed in this volume might be stated:

> Who (if anyone) is *responsible* (morally and legally), and who (if anyone) is *liable* for *compensating* an individual who experiences a *bad outcome* which may have been *caused* by the use of a *medical innovation.*

The terms in the above question are ambiguous; no consensus exists about their meaning. Unfortunately, this is more than a semantic problem. Because of this uncertainty, physicians, patients, lawyers, and the courts are often confused about legal liability and moral responsibility for actions taken in the clinical setting. Thus, throughout this volume, the authors examine the central concepts of causation and responsibility as the basis for developing a sound public policy for compensation.

The general problem of determining responsibility and liability is especially troubling in the United States because of three widely shared, but not always harmonious, societal goals:

1. A commitment to improving the medical care of the American people through biomedical research and through the rapid application of medical advances;

2. An inclination to view individuals who experience such bad outcomes as being entitled to compensation from someone;

3. A reluctance to provide compensation to those who are injured based on an entitlement approach.

At present, an imperfect compromise is struck between these conflicting goals by encouraging the use of innovative medical techniques and then by assigning responsibility for bad outcomes to individual physicians and manufacturers according to traditional tort principles rather than to the collective scientific enterprise.

The underlying objective of this book is to help all parties—patients, physicians, manufacturers of drugs and medical devices, insurance companies, lawyers, and judges—to deal more efficiently and fairly with these conflicts than has been possible in the past. The goal is to ensure both the timely application of medical innovations to improve the health of patients, and also, the appropriate compensation for individuals who experience a bad outcome after receiving innovative medical care.

CASE EXAMPLES

The legal and ethical concepts of causation, responsibility, and liability are the intellectual foundation upon which judicial decisions and legislative policy are built. Case studies of medical innovation are useful touchstones for testing general conceptual accounts of causation and responsibility in the light of real cases which generate practical policy concerns. Reference to a few carefully chosen sample cases of medical innovation (some consequences of which were, in retrospect, adjudged to be "bad outcomes") could serve to: (1) encourage clarification of legal and ethical concepts, (2) indicate the existence of practical problems which had not been anticipated at the level of conceptual analysis, and (3) determine whether improvements in conceptual analysis illuminate social and political debate and assist policymakers.

The two cases presented below represent two types of medical innovation: (1) a *new technique* (that is, tonsillar irradiation) and (2) a *new drug* (diethylstilbestrol, DES). Similar cases could have been chosen to examine *new technologies* (such as nuclear magnetic resonance imaging), *new surgical techniques* (such as implantation of the totally artificial heart), or *new vaccines* (such as measles). Also, we could have considered many other recent medical cases associated with varying degrees of bad outcomes, including the polio vaccine, swine flu vaccine, oxygen toxicity and retrolental fibroplasia, drugs such as Selacryn and Oraflex, the Dalkon Shield intrauterine device, and so on.

CRITERIA FOR CASE SELECTION

The two cases to be commented upon meet many of the following criteria:

1. There was an early stage of relative ignorance during which the association between the medical bad outcomes and the medical innovation was not yet fully recognized.

2. There was a later stage of (relative) knowledge in which the "cause" of the bad outcome was discovered, the use of the medical innovation discontinued, but during which there continued a residual, lower percentage of similar maloccurrences. (Some of the most problematic cases are those in which there remains a residual, background, or baseline level of medical maloccurrences, even when the new intervention is discontinued.)

3. Solid pathophysiological knowledge of the effects of the new technology or drug has become available.

4. The cases have been litigated through the appellate stage, so there has been a legal consideration of issues of causation, liability, and compensation.

5. The medical cases are generalizable to the entire range of scientifically and technologically induced medical innovations.

The cases selected raise problems of causation, responsibility, accountability, liability, and compensation which arise in the diverse contexts of the industrial, manufacturing, construction, defense, and transportation sections of the economy.

CASE 1: TONSILLAR IRRADIATION AND THYROID CANCER

In the pre-antibiotic era, tonsillar enlargement and infections associated with this condition were very serious and occasionally life-threatening problems. By the 1920s, radiation therapy was used to treat a variety of benign conditions, including arthritis, skin problems such as acne, lymph gland enlargement, and enlarged tonsils and adenoids. Radiation therapy was viewed by some physicians as a safer alternative than tonsillectomy, particularly for patients who might be at a high risk with surgery. From the 1930s to the early 1950s, a large number of patients (estimates range from 400,000 to 1,000,000 or more) received external X-ray therapy to their tonsils. In the early 1950s, the association between tonsillar irradiation and the subsequent development some 20 years later of thryoid cancer was first noted and brought to the attention of the medical profession by Duffy and Fitzgerald[1] and was confirmed later in studies by Clark and Hempelmann.[2] Initially, several other studies denied this association. Nevertheless, the use of external X-ray therapy to treat enlarged tonsils generally was abandoned after the early 1950s. In the 1970s, several institutions initiated recall programs designed to find and screen people who previously had received neck irradiation. These recall programs were themselves a kind of medical innovation and were controversial because some thought the medical risks of recall were greater than the medical risks of not recalling patients. The reasons for concern were:

1. Since the incidence of unsuspected thyroid cancer in those nonir-radiated individuals who die of causes other than thyroid cancer and who are autopsied may be as high as 6 percent, perhaps the recall-screening programs were detecting only a baseline level of carcinoma in those individuals who had asymptomatic tumors.

2. Since the thyroid scan, which was part of the recall evaluation, included a dose of radiation, perhaps one was doing more harm than good by performing such a diagnostic procedure and exposing patients to additional neck irradiation.

3. Since some recall patients would require surgery, and some might die at surgery, perhaps the risks of surgery were greater than the risks of undetected thyroid cancer.

4. Further, there were large economic costs associated with recalling a large number of patients who had received tonsillar irradiation.

As a result of the information about the relationship between tonsillar irradiation and thyroid cancer, and partially as a result of recall programs, a large number of malpractice suits against physicians and hospitals have been filed by patients who had received tonsillar irradiation and who were found to have thyroid tumors. Many of these suits remain in litigation.

CASE 2: DIETHYLSTILBESTROL (DES)

The DES example relies on a 1971 epidemiological discovery by Herbst, Ulfelder, and Poskanzer.[3] These authors found a strong association between DES exposure in utero and the subsequent development of a rare form of vaginal cancer, clear cell adenocarcinoma.

DES is a synthetic estrogen discovered in England in 1937. It was approved for human use by the Food and Drug Administration (FDA) in 1941 after clinical trials and in 1947 was given FDA approval as an antimiscarriage drug. Studies concerning its efficacy for preventing miscarriage are controversial, but the 1953 study by Dieckmann[4] generally is accepted as demonstrating its ineffectiveness.

Following the appearance of Herbst's report in 1971,[5] a number of epidemiological investigations have been initiated to study the effects of DES. In 1972, Herbst initiated a worldwide registry of women with clear cell adenocarcinoma. By 1980, the registry had identified 425 such cases, but 33 percent had *not* been exposed to DES in utero.

An organization of DES daughters known as DES/Action has estimated that 3 to 6 million mothers took DES and that 1.5 to 3 million daughters were exposed in utero to the synthetic estrogen. Hundreds of suits against drug companies, hospitals, physicians, and pharmacists have been brought and two such suits, the *Sindell* case in California and the *Bichler* decision in New York, have received considerable attention in debates concerning causation, liability, and compensation involving medical maloccurrences relating to new drugs.

These two examples illustrate that ambiguities and potential difficulties arise on at least five levels:

1. In assessing the *cause* of the bad outcomes: Was the medical innovation the causative factor or was the bad outcome the result of the natural course of the medical problem?
2. In attributing *moral blame and legal responsibility* for the patient's bad outcome,
3. In assigning *liability* for damages,
4. In determining who should *compensate* the injured party, and

    5. In *distributing the risks and benefits* of medical innovation fairly and equitably.

WHY EXAMINE THESE ISSUES IN A MEDICAL CONTEXT?

The essays in this volume focus on the problems of causation, liability, and compensation as they arise in medical contexts. Yet, surely, the class of medical mishaps is not unique in giving rise to such difficulties. It is important to note that these questions about medicine are simply a special case of a more general political discussion about how our society should balance the benefits and risks of technological innovation in any sphere.

    When a society is committed in many fields of personal life and public policy, as American society now is, to putting new technologies to work as rapidly as is safe and prudent, such technological innovations (for example, in the design of nuclear power plants or the use of asbestos as a fire-retardant substance) may easily have unforeseeable side effects.

    Individuals injured by exposure to toxic substances in industrial settings or from environmental sources will then claim compensation from industry or government. The scale of this problem is underscored by the fact that in each of the last three Congresses at least ten separate bills designed to address various aspects of the "toxic tort" have been introduced. (The toxic tort is the issue of compensating people who may have been injured by toxic substances that industry or government or medicine have "exposed them to.") Furthermore, two major corporations have sought protection through bankruptcy procedures from claimants and these same companies have established funds to compensate those injured from exposure to asbestos (The Manville Corporation) and from using the Dalkon Shield (A. H. Robins Company). In recent years, other highly publicized toxic tort cases have come to the attention of courts and legislatures: Agent Orange; cancer in uranium miners and military personnel exposed to radiation; the Union Carbide disaster in Bhopal, India; and the demonstration of unanticipated adverse effects with drugs such as Oraflex, Selacryn, and Bendectin.

THE MEDICAL MODEL

The current project focuses primarily on medical situations in which maloccurrences follow innovative treatment. In contrast perhaps to industrial innovations, where caution is the watchword, the medical enterprise appears to be one in which there is a broad consensus among the public and the profession that new, efficacious, and reasonably safe drugs and techniques should be applied as rapidly as possible. But past experience shows that the application of medical innovations is often associated with unanticipated bad outcomes, at least for some individuals; and there is a large volume of litigation (past and present) associated with these medical cases. Many of the issues raised in these medical cases are generalizable to other large societal enterprises involving innovations and risks; and the way in which society deals with the harms that follow the use of medical innovations can serve as a model for dealing with harms that result from industrial and environmental exposures.

Finally, there is a renewed enthusiasm in medicine supported by a variety of powerful interests, including the Congress, manufacturers of new technologies, and the medical profession, and based largely on issues of medical costs, to develop better approaches to assess the safety and efficacy of new medical techniques and technologies. This new emphasis on technology assessment and the unavoidable linkage of new technologies with cost-effectiveness (which presumably includes safety standards) suggests that the issues discussed in this book are particularly important in the current political climate.

THE ORGANIZATION OF THIS BOOK

This collection of invited essays has been assembled into four sections. In section 1, the American medical and research enterprise is scrutinized. Contemporary medicine is seen as a "progressive" component of a "progressive" society. Section 2 examines fundamental questions about causation and responsibility in medicine and the law. Section 3 explores legal theories to establish liability when bad outcomes occur after the use of innovative medical treatments. Section 4 considers alternative systems of compensation for the injured and the public policy implications of these alternatives.

SECTION 1: BAD OUTCOMES FROM MEDICAL INNOVATION:
IMPLICATIONS FOR SCIENCE, MEDICINE, AND SOCIETY

The social and political significance of medical mishaps associated with innovative treatment are best understood by recalling certain historical developments.

Nowadays we take for granted a very close relationship between medical practice and the biologic sciences, but this is a twentieth-century development. Before American medical education was reformed, in the years immediately preceding the First World War, the clinical practices of physicians were (and were generally expected to be) conservative. The approved treatment for dealing with any medical condition was "the routine and accepted practice," and any departure from that standard— "experimentation," as it was called—was legally frowned upon. Until antibiotics came into general use in the 1940s as a weapon against infectious diseases, practicing physicians retained their traditional attitude of suspicion toward science and scientists—"That's all very well in theory. . . ." So, the standing public expectations that all life-threatening conditions will yield in time to scientific research, and that the novel treatments developed by medical scientists will be introduced to general practice with a minimum delay, are historically new features of the period since World War II. Today, for the first time in history, the demand that the "cause" of all pathological states should be diagnosed in scientific terms is not unreasonable.

Describing these broad developments in social-intellectual history reminds us of the context within which the problem of medical mishaps has taken center stage. Modern industrial societies are committed, as never before, to adopting technological innovations wherever these serve the welfare of the individual members. In accepting this general policy, they inevitably expose these individuals to certain novel risks also. In earlier times, the consistent use of "routine and accepted" procedures in all sectors of life had given some people the assurance of knowing in advance both the limited benefits and the limited risks they could expect. Technological progress has raised the stakes on both sides. The availability of new methods holds out the reasonable pros-pect of major new benefits; but, at the same time, it creates the likelihood that unforeseen hazards will harm some fraction of those people who are on the receiving end of these innovations.

In "Technological Progress and Social Policy: The Broader Significance of Medical Mishaps," Stephen Toulmin considers the implications of defining our society as a progressive rather than as a conservative one. Toulmin argues that if it can be shown that ours is a progressive society, technological experi-mentation and innovation in medicine and other spheres would be sanctioned and encouraged. In a conservative society, where almost all effort is directed toward maintaining things as they are, innovation is viewed not only with suspicion, but a departure from standard practice frequently is judged irre-sponsible. By contrast, in a progressive society those who fail to apply the latest techniques may be judged negligent. Toulmin implies that in a progressive society, medical practitioners are not only pressured to provide the newest (reasonably validated) procedures, but are held accountable when they fail to do so.

The compelling question which emerges from Toulmin's analysis— indeed, a question which recurs throughout this volume—is whether the pro-gressive nature of American medicine and our society should modify our philosophical and legal attitudes toward medical maloccurrences and their compensation. If ours can be shown to be a progressive society, should this incline us to a broader notion of liability and compensation than is represented, for example, by the traditional tort-negligence system?

Baruch Blumberg, in "The Scientific Process and the Development of Medical Innovation: The Daedalus Effect," expresses, as Toulmin did, an essentially optimistic viewpoint. He analyzes the dynamics of scientific research in relation to society's demand for both innovation and responsibility. Using the myth of Daedalus as a metaphor for the complex drama of scientific discovery, he presents his own work with hepatitis (for which he received the Nobel Prize) as an example of painstakingly constructed research which raises ethical issues that have not existed before. Blumberg argues that it is important to distinguish medical problems that result when research is done inadequately or not done at all from problems that are "part of the scientific process itself . . . a consequence of the best-designed and -executed study." Still, he emphasizes that good scientific research remains committed to dealing with ethical dilemmas that arise in the course of the research and often succeeds in resolving these issues through further scientific investigation.

Paul Meier's essay, "The Scientific and Ethical Foundation of Medical Innovations," sounds a cautionary note about applying medical innovations cavalierly. Meier argues that many medical innovations that have become standard practice are not founded on adequate scientific assessment and validation. He suggests that the underlying problem may not be a tension between innovation and standard practice, but rather may be the frequently inadequate scientific validation of *both* sorts of practice. He regards this as both a scientific and ethical failing. Through a series of carefully selected examples, Meier argues that one way out of this dilemma is to fulfill a scientific and ethical responsibility to establish all clinical practice on the basis of well-designed and well-executed clinical trials.

Alvin Tarlov's reflections in the "Microsocial Influences on the Use of Medical Innovations" reinforce the views of Toulmin and Meier. Tarlov describes the many incentives in medical training and practice that traditionally have encouraged medical innovation and the relatively few countervailing forces that have encouraged conservatism. Medicine, in Tarlov's view, clearly conforms to the progressive vision of society developed by Toulmin. Further, Tarlov refers to studies of differences in physicians' practice patterns that suggest that many innovative practices may emerge as local options precisely because they have not been scientifically assessed and validated. Tarlov advocates better outcome studies than are now available for most clinical practices. In this respect, he allies himself with Meier's viewpoint that better clinical science may contribute to the resolution of many of the problems addressed in this book.

SECTION 2: CAUSATION AND RESPONSIBILITY: CONCEPTUAL ANALYSIS

Even in a progressive society, causation and moral responsibility remain the central conceptual issues that determine culpability and liability.

It appears likely, however, that certain changes have taken place in how we establish moral responsibility, culpability, and blame, though these changes have gone further in some modern industrial countries than in our own. On the one hand, in countries such as Sweden and New Zealand society appears to recognize a collective moral responsibility for ensuring that its individual members receive their "entitlements." In these societies, failure by society to provide for the medical needs of the innocent victims of a medical mishap would be an object of public shame. On the other hand, there are countries like the United States where moral responsibility is still attached primarily to individual agents. Here, ideas of collective blame and shame are foreign to the public social philosophy, and liability to provide redress to victims of medical or other mishaps (as much as willful injuries) still falls primarily on the agents whose actions are seen to have "caused" the mishaps.

Leaving aside compensation policy for the moment, one aspect of our moral thinking is unchanged. To the extent that "blame" and "culpability" remain central and active moral notions, their attribution depends, now as much as ever, on evidence of a causal link, or at least reasonable foreseeability between the agent's actions and the consequences to which moral blame is attached.

In America, the issue of responsibility and culpability arises in medical mishaps because these cases are compared to cases of medical malpractice. In both cases, harms occur to patients after medical interventions (diagnostic and therapeutic); it is not surprising that many people see the reasons for physicians' liability as springing in each case from the same considerations. The natural inferences are easily stated. The possibility that matters might have turned out better if the patient had not received the treatment implies that it was an unhappy mistake for the physician to have prescribed. This in turn suggests that the physician made a mistake in prescribing it, and so was at fault, even to blame, in doing so. Where a physician displays a lack of proper professional caution, these conclusions may perhaps be drawn and a genuine case of malpractice may exist; but where (as in many cases) the physician takes proper conscientious care to guard against any foreseeable side effects, claims of malpractice seem out of place.

In the essay "Causation in Medicine and the Law," Kenneth Schaffner provides a detailed analysis of the different meanings of causation in science and the law, and of the ways in which science and law differ in the means they use to establish proof of causation. Schaffner's thesis is that, for good biomedical reasons, we must be content with less than deterministic explications in describing clinical causation and that, for the same reasons, we must interpret biomedical causations primarily as claims about populations rather than individuals. Schaffner relates the practical uses of causation in both medicine and law to recent theoretical understandings of causation as developed by modern philosophers of science. He shows that the less than deterministic explanations of clinical causality, as developed by modern epidemiologists, are similar in many ways to what a number of philosophers have called "probabilistic causality." Schaffner suggests that the recent use by courts and legislatures of epidemiological approaches to causation may be bringing the scientific and legal concepts of proof closer together. He maintains that the epidemiological notion of "attributable risk" is a prime candidate for conceptual elucidation and application to legal cases such as those involving DES and radiation-induced injuries. He further notes that this concept is currently being proposed in legislation as a means of facilitating fair compensation for radiation-induced injuries. He encourages further explorations of these concepts by epidemiologists, jurists, and philosophers.

Kurt Baier's essay, "Moral and Legal Responsibility," analyzes the concept of responsibility by focusing on the nature of harms and on the many different meanings of the concept of responsibility. Baier notes that responsibility has forward as well as backward dimensions. He emphasizes the backward notions of responsibility by exploring ways to answer questions such as: Who did it? and Who is responsible (morally and legally) for the bad outcome? Baier then tests his analytical principles by applying them rigorously to the case of DES and its unintended bad outcomes.

James Gustafson's paper, "A Broader View of Medical Responsibility," argues that a backward notion of responsibility (which includes causal responsibility and liability-responsibility) is an insufficient account of the nature of medical responsibility. Gustafson suggests that responsibility in medicine is best understood as a positive, forward concept that can be elucidated by answering the following questions: To whom is the physician responsible? For what is the physician responsible? Gustafson's remarks support Toulmin's position that medicine should serve as a progressive, *responsible* profession within a progressive society.

SECTION 3: LEGAL FRAMEWORKS FOR PROVIDING COMPENSATION TO THE INJURED

Section 3 discusses the legal basis for establishing culpability and liability when an individual experiences a bad outcome after receiving a medical innovation.

The essays by Capron, Epstein, and Gray should be examined in the context of recent changes in the law of tort. Initially the law of tort was an instrument by which responsibility for personal injuries could be adjudicated communally to prevent the possibility of a vendetta. Many early legal codes embodied a "price list" of penalties for which a defendant was liable if it were proved that he had caused the injury willfully. In the modern era, tort law was first extended to cover injuries resulting from negligence, as much as from willful acts, though in this case, too, liability depended on proof of causation. More recently, the changing balance of technical knowledge and economic power as between, for example, corporate manufacturers and individual purchasers has given rise to the novel doctrine of strict liability. This has made it possible to recover damages under a tort theory without proof of willful injury or even of negligence. The purchaser of a new car who suffers damage because of its defects is seen as deserving to recover those damages from the auto's makers, even when they could not reasonably have foreseen those defects. So, the law of tort has taken a step away from the attribution of blame and redress and toward a philosophy of strict liability and compensation.

In his essay, "The Role of Causation in Several Legal Systems," Charles Gray analyzes the subtle and complex ways in which causation functioned in Greek and Barbarian law. Gray suggests that although both legal systems appear to have been based on a theory of strict liability, in which liability could be determined without recourse to negligence standards, both systems nevertheless examined the cause of the injury in detail before establishing the extent of the criminal and civil liability. Gray's meticulous analysis of the role of causation in several ancient cases provides an historical framework for Alexander Capron's and Richard Epstein's contemporary legal analyses of how liability should be established in medical contexts.

In "Different Compensation Approaches to Bad Outcomes from Standard Treatment, Innovative Treatment, and Research," Alexander Capron focuses on the following central question: Do innovative medical interventions, including formal research projects, have certain distinctive features that would argue in favor of treating bad outcomes outside the traditional medical negligence framework? Through a series of carefully chosen examples, Capron categorizes the critical distinctions among standard treatment, innovative treatment, and research. He concludes by suggesting that in instances of nontherapeutic research and in instances of "socially beneficial research," there may be a limited role for a non-fault compensation system to supplement traditional negligence standards.

Richard Epstein, in "Legal Liability for Medical Innovation," is far more critical of the existing tort system as a useful means for establishing liability in and control over bad outcomes from medical innovation. Epstein notes that there are many institutional arrangements available for minimizing the risks of medical innovation and for providing compensation to those who are injured. These arrangements include: tort law (either medical malpractice or strict liability); direct legislative or administrative standards (for example, controlled by the Food and Drug Administration or by local institutional review boards); and private contracts among parties. The central problem discussed by Epstein is how to determine the mix of available remedies that will be most effective in achieving the dual goals of advancing the quality of medical care (through medical research and innovation) and of compensating the injured. He concludes by suggesting that the role of tort law and the courts should be strictly limited and clearly defined. He prefers a system based upon medical custom, involving individual contracts based on fully informed consent, and some government and local administrative guidelines. Epstein argues that in this system the role of the courts would be to ensure that the standards developed elsewhere were sensibly and fairly applied in individual cases.

SECTION 4: DEVELOPING A PUBLIC POLICY FOR COMPENSATION

This concluding section examines how those who suffer injuries after receiving an innovative medical intervention should be compensated. Two observations are in order:

1. With the rise of strict liability and similar doctrines, tort law today no longer focuses so exclusively on the harms, or wrongs, done by one individual to another; instead, it is possible now, in some cases, to obtain tort remedies with highly attenuated forms of proof of neg-ligence or imputation of personal blame. If this fact is understood, it breaks the existing link in people's minds between liability, negli-gence, and malpractice. In this way, the automatic implication of moral culpability is removed, and people can perceive more clearly the element of consumer insurance involved in current tort practice.

2. As the law of tort has taken a step away from the attribution of blame, alternative methods have emerged in other areas of law and social policy for meeting the socially acknowledged needs of those who are poor, infirm, aged, or disabled. In those areas, what triggers the right to have needs met is not evidence that they spring from harms experienced at the hands of another, whether by willful injury, negligence, or the sale of a defective product. Rather, it is some specific fact about the petitioner's condition of life, such as age or employment-related injury. The very fact that these alternative procedures exist alongside the law of tort for compensating or meeting the specific needs of certain well-defined kinds of petitioners has given rise to a certain tension in both areas of law. Faced with a problematic class of cases such as medical mishaps, it is natural to ask what legal theory is appropriate to them: one derived from the law of tort or one modeled on workmen's compensation.

In the essay "Insurance for Medical Maloccurrences: Are Innovations Different?" Patricia Danzon examines alternative liability rules and compen-sation systems in terms of their prospective impact on incentives for injury prevention, on allocation of risks, and on maintaining the rate of innovation. She notes that liability rules designed to provide optimal incentives for stan-dard care provide suboptimal incentives for innovation. Although first-party and liability insurance markets perform adequately for standard care, they perform poorly for permanently disabling injuries from medical innovation (particularly when the manifestations are delayed) and from vaccinations (in part, because of their mandatory nature). Danzon concludes that a strong case can be made for a special compensation program for seriously disabling vaccine injuries but not for injuries from innovative therapies in general.

Frank Zimring, in his essay "Some Social Bases of Compensation Schemes," concurs with Epstein in arguing that tort law is inadequate and outdated for compensating those injured after receiving an innovative medical intervention. Zimring suggests that once society agrees that those who are the victims of medical mishaps should receive some remedy, redress, or compensation, even in the absence of specific proofs of causation and negligence, the problems of moral culpability and scientific causality can be set aside. Attention can then be focused on developing alternative administrative or judicial procedures for achieving efficient and fair compensation systems.

Zimring notes that if tort law is viewed as one alternative social welfare scheme, a variety of compensation and insurance approaches are available as models for making compensation decisions about medical mishaps. Our social security system pays for the retirement of one generation of workers with pay-roll taxes on the next generation. General tax revenues are used for compensating other harms. Zimring would include the class of persons injured from medical innovation as entitled to some form of no-fault compensation. He concludes: "The most important change relating to compensation for medical mishaps may occur outside both the medical services liability field and the tort system. If we continue to build disability and medical care compensation systems into government and the employment relationship, we may solve most of the problems associated with compensating the losses from medical mishaps without ever specifically addressing them. As both a political and conceptual matter, this would not be wholly unfortunate."

In the book's concluding chapter, "Responding to Biomedical Innovation: A Beginning Synthesis and Modest Proposal," Alan J. Weisbard argues that the "law and economics" perspective advanced in several earlier chapters and the accompanying proposals for incremental changes in the legal system fail to meet the challenge posed by technological innovations in modern society. Weisbard proceeds from the premise that more generous and less adversarial modes of providing compensation to innocent victims of innovative activity are both a social necessity and a necessary foundation to encourage innovation. He argues that no adequate response is possible within the contours of the existing tort law system and calls for major reform in the direction of a non-fault compensation system, suitably modified to provide appropriate incentives for safety. While agreeing with Zimring that legislative approval of such an approach is probably not likely in the near term, Weisbard stresses the need to expand the range of scholarly and policy discourse and urges scholars and policymakers to accept greater personal responsibility for articulating and defending the moral and value premises of their proposals.

CONCLUSION

The issues raised in this volume are multidisciplinary; essentially, they fall across the boundaries that separate medicine from law, the social sciences, and philosophy. The essays assembled are the work of an interdisciplinary team of investigators who have analyzed in a fresh way the complex and multifaceted concepts of causation, responsibility, liability, compensation, and public policy for dealing with medical innovation. We wish to conclude this introductory essay by offering our own views.

Our basic view is reflected in the following account by Mark Siegler of a conversation he had with a medical intern.

> Recently I was asked to give a lecture to the medical staff on the topic: "Bad Outcomes from Innovative Medical Practice: Who is Responsible?" One intern informed me that he would not attend my talk for the following reason: "Why should I listen to a 45-minute lecture when the answer to your question is obvious?" I was eager to learn the "obvious" answer, since I hadn't really made up my own mind about it. I said to the intern: "Who is responsible?" He replied: "The *intern* is responsible. Isn't the intern responsible for everything that goes wrong?"

We consider this an interesting remark. Leaving aside the intern's obvious anger about feeling that the internship process has placed him as the "man on the spot," there is a lot to be said for the intern's underlying conclusion. There is a lot to be said for holding individuals accountable and responsible for their actions, and with respect to bad outcomes from innovative medical therapy, senior physicians (rather than interns) should be held accountable for their actions and should be responsible for them. In fact, many might agree that it may be in the long-range best interest of medicine and of clinical research that this level of personal responsibility for actions and outcomes be maintained. Any replacement of an old-fashioned sense of responsibility by such new ideas as strict liability on the one hand, or no-fault compensation on the other, may lead to worse rather than better results for innovative medical practice, clinical research, and ultimately, for the public.

Thus, our own conclusions regarding physicians' moral responsibility and legal liability for patients' bad outcomes after innovative therapy are as follows:

1. *Cause.* In medicine, the cause of outcomes and the way in which cause is used to establish responsibility are vital. Medicine should defend a negligence approach and resist the movement to a strict (product) liability

standard. By this latter standard, a harm caused is considered sufficient reason to ascribe responsibility for that harm. In order to resist the drift toward strict liability, we must maintain the notion of a responsible action generating a result. Medical practice is based on scientific beliefs in causality and causation, but causation without negligence should not entail responsibility in a medical context. Furthermore, we should not allow shifting legal doctrine to usurp these important scientific attitudes.

2. *Foreseeability.* Physicians must try to keep alive the foreseeability rule. This rule has traditionally determined moral responsibility and is closely associated with a negligence approach. Simply put, one is responsible for a bad outcome only if one could reasonably have foreseen the result. The foreseeability of harms is an essential component of our implied contract with every patient. It is the vital ingredient in the doctor-patient relationship captured in the Hippocratic maxim, which describes the physician's principal obligation as "Help and do no harm." If we abandon this element in medicine, we may soon abandon the primacy of the doctor-patient relationship and we will move medicine further along the road to becoming just another commercial or bureaucratic service. Medicine should remain a human service and not a product. Of course, to what extent physicians are in a position to inform or educate their patients is not always clear, and to what extent patients are in a position to give informed consent is also not always clear. Regardless of these practical difficulties, and particularly, one might argue, in the circumstances involving innovative medical practice, it seems appropriate to hold physicians responsible both for appraising a procedure that is available and for recommending it (or not) to a particular patient. Physicians should remain "on the spot," caught, on the one hand, between the general public's demand for progress and, on the other, a specific patient's demand for professionally sound judgment. As much as the public expects progress, the public also expects individual physicians to stand between the patient and the research community and drug companies—to act as a professional who advises, educates, and advocates for individual patients.

3. *Compensation.* In a limited number of cases of medical innovation (and vaccine) injuries, where all reasonable precautions were taken and where the harm was not foreseeable, and where it is likely that medical actions *caused* the injury, we should explore the possibility of a fair and efficient no-fault compensation system.

NOTES

1. B. J. Duffy, Jr. and P. J. Fitzgerald, "Cancer of the Thyroid in Children: A Report of Twenty-Eight Cases," *Journal of Clinical Endocrinology* 10(1950):1296.

2. C. L. Simpson, L. H. Hemplemann, and L. M. Fuller, "Neoplasia in Children Treated with X-Rays in Infancy for Thymic Enlargement," *Radiology* 64(1955):840.
3. A. L. Herbst, H. Ulfelder, and D. C. Poskanzer, "Adenocarcinoma of the Vagina: Association of Maternal Stilbestrol Therapy with Tumor Appearance in Young Women," *New England Journal of Medicine* 284(1971):878-81.
4. W. J. Dieckmann, M. E. Davis, L. M. Rynkiewicz, and R. E. Pottinger, "Does the Administration of Diethylstilbestrol During Pregnancy Have Therapeutic Value?" *American Journal of Obstetrics and Gynecology* 66(1953):1062-81.
5. Herbst et al. (1971).

Section 1

Bad Outcomes from Medical Innovation:
Implications for Science, Medicine, and Society

2

Technological Progress and Social Policy: The Broader Significance of Medical Mishaps

Stephen Toulmin

The phenomenon that I shall call "medical mishaps" covers those injuries, illnesses, and other bad outcomes which occur in a small number of the patients who receive newly developed medicines or vaccines, or other inno- vative treatments based on current biomedical research. Such occurrences give rise to at least four kinds of problems:

First, there is a *post hoc, ergo propter hoc* question: with occurrences as infrequent and unprecedented as these mishaps, how can we confidently establish genuine causal connections between the innovative treatments and the subsequent outcomes?

Second, there are problems of moral responsibility. Should a physician who prescribes, in good faith, an innovative therapy which backfires reproach himself or be subject to reproach by others?

Third, certain legal issues are closely connected but not identical to the ethical question. What legal liability should attach to the physician, or to the institution within which he works, to pay damages or provide other redress to patients who are the victims of these mishaps?

And finally, these mishaps give rise to questions of social and political policy. Supposing that direct monetary or other damages from the physician or hospital turn out to be an inappropriate vehicle for compensating victims, what alternative methods of compensation might prove more appropriate and how might they be made available?

All these questions will be addressed in this text. Since the issues that arise under each heading can easily become complex and technical, I shall do no more here than acknowledge their existence and importance. Obviously, the issues of medical mishaps associated with innovative modes of medical treatment demand close, careful, and detailed analysis; but those problems— and the very phenomenon of medical mishaps—have a broader context, which provides necessary background to more detailed concerns. That context has several facets: social and political, economic and technological. It is the product of a particular phase in the history of society and technology; of a particular kind of human culture; and, most especially, of a particular set of social attitudes toward the use of new technology for improving the conditions of human life.

Historically speaking, those social attitudes are fairly new, and to that extent the problem of medical mishaps is a problem of our time. Culturally, these attitudes are prevalent only in certain nations and predominate in certain social classes. To that extent, the problem is specifically one for our place. Thus, my aim here is twofold: to show why this problem is so characteristically a problem for the United States in the late twentieth century, and to explain how this fact bears directly on policy questions regarding compensation for medical mishap victims.

To begin, let me broaden the technological picture. Some of you may recall the old lady Michael Flanders quoted in the revue "At the Drop of a Hat" who said, "If the good Lord had intended us to fly, he would have never have given us the railways." In thinking about the problems associated with the innovations available in our present stage of technological development, we should resist the temptation to suppose this current situation is unique. Instead, we must always bear in mind that our present stage is the product of a series of previous steps. The extraordinary technical progress characteristic of the so-called biomedical sciences since the Second World War may so completely engross us that we focus on them in isolation and assume that the problems they give rise to are quite unprecedented.

In fact, however, technological change, and its social impact, had had major effects on other spheres of human life long before medicine seriously joined the "march of scientific progress." Lynn White credits much of the social progress and economic success of medieval society, notably in Northern Europe, to two technological developments: the stirrup—which gave horse-riding knights their military advantage—and the horse collar—which allowed farmers to plow the heavy Northern European plain without strangling the poor beasts that pulled the plow.

Without going back quite so far, it is clear that the social impact of technical innovations in the eighteenth and early nineteenth centuries came primarily in fields other than medicine. Obvious examples are agriculture, industrial production, and above all, as Michael Flanders' old lady said, the railways. Other socially significant areas of technical progress—among them oceanic navigation, improved house building and coal mining, industrial chemistry, the internal combustion engine, and the generation of electric power—also antedated the current phase in the development of medical technology. There are chapters of legal and social history in all of these fields which could throw light on the problems we are addressing in this book. Let us examine a few technological innovations that generated unforeseen—and unforeseeable—bad outcomes.

One spectacular precedent in the field of transportation is the nineteenth-century Tay Bridge disaster, in which the new railway bridge across the River Tay in eastern Scotland collapsed during a violent storm, and a trainload of passengers drowned. Another, more familiar instance is the sinking of the steamship *Titanic*, which was specially—but unsuccessfully—designed to withstand the icebergs in the North Atlantic. A fairly recent example is the failure of the original British supersonic transport aircraft, the *Comet*. This failure had nothing to do with its being supersonic: it was designed to have square rather than round windows, and metal fatigue at the corners of the windows led to explosive decompression of several aircraft, with catastrophic results. Yet other instances are the destruction of the Tacoma Narrows Bridge and, most recently, the collapse of the airborne walkway in a Kansas City hotel.

In all these cases, honest and conscientious attempts had been made to use the latest technical procedures in a manner calculated to withstand reason-ably foreseeable stresses. But in each instance failure resulted—either through ignorance of the actual conditions under which the structure would function, or because those technical procedures had previously unsuspected limitations. In these respects, the examples show clear parallels to the phenomena that concern us.

How did the public respond to questions about the *causation* of such events as the Tay Bridge disaster or *Comet* failure? It is hard to give a general answer since responses varied from episode to episode, and from decade to decade. Still less do we find any common response to questions about the *moral responsibility*, let alone the *legal liability* to pay damages, or the need for other *mechanisms of compensation*. For a long time, the general public understood, quite realistically, that it was impossible to foresee each and every condition to which any novel structure or mechanism might be subjected, once in actual use. In extreme cases, disasters that were evidently beyond all human foresight or calculation, and so not truly matters of human agency, were attributed to a Higher Power; they were known, in insurance parlance, as "acts of God."

Only the increasing ability of twentieth-century civil engineers, physicians, and other users of modern technology to predict the actual outcomes of their work has encouraged people to demand complete and accurate prediction under all circumstances. In discussing the major catastrophe at the Union Carbide plant in Bhopal, India, the one hypothesis no one takes seriously is that the escape of poisonous gas was an act of God. On the contrary, everyone involved clearly agrees that the catastrophe was attributable to human agency. The only question is, Who *exactly* is to blame? Still, we should recognize just how new a development this demand for perfect prediction in technological innovation really is. My primary aim here is to focus attention on the factors that lie behind this historically novel demand.

Let us first draw a distinction between two kinds of societies and cultures. In considering the hopes and expectations around which people have structured their lives in different cultures and societies and at different stages in history, we can recognize a spectrum of attitudes toward inherited forms of life and standard operating procedures. These range from attitudes prevalent in highly traditional (or conservative) societies at one extreme, to deliberately modernizing (or progressive) ones at the other.

In traditional or conservative societies, the existence of a fixed stock of techniques and procedures is now taken for granted. Life is structured around *idées reçus,* now patronizingly referred to as "the conventional wisdom." For people living in these societies, what *ought* to be done about any problem is equated with what *is* done—that is, with "the done thing." There are well-established ways of planting and harvesting grain, of dealing with attacks of hysteria, of celebrating the winter solstice, and so on. No society or culture is equally conservative in all respects, so in speaking of "traditional societies" I am clearly defining what Weber calls an "ideal type." Still, some societies and cultures are highly conservative in a great many respects, and all societies and cultures are somewhat conservative in some respects.

In deliberately modernizing or progressive societies, by contrast, the current stock of techniques is subject to continual refinement and improvement. In transportation, house building, weapons design, or medical practice, people in these societies are continually asking how the same needs might be met more efficaciously, economically, or elegantly. Once again, no society or culture is totally committed to transformation in every aspect of existence and at all times. To that extent, the notion of a modernizing or progressive society is also an ideal type. Still, the contrast between conservative and progressive societies, or between traditional and modernizing ones, turns out to be a useful instrument for analyzing the central issues of this book.

One needs no special knowledge about the history of American medicine to recognize that, in this respect, current medical practice in the United States conforms, and is expected to conform, more closely to the progressive than to the traditional ideal. The public at large, and its political representatives in Congress, have the standing expectation that physicians are continually refining and improving their techniques for dealing with pathologies and injuries of all kinds. Once again, this demand is not carried to an extreme: a certain core of standard medical procedures is more or less well protected from change, partly for technical and partly for more broadly based reasons. Nonetheless, in the United States today, no one equates the way in which a pathology or injury *should* be treated with how it currently *is* treated. On the contrary, the possibility of "a revolutionary new treatment" is never far from people's minds.

The precise manner in which such ideas as causation, moral responsibility, legal liability, and entitlement to compensation are understood is, correspondingly, not entirely universal and invariant. Rather, considering their use in different societies, and at different stages in history, these ideas display at most a family resemblance to one another—a certain common core of understanding surrounded by a range of marginal differences.

In traditional societies we find two contrasting attitudes toward liability for mishaps associated with the use of the established techniques. The attitude in some is that, simply by virtue of being inherited, accepted, and even ancient in origin, the use of these techniques is regarded as generally proper and legitimate, even though the outcome may occasionally be unhappy. Practitioners are thus held either legally liable or morally to blame only when their use of those procedures departs from the "routine and accepted practice" of the art in question, or is plainly negligent.

In other traditional societies, absent explicit indemnification, legal liability for bad outcomes may be complete, unqualified, and unlimited; but in this second case, questions of legal liability are divorced from questions of moral responsibility. Even if one employed the routine and accepted procedure in a conscientious manner, the very fact of a bad outcome may render one legally liable to provide a remedy, although no moral reproach attaches to that liability.

In conservative societies of both kinds, however, the deliberate use of technical procedures (other than those which have an established place in the culture) always carries explicit liability for any resulting injuries. As late as the eighteenth century, indeed, the term "experimentation" categorized a legal offense. The use of nonaccepted medical techniques with injurious results was a recognized ground for civil remedy, and was even considered a crime.

In actively modernizing societies and cultures, the situation is totally different. Experimentation is recognized as a socially indispensable activity, one which provides the best way of improving the available repertoire of procedures in engineering, technology, and medicine alike. In consciously modernizing societies, furthermore, once experimentation has demonstrated the existence of effective and reasonably safe new procedures in any field, there is public support for putting those new procedures to general practical use, as soon as this is politically and economically feasible. Thus, a progressive society like that of the United States commonly deals with the question of moral responsibility for bad outcomes of medical procedures by transforming them into a matter of the level of care exercised in the individual physicians *use* of those procedures. Moral reproach is attached to such injuries only in situations where the physician was careless or even reckless in treatment, or where the routine and accepted procedures of the medical profession were departed from in ways that lacked experimental justification.

That generally progressive attitude also stands behind the theory of medical malpractice, as it operated in Anglo-American common-law jurisdictions until recently, before the near-collapse of the medical compensation system. But I shall resist the temptation to hunt that particular hare. For our present purposes, the theory of medical malpractice is relevant only because it is one route by which trial lawyers have sought to obtain redress for the victims of medical mishaps even when the conduct of the physicians concerned was impeccable by both professional and moral standards.

How, then, does the change from traditional to modernizing attitudes affect ideas about moral responsibility and legal liability? Let me again suggest a general answer before examining medicine in particular. We may begin by considering some respects in which our legal ideas about torts have been affected, and will continue to be affected, by that historical transition.

If we look at the origins of the classical Anglo-American conception of torts, within the framework of sixteenth and seventeenth-century civil law, we shall find that this development took place within a comparatively traditional or conservative context. As a result, our general thinking about tort law tends to take for granted a very simple view about the range of individuals who are the natural parties to any injury. In the case of any tort, it seems, only two sets of parties normally need be considered: the agent or agents who are its authors—that is, the tortfeasors—and the victim or victims who suffer the wrong.

Obviously this paradigm of injury is also an ideal type. In actual cases, the courts are often obliged to extend it to meet the demands of justice. As a result, there are whole branches of the law that are concerned, for example, with what is called "agency theory." There the point at issue is, under what circumstances may legal liability for an injury be extended beyond the person whose physical actions directly injured the victim? The legal answers to the resulting questions will differ in subtle ways, depending on whether, for example, the injury is inflicted by a servant in performing duties on behalf of a master; whether the immediate agent was an independent contractor acting as a franchisee, to whom a franchiser nevertheless gave apparent authority to act in his name or on his behalf; and so on and so on.

As with the traditional model of the physician-patient relationship, in which the doctor acts and the patient is acted upon, this oversimplified model of the relationship between tortfeasor and victim dates from an earlier period, when the typical tort situation may indeed have been as simple as this model implies. But the development of modern societies has more recently obliged lawyers to view the tort relationship in subtler and more complex ways.

In the contemporary practice of medicine, to restrict the basic medical relationship to two parties is clearly artificial. Questions about how a physician and a patient interact are always overshadowed by the presence and influence of other parties: on the patient's side, by the interests and policies of the insurance company; on the doctor's side, by the interests and policies of the institution in which he practices (such as a teaching hospital). Correspondingly, in the contemporary application of tort law, the institutional structures of modern life, the inequalities of power and knowledge, and the larger number of people having legitimate interests in a situation of injury increasingly limit the relevance of the old tortfeasor-victim model.

The part which technological innovation has played in these changes is nicely illustrated by the classic case in which tort liability was extended beyond the scope of "negligence" to embrace so-called strict liability. Edward Levi discusses the case of *MacPherson* v. *Buick* in his *Introduction to Legal Reasoning*. There, he shows how the courts felt compelled to extend liability for an injury suffered by the purchaser of a defective automobile beyond the dealer with whom the actual purchase contract was made to the corporation which originally manufactured the automobile. In earlier times, the purchaser's claim for damages would have gone no further than the dealer. It was considered the dealer's responsibility not to sell a defective automobile, just as it is the responsibility of a fishmonger not to sell rotten fish.

With complex modern machinery such as automobiles, however, considerations based on the differences in relative power and knowledge of all the parties make it unjust to retain this limitation. Clearly, an automobile dealer has to rely in part on the representations of the manufacturing corporation that its automobiles are designed carefully enough and tested stringently enough to insure their safety in normal use. To that extent, whatever the actual contractual position may be, the dealer is willy-nilly put in a position of having apparent authority to act as agent for the manufacturers. Conversely, manufacturers do not escape liability for injuries caused by defects in their products, even when there is no direct contract between the manufacturer and the ultimate purchaser. In such cases, the courts seek to redress the imbalance created by the greater technical knowledge and economic power of the manufacturer. Thus they tear away the veil provided by the simple two-party model of tort injuries, and reveal the other parties who have been *implicit agents* of the resulting injury.

Even before the rise of modern scientific medicine, legal scholars and judges alike had already confronted situations in which reasonable reliance on technological innovations had bad outcomes. As a result, they broadened the scope of moral responsibility and legal liability so as to draw related parties into our thinking about such injuries. And in the field of medicine, too, I would argue that something similar has already happened implicitly—if not in legal theory, at least in political practice.

Recall, for instance, the notorious swine flu inoculation program. When, in its somewhat less than infinite wisdom, the United States government launched a crash program of vaccination for that disease, fearing the onset of an epidemic comparable to the disastrous 1919 pandemic, the available time was too short to permit all the testing required to guarantee the vaccine's safety, or even to give sufficient warning of foreseeable side effects.

The drug companies invited to manufacture the vaccine for mass administration foresaw the likelihood of numerous expensive damage suits. They therefore declined to participate in the program unless Congress indemnified them against such damage suits by assuming legal liability for the consequences of the inoculation program. In a very limited number of cases, vaccination was followed by a form of paralysis which few deny was caused by the inoculation. This unhappy side effect was, I understand, so infrequent that it could not reasonably have been foreseen, especially given the limited test population to whom the vaccine was administered during the very short time it was available before general distribution was deemed imperative.

Why did Congress agree to indemnify the manufacturers, instead of leaving them to take their lumps? In large part it was done to acknowledge that the original pressure for mass inoculation had come not from the makers of the vaccine but from the United States government itself. If the manufacturers had been left to themselves, they would undoubtedly have moved more slowly, and insisted on more stringent testing, before releasing the vaccines for mass use. Having insisted on speed, Congress had to recognize its own implicit agency in the situation. It was accordingly obliged to assume its own share of moral responsibility and legal liability for the ill effects that followed from the widespread use of an inadequately tested vaccine.

Here we see how the use of technical innovations, not all the effects of which can be reasonably foreseen, compels us to broaden our conceptions of moral *responsibility* for injury. It also requires us to extend the range of *implicit parties* who need to be included when we consider issues of *legal liability* and *compensation*.

Let me now present my central thesis about the social and historical context of the current problem of medical mishaps. Within this context, I shall try to show why, and how, we must cast our moral and legal nets more widely than is suggested by the simple model of medical malpractice. My thesis is that, by this time, the American electorate is fully committed to a fully modernizing society. In medicine above all, this ambition carries with it the implication that all the powerful new techniques will be put to use as widely as economically feasible, as soon as there is reason to assume their safety and effectiveness. In this respect, I would argue, the American electorate is in a hurry, just as the federal government was in a hurry when it launched the swine flu inoculation program.

The American electorate has general ambitions for medicine which it is determined to realize; it wants results. Knowledge of this ambition creates pressures on all who are involved in the medical situation. And those pressures have implications with respect to deciding issues of moral responsibility, legal liability, and compensation for the occasional mishaps that inevitably arise from the drive to develop ever more powerful techniques.

Since the Second World War, transactions between physicians and patients in the United States have come to involve—as implicit agents—a whole range of institutions and individuals over and above the doctor and patient directly involved. Those agents include not only the medical research community, the National Institutes of Health, and other federal funding agencies, but also the entire medical profession, Congress, and the electorate itself.

Today, when an American patient consults a physician, that patient expects to benefit not just from the individual doctor's best personal skills. The patient assumes—and is encouraged by the medical profession to assume—that he may expect to benefit from "the best that modern medicine can offer." In this situation, the physician acts not merely on his or her own account, but also as a dealer, distributing products and services manufactured and tested by the entire medical establishment.

It is as though the whole profession were in the business of supplying the product known as modern medicine. As in *MacPherson* v. *Buick*, the individual physician must rely on the representations of those who give new techniques, drugs, and devices their blessing, who vouch that these innovative treatments have been prepared carefully enough, and tested stringently enough, to insure their safety in normal use.

Something of this implicit agency relationship is now recognized in the context of malpractice suits. Indeed, the courts already impose on physicians a duty to do more than their own conscientious best, on the basis of their skill and personal experience. They are required to educate themselves on the most up-to-date procedures available and may be held liable for any injuries suffered as a result of their failure to recommend the most current treatments.

The case of medical mishaps associated with innovative treatments, in other words, has already taken on some of the features that, in the manufacturing industry, led to the doctrine of strict liability. If an automobile dealer supplies a defective automobile, and you are injured as a result, your right of recovery is not dependent on proving that either the dealer or even the manufacturer acted negligently. Instead, you may be entitled to redress without prior proof of anyone's negligence. Yet this parallel faces one seemingly intractable difficulty. If the individual physician today is like a dealer who distributes the products of Modern Medicine, Inc., where exactly are we to look for the *implicit parties* who stand in relation to the individual physician as the automobile manufacturer does to the car dealer?

Notice how completely our medical mishap concerns sidetrack the question of negligence. Suppose that, bowing to the expectations of the courts, a physician prescribes an innovative up-to-date treatment which injures rather than helps the patient. It is quite unrealistic to conclude that those injuries must be effects of the doctor's negligence; on the contrary, the patient may have been injured as a result of the physician's very conscientiousness. It may be just because the doctor made the most thorough possible search of the literature, and came up with the most advanced procedures available, that the patient was injured at all. The doctor may have taken every possible care to inform himself of any known side effects, including all relevant contraindications; yet the injuries to this particular patient may be the first known instance of hitherto undetected side effects. That, after all, is precisely what defines medical mishap in our present sense of the phrase.

We now come to the heart of the matter. Assume that certain medical mishaps are associated with the use of technically innovative treatments, yet no question arises about the care and conscientiousness displayed by the physician who recommends those treatments. What other agents implicitly involved in the medical transaction—the medical research community, the Congress, or the electorate at large—can justly be seen as sharing responsibility for the patient's injuries?

I have chosen to state that question in terms which underline my central point: in any given society, the manner in which physicians practice their art depends, among other things, on the general attitude of the people in that society toward innovation and modernization. The physician acts within a larger social and cultural context which imposes certain legal demands and moral expectations on him. The physician cannot justly be held solely responsible for all consequences of those demands and expectations.

Pressures on physicians may work in either of two ways. In a generally conservative society, doctors are encouraged to practice medicine conservatively. In particular, they are encouraged to view technical experimentation and therapeutic innovation with suspicion rather than enthusiasm. Before 1900, for instance, American physicians viewed innovative treatments with great caution. The medical profession kept itself at arm's length from the scientific eggheads, falling back on such maxims as "It's all very well in theory, but . . . ." Even after experimentation had ceased to be a legal offense, this medical empiricism kept its hold on the profession, so that, in the years before World War I, Abraham Flexner had to plead for the introduction of a larger scientific component into American medical education.

During such conservative periods, doctors may hesitate to employ promising new methods against their own inclinations and even against their own better judgments. They do so from fear of being penalized for going beyond the routine and accepted procedures currently approved by their colleagues, and so for acting unprofessionally. Even without legal penalties for resorting to experimentation, internal professional controls can effectively discourage technical innovation. In such a phase of social history, what would happen if a patient went to court, complaining that he was injured because his physician failed to be sufficiently innovative? The case would, clearly, never get off the ground.

In a society like our own, where people's social attitudes are genuinely progressive—where, without specific evidence to the contrary, people tend to presume that newer is better—doctors are encouraged, if not downright obliged, to keep up-to-date in their methods. This may sometimes mean they will use techniques whose side effects are not yet fully known. In this second situation, physicians may be under pressure *not* to be hesitant, but to employ novel methods of treatment against their own inclinations and even against their own better judgment. They do so from fear of being penalized for *not* going beyond what were hitherto the routine and accepted procedures of the profession.

Where at one time being professional meant being *conservative*, now being professional means being prepared to *take risks*. What are those risks? They are, precisely, the risks we are concerned with here; that there exist side effects unforeseeable not only to the individual physician, but to the entire medical research community.

In short, when we concentrate on the purest cases of medical mishaps associated with the use of technical innovations, one prime factor contributing to such mishaps becomes evident. It is the social and legal pressure to which physicians are subjected by the social demand that they employ all innovative procedures of treatment as soon as these procedures *appear* reasonably safe and effective, rather than waiting until safety and effectiveness are proven "beyond the shadow of a doubt." The external pressure of these social demands, reinforced by current interpretations of medical malpractice law, may impose on many physicians a progressive rather than a conservative mode of practice, even against their own judgment.

This is not to suggest that by protecting physicians from outside pressures, leaving them free to judge entirely for themselves when to employ a technical innovation, we could prevent all medical mishaps. In practice, such a policy might reduce the number of mishaps, but it could never eliminate them entirely. No finite sequence of testing procedures can ever do more than reduce the likelihood that we have overlooked significant side effects; it cannot produce a 100 percent guarantee that we have identified them all.

In any case, the social pressures I refer to are merely one more byproduct of the American public's general commitment to the pursuit of technological progress; and, as such, they are not unreasonable. The basic problem is, simply, that so thorough a commitment to the pursuit of technical progress has a price, a fact not yet generally recognized. So, in the purest case of medical mishap, the injured party is the victim neither of malpractice by an individual physician, nor of the medical research community's lack of caution, but of the nation's social and technological commitments. They are inadvertent casualties of social policies which are supported as vigorously by the federal government and the public at large as they are by the medical profession and the research community of biomedical science.

If this account of the social and historical background of medical mishaps has any substance, it will be clear why the moral, legal, and policy implications of those mishaps are so ambiguous. Nothing I have said here, of course, implies that biomedical research scientists can never be enthusiastic to the point of rashness in their use of novel and experimental therapies; nor am I implying that practicing physicians can never be reckless in their employment of innovative treatments. But there are ways to correct that type of error, at least within practical limits.

Our concern here is with a deeper problem of medical mishap. In the rush to compensate victims, even in situations where no moral blame attaches to the physicians or scientists involved, lawyers and juries have too readily assimilated these outcomes—which, in earlier times, would have been set aside as acts of God—to those more familiar and straightforward injuries which can fairly be attributed to negligence or recklessness.

Recognizing the softheartedness of juries, and wishing to keep their legal expenses under control, the insurance companies that write malpractice policies for physicians tend to settle these claims, rather than fight them. Yet, to the extent that most of the medical actions which lead to such mishaps are performed carefully, conscientiously, in good faith, and with the patient's consent, equating claims to compensation on behalf of the victims with cases of downright malpractice is morally inappropriate. Physicians and medical researchers understandably resent the moral reproach implicit in consenting to findings of malpractice in situations where they find themselves penalized *despite*, or even *on account of*, their careful and conscientious use of up-to-date medical treatments.

Current judicial practice is moral nonsense and, to the extent that that is so, the problem of devising alternative methods to compensate those victims becomes an active field for new social policy. Social and historical experience in other fields of technology indicates more than one new direction in which legal theory and judicial practice might move.

One possibility is that claims for redress arising out of medical mishaps associated with the use of innovative medical treatments might be kept within the general ambit of tort law, but brought explicitly under the doctrine of strict liability. That doctrine was introduced to insure that those agents with greater economic power or more detailed technical understanding should compensate those who—out of comparative weakness or ignorance—are in no position to protect themselves against injury by the actions of such agents or through defects in their products, *even in cases where there is no imputation of negligence.* If that became the general policy over medical mishaps also, research hospitals and medical clinics would no doubt seek to insure themselves against the risks arising from such damage claims. Conversely, insurance companies issuing such policies might reserve the right to withhold payment in situations where actual negligence was in fact established. Such insurance policies would then be parallel to, but independent of, regular malpractice coverage. My guess is that the premiums would be comparatively low.

Another possibility is to take the victims' redress for injuries arising out of medical mishaps out of the scope of tort law entirely and deal with it on some alternative model. A range of plausible analogies (for example, workmen's compensation law) will be discussed in other chapters.

There is another topic I might have addressed here in considering the social policy aspect. The attitudes that Americans today adopt in thinking about injuries born of interactions with professional advisors and with suppliers of new products, new techniques, or new medical treatments are strikingly risk-aversive. Having abandoned the notion that humanly unforeseeable mishaps are acts of God, we are quick to look for humans to blame. (In what other country, in what other time, would champagne makers wrap their corks in a label warning purchasers not to point the cork at their own or anyone else's eyes?) I doubt, therefore, whether the American electorate is in a mood to welcome my message—that any deliberate pursuit of medical progress through the use of innovative therapies is bound to produce a certain number of casualties, for which no individual physician can fairly be blamed. In the medical as in the manufacturing field, the public wants the kind of guarantees that are implicit in the legal theory of strict liability. The only question is, How are we most justly and efficiently to give them those guarantees?

Medical mishaps occur from time to time, despite everyone's best efforts. These mishaps pose difficult problems of statistical judgment, causal analysis, moral responsibility, legal liability, and social policy. In other chapters, we shall consider and discuss all these issues in greater detail. For the moment, my survey of the social and historical background of these mishaps leads me to make three linked claims:

1. The public expectation that medicine be practiced in a progressive rather than a conservative manner and that every opportunity be taken to employ the most up-to-date and effective medical procedures and techniques has become an integral part of America's current social and political consensus.

2. To the extent that this is so, some minimum rate of medical mishap, without any human agent being to blame, is the unavoidable price to be paid for maintaining the socially desired momentum of medical advance.

3. The American electorate at large, and the U.S. Congress in particular, will eventually have to acknowledge this price, accept their mutual responsibility for the resulting bad outcomes, and modify their attitudes and policies accordingly.

3

The Scientific Process and the Development of Medical Innovation: The Daedalus Effect

Baruch S. Blumberg

In this essay, I will examine the following topics:

1. The features of the scientific process which, according to certain views, preclude the possibility of perfect knowledge. From this interpretation not only is it impossible to know everything about everything, but it is impossible to know everything about anything.

2. The story of the mythic figure Daedalus will be summarized. An architect, sculptor, engineer, and problem solver, Daedalus can be viewed as a metaphor for the contemporary scientist and physician who is, at the same time, a problem solver and problem creator.

3. An example of problem solving and problem creation provided from the experience of the discovery of the hepatitis B virus and its applications. The solutions of an important medical problem, how to detect blood donors who carry the hepatitis B virus and thereby prevent post-transfusion hepatitis, led to the development of social, psychological, and personal problems: namely, how to deal with the people who were identified as carriers. (Items 2 and 3 are adapted from an earlier publication.[1])

4. A discussion of the relation of these observations and concepts to the topics selected for analysis. The Daedalus effect, which is an inherent characteristic of the scientific process, can be distinguished from problems in which the scientific process has been misapplied. In many cases, medical procedures come into use without adequate scientific investigation; this can lead to profound problems.

This work was supported by USPH grants CA-06551, RR-05539, and CA-06927 from the National Institutes of Health and by appropriation from the Commonwealth of Pennsylvania.

Adapted, in part, from B. S. Blumberg and R. C. Fox. "The Daedalus Effect: Changes in Ethical Questions Relating to Hepatitis B Virus," *Annals of Internal Medicine* 102(1985):390-94.

Scientific Process in Clinical Research

A hypothesis is a declarative statement concerning the scientist's view of a state of nature confined to the subject matter of a project. In the inductive phase of scientific process, the data are collected first and the hypothesis induced from it. In the deductive phase, the hypothesis is stated first, and then data is collected to test it. After the hypothesis is stated, a study is designed to test the hypothesis (usually an attempt is made to reject the hypothesis), and during the course of testing, a body of data accumulates. Irrespective of the support or rejection of the hypothesis, the data can be used to generate other hypotheses. These, in turn, can be tested by additional data. Again, a decision can be made as to whether the hypotheses of the second cycle are supported or rejected and the data used to formulate a third series of hypotheses, which are also available for testing. This process may be continued through many cycles. As the process proceeds, more and more hypotheses are tested (that is, more and more questions are answered), but at the same time, an even greater number of new questions are asked. The more that is known, the greater is the number of unknowns, and it becomes clear that total and perfect knowledge about the project may not be possible. If a perfect solution means that the investigator knows everything about a subject, then, if this model is valid, solutions will always be imperfect.

The Daedalus Myth as a Metaphor
of Scientific Process

Models, analogies, metaphors, parables—all are valuable not only because of their similarities to the real observations and events which they model, but because of their dissimilarities. The theologian I. G. Barbour, in his fascinating book *Myths, Models and Paradigms*,[2] states, "There is a tension between affirmation and negation, for in analogy there are both similarities and differences." The complex and rich myth of Daedalus, when used as an analogy for scientific process in clinical research, can generate a host of instructive and useful ideas.

Daedalus, the legendary builder, designer, and inventor of the ancient Greek world, murdered his nephew Perdix, probably because of his jealousy of the young man's skills. To escape punishment, Daedalus fled Athens, went to Crete, and was employed at the court of King Minos. Known for his ability to make clever images of animals, Daedalus was employed by Pasaphae, Queen of Crete and wife of Minos, when she became hopelessly enamoured of a great white bull presented to her and her husband as a gift by the god Poseidon (the mythic father of Minos). Daedalus designed and built a life-sized, hollow, upholstered cow. The queen positioned herself in the model, which was placed in a seductive situation in a field, and eventually she was impregnated by the white bull. Her problem, her desire for the bull, was solved, but it created another: the offspring of this unfortunate union was the half-beast, half-human Minotaur. This awful animal terrorized the citizens; the noise it created was like thunder, when it stamped its feet the earth shook, and it was a nuisance and danger in other ways as well.

To solve this problem, Daedalus designed and built a labyrinth in which the Minotaur could be isolated. However, the Minotaur also required the sacrifice of young men and women. Each year, youths were sent from Athens to be offered up to his insatiable appetite. When Theseus, the son of the King of Athens, was sent with the sacrificial youths, Daedalus told him and Ariadne (the daughter of Minos and Pasaphae, thus half-sister of the Minotaur) of a secret door by which they could enter the labyrinth to slay the Minotaur. He also gave Ariadne a magic spool of thread that would unwind and show them the way to escape the labyrinth after they had slain the beast. Theseus and Ariadne killed the Minotaur and fled Crete, with many adventures along the way. Ariadne was eventually abandoned by Theseus on the island of Naxos.

Hence, another problem was solved but others developed. Minos imprisoned Daedalus and his son Icarus in the labyrinth for their part in the death of the Minotaur and the escape of the killers; the mazemaker was trapped in his own maze—an ironic metaphor within a metaphor. But the imprisonment had its solution. Daedalus invented wings and fashioned them from feathers and wax. He and his son escaped their jailers, but, in the ensuing flight, against paternal advice, Icarus flew too high. The heat of the sun melted the wax, the wings came away, and Icarus fell to his death in the sea that now bears his name. (This also provides an additional metaphor for scientific process. The misuse or misunderstanding of knowledge can lead to unwholesome effects: the Icarus effect.) Daedalus flew on to the Greek colony of Cumae, south of Naples (or, in some versions of the myth, to Sicily), and additional problems and solutions ensued.

The sun and its heat, the wings and their wax, the sea into which Icarus plummeted, his attitudes and his death, all became part of the continuing cycle of questions and answers, problems and solutions that are inherent to creative and responsible science and to human questing.

THE DAEDALUS EFFECT AND THE HEPATITIS B VIRUS

Many examples of the Daedalus effect can be found in the history of medical research. An application with which I have had personal experience will be used to show how a major medical problem was solved, and how it, in turn, generated a problem which had not been fully perceived before the solution was in progress. In this case the problem was bioethical. Continuing research has, in part, mitigated the original problem but added additional complications.

The test for what was then known as the Australia antigen, a proteinlike material present in the blood, was reported in 1964. By 1966, there was substantial evidence that Australia antigen was on the surface of hepatitis B virus. In 1967, screening of blood donors for occult carriers of hepatitis virus was routine in some hospitals in Philadelphia, and by 1970 it was widely applied in the United States and other countries. [3]

In 1968, reports were heard from persons, usually health care personnel, who had been identified as carriers as a result of a blood donor or hospital staff testing program. For example, a hospital nurse identified as a carrier was told that she would be fired because she might infect people by personal contact. An applicant for a hospital position was deemed ineligible for employment because he was a carrier. A homosexual was informed that he was a carrier but was given no instructions on how to conduct himself socially.

Along with many incidents of this nature, policy questions about hepatitis B virus carriers were raised by institutions. Military medical authorities in a foreign country where hepatitis B virus carriers were commonly asked if they should screen applicants for admission to medical school and disqualify those found to be carriers. The same question was raised with respect to admission to officers' training school and to graduation from nursing school: should these applicants and graduates be screened for the carrier state to determine if they should be allowed to enter or undertake the practice of their chosen profession? (We recommended that screening not be done.) Still another difficult policy problem arose in relation to the adoption of Southeast Asian refugee children. In the mid-1970s, many children from Indochina were placed for adoption. Because hepatitis B virus carriers were known to be prevalent in Vietnam, the advisability of screening these children for the virus became an issue. Should the results of this screening test determine who would be accepted for adoption and who would not? (U.S. health officials decided that carrier testing should not be done as a qualification for immigration to the United States from Southeast Asia.) These carrier-related questions surfaced in increasing numbers as the hepatitis B virus test became more widespread.

What appeared to be emerging was the possibility that a new class of stigmatized persons and groups—hepatitis B virus carriers—was being created by the introduction of a single laboratory test. [4] These people did not have any recognizable external characteristics. Their carrier state was occult, that is, discernible only by use of a blood test. Many carriers already had been, and even more would be, identified as a result of the donor and other blood-testing programs that had been launched. (Tens of millions of donor blood samples are collected each year, and, in due course, most of these would be tested.)

It was known that some carriers could transmit hepatitis readily by blood transfusion. From this knowledge, but without quantitative data on actual transmission, it was inferred that carriers could also convey hepatitis through social interaction. This assumption began to take hold despite the fact that it was apparent that most carriers were not very infectious. It had been estimated that there were about 700,000 carriers throughout the United States. If they were infectious—for example, to the degree that people infected with smallpox are—there would have been far more hepatitis in this country and elsewhere than there is known to be. Furthermore, several preliminary studies of health care workers known to be carriers showed that they had not transmitted hepatitis B virus to their patients. The scientific evidence strongly suggested that, although some carriers might be infectious, many were much less so, if at all, and that the danger to public health was probably not immediate or enormous. Nevertheless, persons who had been identified as hepatitis B virus carriers were being medically and socially marked in potentially disadvantageous ways. They were having personal, family, and career difficulties as a result of their disclosed carrier status.

Consideration of these problems made it clear that an evaluation of a general screening program should be done before any such program was executed. (This program refers to the screening of persons other than blood donors. Blood donor screening had been evaluated, found to be justified, and accepted.) What was called for was a judicious, well-informed set of decisions about screening that would potentiate its public health benefits and protect individual hepatitis carriers from undue economic, psychic, and social harm. It became apparent that there were not sufficient data on which to make sound decisions that would appropriately balance collective needs and individual rights. It was not at all clear what the rules for a screening program ought to be. Should screening be compulsory? Should the activities of carriers be distinguished from those of people who were not infectious? What instructions should be given to identified carriers? What kind of protection could and should be offered to those with whom carriers come in contact? The history of previous medical applications strongly suggested that these issues should be addressed before the screening procedure acquired the routine familiarity and authority of an established practice; once a procedure has been instituted it becomes increasingly hard to question or freshly evaluate it.

There were also broader issues that had been raised and required consideration. Most of the infectious diseases that people contract are transmitted either directly or indirectly from other people, in many cases from carriers. However, screening for these agents is difficult and not done routinely on large segments of the general population. For example, *Staphylococcus aureus* carried on skin surfaces may be spread from person to person and has caused large and calamitous epidemics in hospital nurseries. Nevertheless, routine screening is not done for this bacterium except after infection has been found. *Salmonella* species may be spread by food handlers and cause serious epidemics of diarrheal disease, but routine screening is not done because of its expense and difficulty. Should hepatitis carriers be targeted for screening simply because the test is easy to do and widely available? Beyond this, how much should biological knowledge be allowed to influence and control our social relationships? To what extent should medical and public health practices be allowed to affect our social behavior—particularly in the face of the inadequate information regarding hepatitis B virus carriers and the infectious risk they constitute?

For various reasons, hepatitis screening for blood donors was accepted quickly, whereas screening for many other infectious agents has not been accepted. There was an unambiguous, long-standing need to screen blood donors for hepatitis. Post-transfusion hepatitis was a real and significant problem that had been recognized for years, and any solution was bound to be accepted quickly. The tests for hepatitis B virus (particularly the radioimmunoassay that was introduced relatively early in the program) were sensitive and specific. There was a large commercial interest in these tests. Test reagents for hepatitis B virus to the value of tens of millions of dollars are sold yearly, aided by extensive advertising and skilled promotion. Further, several lawsuits had been brought against hospitals, blood banks, and physicians by defendants who developed post-transfusion hepatitis and claimed that the institution and health care workers were liable because they had not used the screening test for hepatitis B virus. In addition, blood has a powerful symbolic meaning in our culture. It is associated with life and vigor, lineage and kinship, and sacrifice, and is sacred in ways likely to confer special positive significance on technical procedures that guarantee its "purity."

The question of a general screening program (the testing of persons who are not blood donors) had to be viewed very differently. We, and others in the field, took the position that there had not yet been enough research on hepatitis B virus carriers to justify general screening programs, except for those that were part of a research protocol. It was obvious that additional research was necessary to resolve these medical and bioethical problems.

ADVANCES IN RESEARCH
AND THEIR IMPACT ON ETHICAL QUESTIONS

Since our original publication on these issues, there have been scientific and
technical advances that have changed the ethical issues in hepatitis B virus
carrier screening, and altered our views in the process. In 1972, Magnius
and Espmark[5] reported their finding of the hepatitis B e antigen (HBeAg).
This antigen appears to be a part of the core of hepatitis B virus, and its
presence in a carrier indicates that significant amounts of whole infectious
virus are present in the blood.[6,7] Mothers who are hepatitis B surface
antigen (HBsAg) and HBeAg positive can transmit hepatitis to their
offspring, particularly in Asian populations. Carriers in general with
HBeAg are more likely to transmit the virus than those without.
Furthermore, HBsAg carriers who also have antibody to hepatitis B e
antigen (anti-HBe) in their blood are much less likely to transmit the agent
than those with HBeAg or those without any sign of HBe antigen or
antibody. By separating the carrier group into those who are potentially
infectious and those unlikely to transmit hepatitis, the problems of screening
were narrowed and focused.

In 1969, Millman and Blumberg introduced a unique method for the
production of a vaccine to prevent infection with hepatitis B virus.[8] The
vaccine has been tested,[9] accepted by government agencies, and is now
widely used by individuals and for public health projects in this country and
abroad. Since it is now known that the vaccine is safe and effective, it will
be possible to protect persons with whom carriers come in contact. In time,
in some regions of the world where hepatitis prevalence is high, all or
nearly all of the population will either have natural protection against
hepatitis B virus (they will have developed the antibody to hepatitis B
surface antigen [anti-HBs] after natural infection with the virus), or they will
have been vaccinated. When this happens, the public health impact of the
carriers will be greatly minimized. As a consequence, the chief ethical
problem of the carrier will have been eliminated.

In areas with low intensity of hepatitis B virus infection, the vaccine
will probably only be used in high-risk populations, including health care
personnel, travelers, military personnel, blood handlers, homosexual men,
drug abusers, family members of carriers, and certain other groups. In
some of these high-exposure populations, the frequency of naturally
occurring anti-HBs may be common (15 to 50 percent). Because the cost of
vaccine is high, it would be prudent in some areas to screen these
populations for the presence of anti-HBs (and possibly HBsAg), because
they would not profit from vaccination. Under these changed circumstances,

the screening of general populations would be warranted. The initial concerns about general population surveys would be set aside, because measures of known value could be taken as a consequence of the survey.

There are other situations in which screening surveys may be warranted. Current policy encourages the "mainstreaming" of mentally retarded children by placing them in small, homelike settings in the general community and in regular schools with other children. There is a relatively high frequency of carriers among children and young adults with Down's syndrome, who make up a sizable portion of deinstitutionalized, mentally retarded people. Research should continue to determine the risk that these children may impose on their classmates, and on the feasibility of vaccine protection. Similarly, adopted children from communities with high frequencies of carriers (for example, Southeast Asians) may also be screened after adoption has occurred. Vaccine could then be recommended to family members if the adopted child is found to be a carrier and have HBeAg. In selected cases, connubial partners may request screening tests in order to decide if an uninfected partner should be vaccinated.

Nevertheless, these screening procedures will continue to raise ethical problems. Although there is now a more obvious public health value that would derive from screening in certain populations, the identification of hepatitis carriers still involves some degree of individual and group stigmatization and is a potential disadvantage.

Other advances that would further alter the ethics of screening are likely to occur. Research is now being directed toward an understanding of how to either eliminate hepatitis B virus from carriers, or affect virus replication so that the amount of virus produced and excreted is so low that the carrier is no longer infectious.[10] If such measures become possible, they would probably also decrease the likelihood of the carrier's developing chronic liver disease or primary cancer of the liver. Under these conditions, identified carriers could be offered a therapeutic procedure. This would provide a powerful new medical and moral rationale for general hepatitis B virus carrier screening that might further offset the negative personal, social, and cultural side effects associated with it.

INAPPROPRIATE BIOMEDICAL APPLICATIONS

We can now examine medical problems which have been recommended as case studies for this seminar. Most of these problems have arisen because research has either not been done or has been done inadequately before the procedures were applied. These may not be examples of the Daedalus effect, which is, in a sense, a part of the scientific process itself and can be a consequence of the best-designed and -executed study.

Research is often adopted in clinical practice before it is actually completed. When the possibilities of a scientific advance are perceived, they are frequently applied to clinical practice as if their value had already been tested. Or, to put it in a more formal statement, a distinction is not made between the hypothesis when it is first stated ("Based on laboratory observation, the hypothesis is made that drug Alpha is beneficial for cardiac arrhythmias"), and the hypothesis after it has been adequately tested and supported ("We have already tested Alpha in a series of controlled trials and find it to be better than the previously available therapy"). In the early phase of research there often appears to be greater awareness of and more frequent and enthusiastic reporting on the problem-solving (beneficial) consequences of the discovery than on its problem-creating consequences (side effects). It is a common experience to read the glowing first accounts of a newly introduced procedure or therapy proclaiming its effectiveness and nearly trouble-free character. Only later one learns that the procedure is not as effective as first thought and carries with it significant toxic or undesirable consequences.

We can now consider some of the examples. In the pre-antibiotic era, there was a prevalent medical notion that enlarged tonsils were injurious to a child's health, and removal was widely practiced. In the 1920s, irradiation of the tonsils was introduced as an alternative to surgery and some 400,000 to 1,000,000 individuals received this treatment. In the 1950s, an association between irradiation and the subsequent (about 20 years later) development of cancer of the thyroid was noted; the use of irradiation dropped dramatically. In this case the effectiveness of removal of tonsils was never fully evaluated; that is, the research to determine the medical value of the procedure was never completed. In addition, it became extremely dfificult to evaluate the side effects of the irradiation, and this has not been determined with great accuracy or assurance. The failure to do adequate research led to a serious misapplication of technical knowledge.

Silverman[11] has given a graphic description of the development of retrolental fibroplasia in premature infants as a result of the use of hyperbaric oxygen in children with respiratory distress. Later, the therapy was used in premature children even without severe respiratory symptoms but without any evaluation of the value of the therapy. The unfortunate consequences of an inappropriate treatment were not recognized for many years.

Other examples, such as irradiation of the scalp for infections leading to the development of cancer, and the use of DES (diethylstilbestrol) to prevent abortion, which in some cases resulted in clear cell tumors of the vagina, will be discussed in later chapters.

In all of these, the value of a procedure and its possible hazards were not determined before the procedure was applied. This differs in some respects from the hepatitis example, in which the results of the initial studies were scientifically valid, but their consequences could not be recognized before they were in use.

NOTES

1. B. S. Blumberg and R. C. Fox, "The Daedalus Effect: Changes in Ethical Questions Relating to Hepatitis B Virus," *Annals of Internal Medicine* 102 (1985): 390-94.
2. I. G. Barbour, *Myths, Models and Paradigms: A Comparative Study in Science and Religion* (New York: Harper & Row, 1974).
3. B. S. Blumberg, "Australia Antigen and the Biology of Hepatitis B," *Science* 197(1977): 17-25.
4. _____, "Bioethical Questions Related to Hepatitis B Antigen," *American Journal of Clinical Pathology* 65(1976): 843-53.
5. L. O. Magnius and J. A. Espmark, "New Specificities in Australia Antigen Positive Sera Distinct from the LeBouvier Determinants," *Journal of Immunology* 109(1972): 1017-21.
6. E. Nordenfelt and M. Andern-Sandberg, "Dane Particle-Associated DNA Polymerase and e Antigen Relation to Chronic Hepatitis Among Carriers of Hepatitis B Surface Antigen," *Journal of Infectious Diseases* 134(1976): 85-89.
7. S. H. Hindman; C. R. Gravelle; B. L. Murphy; D. W. Bradley; W. R. Budge; and J. E. Maynard, " 'e' Antigen, Dane Particles and Serum DNA Polymerase Activity in HBsAg Carriers," *Annals of Internal Medicine* 85(1976): 458-60.
8. I. Millman, "The Development of the Hepatitis B Vaccine," in *Hepatitis B, The Virus, the Disease and the Vaccine,* ed. I. Millman, T. K. Eisenstein, and B. S. Blumberg (New York: Plenum, 1984), pp. 137-47.
9. W. Szmuness; C. E. Stevens; E. J. Harley; E. A. Zang; W. R. Oleazko; D. C. William; R. Sadovsky; J. M. Morrison; and A. Kellner, "Hepatitis B Vaccine: Demonstration of Efficacy in a Controlled Clinical Trail in a High-Risk Population in the United States," *New England Journal of Medicine* 303(1980): 833-41.
10. B. S. Blumberg and W. T. London, "Hepatitis B Virus and the Prevention of Primary Cancer of the Liver," *Journal of the National Cancer Institute* 74(1985): 267-73.
11. W. A. Silverman, "Retrolental Fibroplasia Neonatal Respiratory Distress," *Perspective in Biology and Medicine* 23(1980): 617-37.

4

The Scientific and Ethical Foundations of Medical Innovations

Paul Meier

It is not unusual, or even reprehensible, for an individual—or a whole society—to have desires that are not mutually compatible. It becomes unfortunate, however, when such incompatibilities are not recognized and when public policies come to be based on false models of reality.

Our society values highly the exploration of new modes of medical therapy and commends the research required to validate their efficacy. Enthusiasm extends even to innovations some consider bizarre: witness the evident approbation for trials of the Jarvik mechanical heart.

At the same time there is a comparable commitment to the protection of individual patients who participate in clinical research. Ever since the postwar exposure of Nazi medical research on prisoners, we have engaged in elaborate analysis and have set up administrative procedures to try to prevent such abuse. And, recognizing that inevitably some patients will be harmed in the course of research, we are particularly concerned to identify those persons responsible for causing such harm and to see that there is special compensation for the victims.

It is my claim that these highly commendable objectives are not commonly attainable. More specifically, I put forward three provocative propositions:

1. The above stated objectives are mutually inconsistent.
2. The patient's interest in optimal treatment does and should yield, in some degree, to other interests.
3. Provision of special compensation for harm which occurs in a research setting is generally unworkable and unjustifiable.

It is my view that all of us—ethicists and statisticians even more than clinical investigators—have been avoiding these inconsistencies rather than facing them and that this failure has led us into unproductive and strident debate rather than toward the development of a badly needed consensus.

The choices we need to make are neither easy nor entirely pleasant, but they cannot be avoided. Certainly they should not be made by the courts alone.

We may take some consolation, I think, in the often affirmed fact that patients treated in a research setting are generally far better protected from abuse than those receiving care in the normal course of therapy; this is an issue I shall return to later.

EXAMPLES

DES AND FETAL WASTAGE

In the early 1970s, a group of physicians in Boston reported a strange and unsettling phenomenon.[1] A rather uncommon form of cancer in young women seemed related to exposure to diethylstilbestrol (DES), which had been popular 20 years earlier as a treatment for pregnant women. The mothers of most of these women had been given DES while the subjects were in utero. At that time no one thought that modest doses of DES, then a newly discovered substitute for normal female estrogen, could cause harm. The new finding was both surprising and alarming.

A few days after that first report, there was another. It seems that in the early 1950s the University of Chicago had carried out an experiment testing the value of DES in maintaining pregnancy, and had announced that it was seeking to trace the children born from such pregnancies. So far as I know, no vaginal cancers have been discovered in the Dieckmann study group,[2] but there were other, less drastic effects and, of course, considerable distress. The university has been put to great expense to defend, and in some cases settle, multiple lawsuits.

But the significance of the Dieckmann study lies as much in its origins as in its outcome. The use of DES as a prophylactic to reduce the incidence of fetal wastage in high-risk women experiencing a first pregnancy was initiated and promoted in the late 1940s by a respected Boston clinic. The results reported by that clinic and by the prestigious Joslin Clinic for the Treatment of Diabetes were highly favorable, and the use of DES became very popular, especially in the Boston area. However, the quality of the supporting data seemed questionable to some, and the theory of why DES should help prevent premature termination of pregnancy seemed farfetched. Dieckmann had made the problem of successful pregnancy a major line of research and had not yet found a therapy that had any noticeable benefit. He thus determined to subject the DES treatment to careful study. Shortly thereafter, several other well-controlled studies, similar to Dieckmann's, were carried out.[3] All found the DES therapy to be without value.

It can be argued, and I do so argue, that we should like political and social incentives to favor such research as Dieckmann's. But for studies of this type, there would have been no persuasive evaluation of DES, and it seems at least plausible that its use would have become far more widespread than it actually became. Since at the time of this study DES was already regarded as established therapy in New England, its use by Dieckmann could scarcely be deemed improper in any event.

ABUSIVE EXPERIMENTS

There are, of course, genuine abuses of patients in experimental situations, and mechanisms are needed to identify, terminate, and, when appropriate, to punish those who conduct them.

The Tuskegee study on the "natural history" of syphilis is, by common consent, a case in point.[4] It does not compare, as some have claimed, to the Nazi experiments, but the long-term withholding of treatment from uninformed patients is impossible to condone. Likewise, the Willowbrook study of hepatitis vaccine is also widely condemned.

ORAL DRUGS AND DIABETES

A now classic and still controversial study is the University Group Diabetes Program (UGDP), started in the mid-1960s.[5] This was a cooperative, randomized, double-blind study of therapies for mild diabetes in the middle-aged and elderly. A few years earlier compounds had been discovered which, unlike insulin, could be taken by mouth, and which have a modest ability to lower blood sugar; these oral hypoglycemic drugs had been widely adopted. In addition to two insulin regimens, the study included one of these oral agents, tolbutamide, and a placebo. As time went on, it appeared that tolbutamide was associated with excess mortality, particularly from heart disease. Since this excess appeared to increase steadily, there came a point at which the investigators judged they had to stop using that drug, and the decision was duly announced, to the dismay of manufacturers and diabetologists alike. After all, tolbutamide (and its close chemical relatives) had become a mainstay of treatment for mild diabetes. Diabetologists would hardly welcome being told that they must confess error to their patients, withdraw what they had prescribed as helpful medication, and advise these patients to go on a stringent diet—all this on the basis of very marginal evidence. (The difference in total mortality was about 1 standard error; that for coronary mortality, only a little over 2 standard errors.) The early termination, based on suspicious but far from convincing evidence, proved to be a disaster in many ways. Quite apart from what I believe to be generally misguided attacks on the study design, the evidence against tolbutamide was just too thin to support a conclusion so unwelcome on other grounds. Nonetheless, the investigators were persuaded that their responsibility to the patients in the study compelled them to terminate it.

CLOFIBRATE IN CORONARY DISEASE

Not long after the UGDP, the National Heart Institute initiated the Coronary Drug Project (CDP) to ascertain the possible benefits of lowering blood cholesterol by pharmacologic means.[6] It had been established by the Framingham study that individuals with a higher level of cholesterol were at higher risk of heart attack,[7] but it was not established that high cholesterol actually *caused* the disease: it might be merely a symptom of a more complex process. In any event, it was not at all clear that the lowering of cholesterol by use of drugs would be beneficial. However, early in the conduct of the CDP one drug, clofibrate, seemed likely to be a winner. The death rate was substantially and consistently lower in the clofibrate group than in the placebo group, and the difference soon came to approach 2 standard errors. This evidence of a difference was even more potent than in the UGDP, of course, because the endpoint in view was total mortality, not merely coronary death. Were the difference to become clearly greater than 2 standard errors the investigators knew they might be obliged to terminate the study and recommend clofibrate, an easily administered pill with no evidence of uncomfortable side effects, as an effective prophylactic against death from recurrent heart attack. As it happened, however, the death rate for the clofibrate group began to increase at that point and thereafter was somewhat higher than the death rate in the placebo group. The issue of termination had come close, but it had never been reached. At the end of the study, the cumulative mortality in the two groups was virtually the same.

Shortly thereafter a much larger clofibrate study sponsored by the World Health Organization again pointed to early benefit.[8] Unfortunately it later emerged that clofibrate is a toxic drug; the total mortality of the clofibrate group after eight years proved to be about 25 percent higher than in the corresponding controls. Had the early results in the CDP been just a little more favorable, and had a "significant" benefit been seen as sufficient to preclude further experimenting, clofibrate would likely be in widespread use today, its toxicity hidden in the inherent variability of coronary artery disease.

My list of provocative cases is long, but these will serve for a beginning. Let me turn now to the mechanisms we have evolved in attempting to avoid abuse of patients, apart from lawsuits, and weigh their pros and cons.

ETHICAL CODES

It is scarcely surprising that after exposure to the horrors of Nazi medical experimentation there should have followed a sequence of attempts to codify the principles of decent behavior on the part of clinical researchers. This was attempted in the Nuremberg Code (1947), the Declarations of Helsinki (1964) and Tokyo (1975), U.S. Department of Health, Education, and Welfare guidelines (1971, 1974), and others as well.

More recently, building on this background the National Commission for the Protection of Human Subjects issued the Belmont report, in which the commission undertook to lay out general principles of ethical research, from which more specific practices should be derived.[9]

The three general principles—respect for persons, beneficence, and justice—are commendable but a bit diffuse, and the report goes on to detail the familiar list of particulars, which I summarize as follows:

1. The choice to participate in the experiment, which may involve randomized assignment to one or another treatment, should be one that a rational and informed person might reasonably make—for example, the investigator, on behalf of himself or a family member.

2. The relationship should be explicit. It is in the nature of things that the patient cannot understand everything the investigator understands, but he can usually be made reasonably well informed in layman's terms.

3. The patient should have a real option to refuse. That is, the opportunity should be more than formal. It would be meaningless, for example, if the doctor made it clear that without participation in the study, the doctor would no longer be concerned about that patient. The latter needs the doctor's goodwill, and should not be pressured by the threat of losing it.

4. At any time that there is a clear indication that the patient's best interests call for removal from the study, the patient's interests must be paramount.

Appealing as these guidelines are, there are sharp limits to their applicability.

There appears to be common agreement on the first: participation had better be something the investigator personally believes makes sense for an informed, intelligent person. But despite the reverential attitude commonly taken toward informed consent, points 2 and 3, it is by no means uniformly applicable. There are many who consider it inappropriate, even in cases where it could be applied. Thus, research on trauma patients (for example, head injury) involves comatose patients, often unaccompanied by family, and in urgent need of prompt intervention. Informed consent is simply not obtainable in such situations, and the various codes make appropriate exceptions for them.

Most American commentators would be shocked at a proposal to randomly assign women with breast cancer to a recommendation for simple or radical mastectomy without full explanation of the pros and cons of each procedure. Nonetheless, Sir Hedley Atkins, a distinguished, humane, and deeply thoughtful London surgeon, judged that the patients in his study of primary breast cancer therapy would *not* benefit by a discussion of the myriad uncertainties in choice of therapy, and he persuaded his local Institutional Review Board that it was proper to proceed without it.[10] Richard Peto, the outstanding (if cantankerous) British statistician and epidemiologist, speaks for many when he says that informed consent is "a legalistic trick to devolve what should properly be the doctor's responsibilities onto the patient."[11] (Peto supposes that informed consent may be useful in warding off American lawyers, but he considers it a good deal less useful in countries of more rational persuasion.)

No one disagrees in principle with the proposition that the patient should have a clear option to refuse participation without penalty, but many regard it as largely a sham in practice. In cases of serious illness few patients are likely to believe that refusing the doctor's invitation is an option without probable adverse consequences. Freedom of choice, in these circumstances, is limited to those of strong ego and unusual courage.

Our concerns about these first three principles will vary from one situation to another but, by and large, they seem not to face us with any insuperable obstacles to the initiation and conduct of clinical research. The real dilemma arises from interpretation of the last criterion. In one sense the paramount concern for the patients' interest is indeed obvious and noncontroversial. If we find that a particular patient cannot tolerate the assigned treatment, that his blood pressure drops to dangerous levels each time he takes the pill or that he breaks out in severe and agonizing rashes, his interest is clearly not served by continuing with that treatment, and so treatment must be withdrawn. If, however, the paramount concern with the interests of the patient is given a more general interpretation, we may be in serious difficulty.

A great many commentators, for whom Chalmers is an articulate spokesman, hold the view that, once we have grounds for even a modest presumption in favor of one treatment over another, we may not ethically conduct a clinical trial.[12] Thus, he argues, when a new therapy is proposed, the very first patients should be randomized, lest we prejudice ourselves with evidence of poor quality and lose forever the opportunity of getting good evidence. Although I share the view that even the earliest evidence should be gathered in a careful experimental mode, I have some difficulty with the rest of the argument. It is certainly natural, and even appropriate, to develop some hunches about how things are going long before the evidence warrants assurance. These hunches are often wrong, of course, but if a modest hunch is enough to proscribe further experiment, then a modest hunch is about as far as we will ever get.

The claims of the community at large, as opposed to those of the individual patient, lead to comparable avoidance. The same Hedley Atkins quoted above has also written of his anxieties about continuation of his study of surgical alternatives for primary breast cancer.[13] (Unlike most investigators, who rarely give more than a formal acknowledgment of ethical problems, Atkins has written widely on the subject.) There came a time, he says, when one of the therapies was trending more favorably than the other, and he and his colleagues could no longer say that they would willingly advise members of their own families to accept a random choice of therapies. Now Atkins was a friend and admirer of Sir Austin Bradford-Hill, the highly regarded initiator of large-scale randomized clinical trials, and Atkins took the problem to him. He reports that Bradford-Hill explained that, once having committed oneself to a study which was at the start entirely ethical, the failure to carry it through to a definite conclusion would be an unethical act, since it would preempt further study without itself answering the question posed and would render fruitless the contributions of the earlier patients. Atkins found this rhetoric persuasive, or at least comforting, but he fails to note that he has shifted focus from ethical responsibilities to the incoming participant to ethical responsibilities to the community. Atkins does not answer his own original question. Apparently he still would not feel easy about randomizing his sister, and it is not at all clear what his ground may be for continuing to randomize others.

An articulate argument in support of individual over group ethics is that of T. B. Schwartz, a participant in the UGDP. After discussing the original selection of patients, Schwartz continues:

> What, then, were we to do? It was not necessary for me to remind myself that the mortality curves represented the deaths of patients in our own clinics. Were we justified in continuing the study, or should tolbutamide be discontinued as a form of treatment? Let the reader forget about the reactions of drug companies and diabetologists. . . . Could he justify the continued use of tolbutamide? I could not.

> The decision to discontinue tolbutamide therapy was not unanimous. The reactions ranged from an unwavering insistence on discontinuance to total opposition to the decision. . . .

> The less rigid opponents to the decision marshaled two main arguments. There was the "scientific" notion that the discontinuance of the tolbuta-mide therapy was an unplanned break in the original protocol. We had set

out to study these patients for 10 years, and we should do so. The fact that the data were frightening should not intimidate "scientists." The second argument was "humanitarian." It ran that, should the study be continued, results would likely be more convincing, and, although a few more patients may die, more convincing results might save thousands of lives, since they would brook no argument. Those in favor of discontinuance pointed out that continuance of the study would in no way change baseline uncertainties. These were built in at the time the study started. Most telling, however, was the counter-"humanitarian" argument. It was pointed out that sacrifice of the few without their knowledge and consent in order to save the many is the height of medical immorality. It was this immoral premise that served as the main line of defense at the Nuremberg trials. It seemed to me that, as a physician-investigator, I could not, and must not, sacrifice the life of a single patient, even though it might save the population of the entire world. As an operational principle, this is not hyperbole; it is a crucial . . . tenet of the medical profession.[14]

What Schwartz fails to consider is the problem of initiating a study when we know that, for ethical reasons, we will have to stop it before its results are substantially informative, the problem of the "modest hunch" discussed earlier.

SPECIAL COMPENSATION

I have suggested that the social objective of scientific evaluation of medical innovations is not easily reconciled with an extreme position on the dominance of the patient's interests over those of research. It is, perhaps, in recognition of this problem that we seek to elevate the claims of patients injured in a research setting above those of patients injured in other ways. The injured research patient, we may feel, has been a sacrificial lamb. He gave up his claim on an undivided commitment to his personal benefit and, now that he is injured, he has a special claim on us for compensation.

Whatever one makes of the sacrificial lamb model, the principle of special compensation can at best have only limited application. Where untoward outcomes can be uniquely, or at least dominantly, connected to a specific therapy, as vaginal cancer is connected to prenatal exposure to DES, special compensation may be a realistic option. But for the vast majority of clinical studies, the link between specific therapy and bad outcomes is weak and entirely statistical.

Consider again the UGDP, and suppose for the moment that we regard the evidence of an increase in mortality as persuasive. Who is to be compensated here, and on what basis? As a crude estimate, we may judge that, of the 30 deaths in the tolbutamide group (compared to 21 in the placebo group), 9 are "excess" and 21 are "expected." Which 9 are "excess" one cannot say. Supposing there is no issue of blame, but only a desire to compensate for unforeseen harm: it is indeed difficult to see a rational basis for deciding whom to compensate and for how much. To this add the considerable uncertainty as to whether there really was any drug-induced bad effect at all. It is this sort of bad outcome situation which is most often faced. The case of bad outcomes clearly and directly linked to specific therapy is relatively rare.

Consider also the *Reyes* case.[15] Here a little girl in south Texas came down with paralytic polio two or three weeks after being given oral polio vaccine, and the parents sued the drug manufacturer for damages. There was no evidence of error in the manufacturing process or contamination of the vaccine. There was evidence that properly prepared vaccine can, very rarely, cause paralytic polio in immunosuppressed individuals. There was considerable evidence that wild-type polio was endemic in that region because of the ineffective vaccine program in Mexico. One may sympathize with Judge John Minor Wisdom, who, on appeal from a large jury award, determined to hold the manufacturer to account on a theory of strict liability for the consequences of administration of an "inherently unreasonably unsafe" product. Judge Wisdom did not argue that the evidence really pointed to vaccine causation. He argued, rather, that this child had been severely injured and would need the money, and that the only deep pockets in sight belonged to the manufacturer. The problem I see with this type of argument, even apart from the incentives it provides potential litigants, is this: the Reyes child was by no means the only one seriously affected by paralytic polio in south Texas, and the others were equally in need. If the desire to help the unfortunate is the dominant motive, that law seems to be a peculiarly ineffective way to satisfy it.

The distortion of incentives induced by relying on a theory of blame where none, in fact, exists, has been brought sharply into focus in the current crisis concerning the manufacture of pertussis vaccine. In a very few individuals a properly made vaccine may induce severe brain damage. Damage awards are high and, above all, variable, and only a few manufacturers have cared to stay in the field. Recently two of the remaining three have decided to withdraw, and, since a population unprotected by vaccine would be subject to severe epidemics, there is much wringing of hands in public health quarters over what to do about it.

AN ALTERNATIVE FRAMEWORK

It seems that there does not exist common consent on a set of principles adequate for guidance, if we believe both in the importance of scientific clinical experimentation *and* in the protection of the individual.

To make headway in dealing with these problems we have to put aside our aphorisms. We can accept all of the above principles *to a degree*, but—unlike Schwartz—far from absolutely.

The key to what I think is wrong with most arguments on the ethics of clinical experiments lies in the notion that it is unethical to deny an individual *any* expected benefit of treatment A over treatment B, regardless of how small that benefit may be or how uncertain.

Neither in setting our own patterns of behavior nor in fashioning general societal rules do we behave this way in other areas. The breast cancer surgeon who claims that a 1 percent improvement in survival probability is a pearl beyond price is simply wrong. As individuals, many of us accept an increased risk of death by auto accident in exchange for the privilege of living in pleasant surroundings a 20-minute drive from work, rather than taking less pleasant accommodations within walking distance. As a society we impose survival losses on ourselves for convenience, as when we fail to lower speed limits on city streets, or for economy, as when we fail to eliminate grade crossings.

In fact, of course, all innovation in medicine is experimental, admitted or not, and it involves some loss of expected benefits, if only because we know that most innovations, like most mutations, are failures. We continue to innovate, not because the odds favor any particular innovation, but because we value the long-range progress that goes with that course of action. The fact that informal innovation can often be disguised and the practitioner thereby protected from charges of misbehavior should not make us as potential patients prefer the hidden experiment to the explicit one.

As a matter of ordinary social behavior, most of us would be quite willing to forego a modest expected gain in probability of cure in the general interest of advancing the science of therapeutics. However, we should want to be assured that what we agree to give up is indeed modest. And no matter how small the loss, we should also want to be assured that we are not being singled out for special sacrifice.

Not everyone accepts this outlook, but for those who do there is still the problem of distinguishing a "reasonable loss of benefit" from "abuse." I do not suppose this will be easy, but I do believe it is the only way to find an ethical basis for the conduct of clinical research.

To be specific, suppose we are comparing, as Atkins did, two surgical treatments for cancer of the breast (lumpectomy and radical mastectomy). Consider once again the objectives of the clinical investigator. If possible, he should like to determine the difference in treatment effects with a suitably high precision. In statistical terms, he would like an estimate of that difference with a decently small standard error. At the same time, this object must yield to a decent regard for his patients' well-being. If the claim that "small differences do not matter much" is valid, there may be room to cope with both requirements at the same time.

Suppose we decided that, if we could be sure that the difference in treatment effects were *no more than* 10 percent, we should admit that the vagaries of the different populations at issue are such that we would not think it essential to insist that the apparently better treatment be uniformly adopted. Suppose, at the same time, that if we could be sure that the difference were *at least* 5 percent, we would think it fair to assert that a potentially worthwhile difference *had* been detected. Clearly, with a finite effort we could establish *at least one* of these conclusions, perhaps both, with strong assurance and without running into either statistical or moral paradoxes.

I propose, then, that we frame our problem as follows. We must identify a scale for comparison of the treatments, say the proportion surviving a fixed time. Using whatever philosophical, social, and political tools at our command, we must identify a maximum acceptable difference (*MD*) in the treatment effects such that we think it would *not* be abusive to patients to deny them that much benefit in the societal interest of obtaining useful information. We need also to decide upon a least interesting difference (*LD*) such that a difference that large or larger, if established, would be enough to justify a decision in favor of the winning therapy. And suppose, finally, we can agree on some method of setting an allowance for error in measuring the average difference at each time. Then our situation can be described graphically, as in figure 4.1.

However we set allowances for error, continued recruitment and follow-up will narrow the range of uncertainty, as shown in the upper graph. Meanwhile, the estimated difference fluctuates and is subject initially to a large error allowance. Our stopping rule has some flexibility, but it can be stated this way. Should the range of uncertainty ever show that we are clearly outside the maximum acceptable difference, we have gone too far and we must stop, because we now judge that further experimenting would be abusive.

But before that happens, the range of uncertainty will have to show that we are beyond the least interesting difference level, a point at which we might be content to stop and declare a winner. In between, we have room for judgment. Further experimenting might not be abusive, but it would have to be justified on the basis of expected additional knowledge.

Finally, of course, neither condition may be met. The estimated difference may remain fairly small, and we may not find an interesting difference and not feel compelled to bring the study to an early termination.

The framework currently popular for assessing treatment comparisons is a special case of the one described. What it does is to declare the maximum

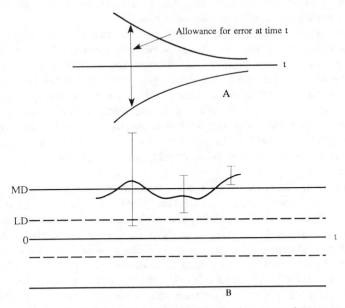

A, allowance for error in the estimate of difference in outcome between two treatments as a function of time. B, estimated difference in outcome as a function of time. Vertical bars represent the allowance for error. *MS* is maximum acceptable difference. *LD* is least interesting difference.

Figure 4.1: Framework for Conceptualizing Stopping Rules for a Clinical Trial.
Source: Paul Meier, "Terminating a Trial—the Ethical Problem," *Clinical Pharmacology and Therapeutics* 25, no. 5, part 2 (1979):663-40.

acceptable difference (and, consequently, the least interesting difference) to be zero, and this choice has two quite unattractive consequences: (1) the transition from "nothing of interest" to "unethical" is instantaneous, and (2) we promise to stop before we learn anything of real interest, that is, anything more than that the treatment difference is not zero. Once we know with reasonable assurance that the difference favors one of the treatments, by no matter how small an amount, we are ethically bound to declare that treatment the winner and forego the use of the other. By the same token, the current framework regards any difference which is not statistically significant at some specified level to be effectively zero, at least for ethical purposes. It seems that this convention allows the experimenter to escape responsibility for continuing an experiment which trends in favor of one treatment so long as the difference does not reach statistical significance. But in the course of real studies, reality obtrudes. Atkins wrote about this problem with a frankness rarely shown in medical publications, but he did not solve it.[16] Anyone who has sat on data monitoring and policy boards for cooperative clinical trials is aware of the unease felt when one treatment seems to be showing clear signs of benefit compared to the other; debates rage over which particular analysis should be relied upon to declare the result significant or not and thus determine the legitimacy of continuing the study.

I make no claim that the framework I propose would be easy to apply. I see no escape, however, from the fact that the acquisition of substantial knowledge of treatment differences is possible only if we are prepared to deny some patients the benefit of less than conclusive, but nonetheless substantial, intermediate findings.

Indeed, it seems to me within the ethos of modern American society to recognize that technology changes continuously and that, in one aspect or another, most of medical practice is innovative and therefore experimental. An environment in which, as a matter of course, unresolved questions of therapeutic choice are subject to experimental test might be accepted as entirely welcome. Such an environment could, as at present, invite a patient with particular preferences to make those preferences known and to opt out of a randomized allocation. But if experiment is the norm instead of the exception, the problem of the sacrificial lamb essentially disappears.

INNOVATION VERSUS ESTABLISHED PRACTICE

The Belmont report draws a sharp distinction between *research* and the *practice of accepted therapy*, reserving for research alone the requirement for review to protect human subjects. It turns out that "practice" refers to interventions that are "designed solely to enhance the well-being of an individual patient . . . and that have a reasonable expectation of success," and that "the fact that a procedure is 'experimental' in the sense of new, untested, or different," does not automatically remove it from the realm of practice. Thus, it would appear, the Boston obstetricians who introduced DES need not have had their innovation made subject to review, because, having become convinced of the benefits of their intervention on prior grounds, they saw no need for "research" thereon. Dieckmann, on the other hand, who was explicitly evaluating the same therapy in comparison to a placebo, should have had his plans scrutinized and held to a far higher standard.

Whether a structure so heavily weighted *against* evaluation and *toward* casual innovation meets contemporary needs and desires is a political question, but review of a number of initially untested innovations gives reason to question the desirability of such a bias.

CORONARY ARTERY SURGERY

When coronary artery surgery was first introduced, the benefits were seen as obvious. It proved to be moderately safe—5 percent operative mortality in the early years, and much lower since—and the procedure spread rapidly. Happily, the Veterans' Administration promptly initiated a randomized trial of this intervention and presently demonstrated that, so far as survival was concerned, only a small fraction of those being operated on stood to gain. The later and larger Coronary Artery Surgery Study confirmed these results.[17] Meanwhile, the surgeon who had invented the procedure had formed a surgical group which practiced in a number of hospitals in the Boston area, including one in the suburb of Malden. Some time later, a technician at the hospital resigned and set out on a year-long effort to bring administrative attention to what he claimed was an outrageously high operative mortality. Neither the hospital administration nor the county medical society cared to go further than to refer the complaint to the surgical group itself. It was only when the story was ultimately brought to the *Boston Globe* that a serious investigation was made. It emerged that essentially *half* of all patients operated on at Malden had died promptly after surgery, a result attributed to lack of adequately practiced adjunct staff.

LIPID-LOWERING DRUGS

Early in the period when epidemiologic studies were pointing to the association of high cholesterol with heart disease, drugs which lowered cholesterol, and which might therefore help protect against heart disease, were widely marketed. In the 1960s, the Coronary Drug Project undertook a randomized study of mortality for groups using different lipid-lowering drugs or placebo. Most of these drugs were found to be toxic, that is, they caused excess mortality; none was found to extend longevity.

HEART SOUNDS

One need not relive the harrowing night of the dying physician with the imperturbable intern so evocatively described by Martha Weinman Lear[18] to realize that there is a sharp limit to the priority of the patient's well-being over other interests in the ordinary practice of medicine. It is no criticism of physicians in general to note that their need for a private life may not always be consistent with the best interests of a seriously ill patient, or that the ponderousness of modern medical establishments may sometimes work to a patient's disadvantage.

The point of these three examples is simple: the priority of the patient's interest over other claims is far from unconditional in ordinary clinical practice. Is it desirable that the standard be made exceedingly more rigorous when we are dealing with clinical research?

FORM AND SUBSTANCE

It may be, as many practitioners of clinical research aver, that the healthiest situation for a patient is to be positioned as a participant in a clinical trial. In that role he will be carefully monitored, frequently examined, and generally fussed over. Deterioration in health is likely to be noticed early and dealt with promptly.

But while the assertion may be true as a matter of fact, there may well be concerns that are special to the relationship and that must be weighed above and beyond the question of medical outcomes itself. The patient wishes, and is entitled, to see the physician as a devoted healer whose interest in the patient's health is uncontaminated by competing interests. The investigator's dual role when the patient is a research participant is threatening to that perception, and, it may be argued, the threat must be compensated for by taking special pains to be sure there is no abuse.

RESCUE OPERATIONS

Consider, in a different domain, the mountain climber who has slipped and dangles helplessly over a crevasse, in full view of vacationers' telescopes. Past experience may tell us that any attempt at rescue will be so risky in terms of expected loss of life that it would be better not attempted. A generally accepted view, I believe, is that the abandonment such a calculus implies is socially more costly than the excess risk and that the rescue effort should be made.

BABY FARMING

Paul Ehrlich alleges that, far from being inconceivable in Western societies, infanticide as a means of controlling family size was practiced in nineteenth-century England.[19] He was referring to baby farming. Parents wishing to rid themselves of unwanted infants delivered them to poor women who, for a pittance, undertook to provide food and care. In fact, well understood by all concerned, the food was meager, care limited, and infection rampant. Such infants generally died in a short time, and it was expected that they would.

The practice died, I presume with improvements in the condition of the poor, but it may be argued that, dismal as it may have been, baby farming was less socially destructive than direct infanticide would have been.

I do not suggest that such preferences for form over substance lack legitimacy. I do suggest that our concern to guard the patient participating in a research program so much more zealously than a similar patient subject to the ordinary practice of medicine has a large component of this type in it.

CONCLUSION

In sum, no reasonable person wants to allow unrestricted research on human subjects; nor does any reasonable person want to restrict it entirely. There is no happy middle ground, and the choice between more science and less abuse is not an easy one. That choice is not properly scientific, nor legal, nor even, I think, ethical. It must ultimately be a political choice about the kind of society we wish to have, and to that end it is essential to focus discussion on real choices rather than idealized ones.

NOTES

1. A. L. Herbst, H. Ulfelder, and D. C. Poskanzer. "Adenocarcinoma of the Vagina: Association of Maternal Stilbestrol Therapy with Tumor Appearance in Young Women," *New England Journal of Medicine* 284(1971):878-81.
2. W. J. Dieckmann, M. E. Davis, L. M. Rynkiewicz, and R. E. Pottinger. "Does the Administration of Diethylstilbestrol During Pregnancy Have Therapeutic Value?" *American Journal of Obstetrics and Gynecology* 66(1953):1062-81.
3. Thomas C. Chalmers, "The Impact of Control Trials on the Practice of Medicine," *Mount Sinai Journal of Medicine* 41(1974):753-58.
4. James H. Jones, *Bad Blood: The Tuskegee Syphilis Experiment* (New York: Free Press, 1981).
5. Thaddeus E. Prout, "A Prospective View of the Treatment of Adult-Onset Diabetes," *Medical Clinics of North America* 55(1971):1065-75.
6. "The Coronary Drug Project: Design, Methods and Baseline Results," *Circulation* 47, suppl. 1 (1973).
7. Thomas R. Dawber, *The Framingham Study: The Epidemiology of Atherosclerotic Disease* (Cambridge, MA: Harvard Unviersity Press, 1980).
8. World Health Organization Cooperative Trial on Primary Prevention of Ischaemic Heart Disease Using Clofibrate to Lower Serum Cholesterol; Mortality Follow-up. *Lancet* 2, 8191(1980):379-85.

9. National Commission for the Protection of Human Subjects of Biomedical and Behavioral Research, *Ethical Principles and Guidelines for the Protection of Human Subjects of Research* (Belmont report), DHEW publ. no. (OS) 78-0012 (Washington, D.C.: Government Printing Office, 1978).
10. Hedley Atkins, "Conduct of a Controlled Clinical Trial," *British Medical Journal* 2(1966):377.
11. Marc E. Buyse, M. J. Staquet, and R. J. Sylvester, eds., *Cancer Clinical Trials: Methods and Practice* (New York: Oxford University Press, 1984), p. 17.
12. T. C. Chalmers, "When Should Randomizing Begin?" *Lancet* 1, 7547(1968):858.
13. H. Atkins, J. L. Hayward, D. J. Klugman, and A. B. Wayte, "Treatment of Early Breast Cancer: A Report after Ten Years of a Clinical Trial," *British Medical Journal* 2(1972):423-29.
14. T. B. Schwartz, "The Tolbutamide Controversy: A Personal Perspective," *Annals of Internal Medicine* 75(1971):303-6.
15. *Reyes* v. *Wyeth Laboratories, Inc.* 498 F. 2d 1264 (5th Cir. 1974).
16. Atkins, Hayward, Klugman, and Wayte, "Treatment of Early Breast Cancer."
17. "National Heart, Lung, and Blood Institute, Coronary Artery Surgery Study (CASS)," *Circulation* 63, no. 6, part 2 (1981):1-81.
18. Martha Weinman Lear, *Heartsounds* (New York: Simon and Schuster, 1980).
19. Paul Ehrlich and J. Holdren, "The Impact of Population Growth," *Science* 171(1971):1212-17.

5

Microsocial Influences on the Use of Medical Innovations

Alvin R. Tarlov

In "The Scientific Process and the Development of Medical Innovation: The Daedalus Effect," Baruch Blumberg reminds us of the inevitability of medical mishap. Blumberg's model suggests that the rate of medical mishap might even serve as one measure of the rate of a society's progress.

Paul Meier's analysis concludes (although of this I am not entirely convinced) that most patients would be willing to sacrifice a small probabilistic therapeutic gain for the benefit of advancing therapeutics for the whole society. Meier seeks to establish both practical qualitative limits to the allowable sacrifice, and quantitative endpoints to identify with confidence a true therapeutic advance.

Meier further asserts that research and clinical practice are similar in their experimental nature and in their potential for favorable outcomes. The point should be emphasized. The work of Wennberg and Gittelsohn[1] over the last 15 years has demonstrated wide variation in the use of tests and procedures in different geographic areas, and even in adjacent communities within a single area. The rate of performance of surgical procedures such as cholecystectomy, prostatectomy, and hysterectomy varies three to five times among communities matched for demographic and epidemiologic characteristics. Similar findings have been reported from Western European countries. Although many explanations have been offered, the underlying cause for these variations is explained best by a lack of agreement about what practices represent "standard" medical practice. The efficacy, or worth, of three-fourths of what physicians do in standard practice remains uncertain. The wide variation in utilization rates from one area to another is based on this uncertain efficacy. In this sense, I agree with Meier that clinical practice, like research, is largely experimental. Tacit acknowledgment that medical practice is largely experimental should have significant implications for deliberations on the moral and legal responsibility of physicians.

Stephen Toulmin, in "Technological Progress and Social Policy: The Broader Significance of Medical Mishaps," indicates the clear predominance of social influences in determining the extent to which innovations are accepted or demanded by a particular society. Toulmin characterizes the attitudes of a society toward medical innovation as falling on a continuum between conservative and progressive. Physicians in different societies act within a larger social and cultural matrix that imposes certain expectations.

Toulmin believes, and I agree, that in late twentieth-century America the external pressure of social demands imposes on physicians a progressive rather than a conservative mode of practice. The social matrix within which medicine is practiced in America encourages (often implores, even under threat of punishment, such as malpractice claims) physicians to employ the most up-to-date medical procedures and treatments—often before their adverse side effects have been discovered and, increasingly, even before the possible benefits of the new drug or procedure have been established.

For example, on May 14, 1985, the Food and Drug Administration, compelled by a perception of political urgency, approved the use of a drug for acquired immunodeficiency syndrome (AIDS) before its effectiveness

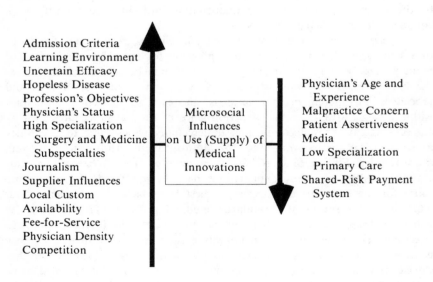

Admission Criteria
Learning Environment
Uncertain Efficacy
Hopeless Disease
Profession's Objectives
Physician's Status
High Specialization
   Surgery and Medicine
   Subspecialties
Journalism
Supplier Influences
Local Custom
Availability
Fee-for-Service
Physician Density
Competition

Microsocial
Influences
on Use (Supply) of
Medical
Innovations

Physician's Age and
   Experience
Malpractice Concern
Patient Assertiveness
Media
Low Specialization
   Primary Care
Shared-Risk Payment
   System

Figure 5.1: Microsocial Influences in Medicine on the Use of Medical Innovations.

had been proved. Thus, for the second time in a decade (the first occasion being the swine flu situation) and on both occasions propelled by fears of an epidemic, our profession has been encouraged for social and political purposes to use a drug prematurely. I suppose physicians who prescribe the drug are absolved of legal responsibility for mishaps because they have been empowered and encouraged by the government and the FDA to do so, but I wonder about their moral responsibility for such actions.

Unquestionably, on a conservative-progressive scale, the United States is far over into the progressive side. So is its medical system. Broad social and political influences—the *macrosocial* environment—exert a powerful influence on medical practices and increase the demand for medical innovation. A second, and parallel, influence on the use of medical innovations derives from the *microsocial* environment—the medical system—in which physicians are educated and trained, and in which they practice.

In figure 5.1, I focus on the many elements in the microsocial environment that encourage medical innovation and the relatively few elements that constrain it. The many factors noted on the left side of figure 5.1 tend to increase the supply and use of medical innovations. The relatively few factors on the right side of figure 5.1 serve as moderating influences.

FACTORS IN MEDICINE
THAT ENCOURAGE THE USE OF INNOVATIONS

1. *Admission Criteria for Medical School.* Individuals favored for admission are likely to be experimental, innovative, and willing to take risks during their careers.

2. *The Learning Environment.* In medical schools, teaching hospitals, and community hospitals—wherever medical students and house officers are trained—the learning environment encourages the application of new techniques and procedures in medical practice.

3. *Uncertain Efficacy.* As Meier notes, much of "standard" medical practice is based on untested hypotheses. This level of uncertainty which operates in ordinary practice further encourages the use of medical innovation.

4. *Hopeless Disease.* Unestablished innovations are often acceptable and are frequently encouraged for conditions that are regarded as untreatable, terminal, or hopeless.

5. *The Objectives of the Medical Profession.* In the latter part of the twentieth century, the primary objectives of the medical profession in America remain to prevent disability and death. The ultimate

enemy in medical practice still is death. As a result, these objectives encourage the relaxation of conservative standards of practice and encourage the application of experimental innovations.

6. *Physicians' Status.* Physicians with the highest status within the profession tend to be those who use high technology.

7. *Specialization.* Specialization and subspecialization in medicine and surgery also favor the application of new innovations.

8. *Medical Journalism.* In December 1983, a five-minute film was shown on a San Francisco television station on the subject of mitral valve prolapse in women. Middle-aged women with certain symptoms were urged to see their physicians and have an echocardiogram done. The Kaiser Family Foundation monitored the subsequent rate of use of echocardiography in middle-aged women in the six counties around San Francisco. It determined that the rate of echocardiography increased threefold and was sustained at that high level for about three months before gradually returning over the course of the next five months to the baseline rate.

9. *Supplier Influences.* Drug companies and manufacturers of medical technology encourage physicians to adopt the latest innovations.

10. *Other Factors.* The availability of high technology and the subsidization that hospitals provide doctors and their practices (for example, by amortizing expensive equipment) favors the application of medical innovations. Hospital administrators sometimes pressure physicians to use available and expensive equipment. The fee-for-service system, which even today remains the predominant mode of reimbursement for medical costs, favors the application of new medical technologies. Physician density results in increased competition for the patient, and this too may encourage the use of sophisticated and innovative technologies. Several additional factors are noted in figure 5.1

FACTORS IN MEDICINE
THAT ENCOURAGE CONSERVATIVE PRACTICE

The factors encouraging conservative practice traditionally have not been as powerful within the profession as those that encourage innovation.

1. *The Physician's Age and Experience.* In 1976, we collected data which showed that more experienced physicians are less likely to use high technology and that the frequency of use of CAT scans to evaluate patients' complaints of headache declines as physicians get older.

2. *Malpractice Fears.* In general, concerns about malpractice tend to discourage physicians from using technology which may be associated with patient risk.

3. *Patient Assertiveness.* Greenfield has shown that providing patients with assertiveness training leads to greater patient participation in the management of their care and, interestingly, to a decline in the use of high technology.[2]

4. *Primary Care Physicians.* Compared to subspecialists, primary care physicians use less high-cost technology.

5. *Shared-Risk Payment System.* There is no doubt that the shared-risk payment system—including copayments, deductibles, prepayment and HMOs—indeed, all systems that have economic incentives to reduce utilization of medical technology, are an important restraining influence.

CONCLUSION

In American medicine of 1985, and probably for the remainder of this century, I believe that the net effect of the microsocial influences will continue to encourage the use of medical innovations. In the near future, we can expect more rather than fewer applications of medical innovations.

The macrosocial environment described by Stephen Toulmin has created a progressive thrust which establishes a high demand for medical innovation. At the same time, the microsocial environment powerfully encourages high supply and high readiness to apply medical innovation. This high-demand and high-supply state is not likely to abate in the near future.

NOTES

1. J. Wennberg and A. Gittelsohn, "Small Area Variations in Health Care Delivery," *Science* 182(1973):1102-8.
2. S. Greenfield, S. Kaplan, and J. E. Ware, "Expanding Patient Involvement in Care: Effects on Patient Outcomes," *Annals of Internal Medicine* 102(1985)520-28.

Section 2

Causation and Responsibility: Conceptual Analyses

6

Causation in Medicine and the Law

Kenneth F. Schaffner

In this chapter I want to develop the outlines of a probabilistic explanation of the expression, "agent A caused result D in person P." Generally we can think of D as a disease, an illness, or an undesirable condition. I shall focus my analysis on one biomedical illustration, and will relate my explication to the domains of tort law and product liability theory.[1] This essay is a synthetic investigation attempting to identify developing similarities in causal concepts arising in medical epidemiology, philosophy of science, and tort theory.

Among my theses are (1) that the existence of significant genetic and environmental variation, widespread multifactorial causation, and inadequate (and for all practical purposes irremediably incomplete) data at the individual level in the biomedical area requires that we be content with less than deterministic explications in describing clinical causation and (2) that for the same reasons we must interpret biomedical causation primarily as a claim about populations. Clinical researchers, biostatisticians, and epidemiologists have developed criteria and methods for testing such claims. I will review Evans' recent generalizations and modifications of the well-known Henle-Koch postulates for evaluating a putative infectious cause of a clinical disease. I shall also comment on Lilienfeld and Lilienfeld's minor modifications of these criteria and consider their application to drug product and radiation injuries. These discussions will require a necessarily superficial account of experiments, randomized clinical trials, cohort, and case control studies. The philosophical foundations of such methods will be discussed, including notions of probabilistic causation, following which legal concepts of causation will be considered. An explication of causation derived from epidemiological, philosophical, and legal principles will then be applied to diethylstilbestrol (DES) and, implicitly because of time constraints, to radiation-induced injuries. I shall argue in these cases that a two-stage probabilistic inquiry needs to be pursued in order to determine fair compensation for injuries associated with such products and processes.

Supported by a grant from the EVIST program to the University of Chicago.

Let me also say a few words about what I shall not be discussing. I believe that deterministic as well as stochastic mechanisms are most important features in biomedical science. I have in mind as illustrations of such mechanisms the operon model of genetic control, the actin-myosin mechanism of muscle contraction, and a two-hit theory of carcinogenesis. These types of mechanisms, often articulated at the molecular level, have been discussed in an article I published in 1980. I shall not be discussing causation in association with these types of mechanisms, though the existence and centrality of such mechanisms will exercise an important conceptual constraint leading me away from the more standard interpretation of probabilistic causality toward one more congruent with both deterministic and stochastic mechanistic causation.

CLINICAL PROBABILISTIC CAUSATION

In this section I begin to examine the methods of the epidemiologists and biostatisticians for attributing causation in a clinical context. I start by considering a more traditional notion of essentially deterministic causation, which is exemplified in what are usually termed Koch's postulates.

THE HENLE-KOCH-EVANS POSTULATES

In 1884 Robert Koch proposed four postulates which needed to be satisfied in order to claim that an infectious agent, A, was the cause of a specific disease, D.

1. A must be present in every case of D.
2. A must be isolated and grown in pure culture.
3. A must, when inoculated into a susceptible animal, cause D. (It would be better, in order to avoid any circularity here, to rewrite this as: D must always be present in the animal after such inoculation.)
4. A must then be recovered from the animal and identified.[2]

These postulates, which Evans (1976) indicates were first developed by Koch's teacher, Henle, are both too strong and too simple. They have had and continue to have a powerful salutary influence in bacteriology, but they overemphasize a universal and deterministic experimental situation, for not all virulent inoculated agents will always cause a clinical disease. Nowadays, we are more familiar with the complex web of causation, including respiratory, endocrine, and immunological protective mechanisms. In addition, Koch's work took place at a time when the focus was on acute bacteriological diseases; later, viral, immunological, and chronic diseases became more important, and more sophisticated biochemical and epidemiological methods of assessing disease causation became available.

Evans (1976) outlined several generalizations of the Henle-Koch postulates to accommodate these advances, and, by way of summary, proposed ten joint criteria as an explication of a "Unified Concept of Causation." These criteria were accepted with only minor modifications by Lilienfeld and Lilienfeld as a kind of "summary of the methods and reasoning presented" (1980). These criteria of causation are:

1. Prevalence of the disease should be *significantly higher* in those exposed to the [putative] hypothesized cause than in controls not so exposed (the cause may be present in the external environment or as a defect in host responses).

2. Exposure to the hypothesized cause should be *more frequent* [present more commonly] among those with the disease than in controls without the disease—when all other risk factors are held constant.

3. Incidence of the disease should be *significantly higher* in those exposed to the cause than in those not so exposed, as shown by prospective studies.

4. Temporally, the disease should follow exposure to the hypothesized causal agent with a distribution of incubation periods on a log-normal-shaped curve [bell-shaped curve].

5. A spectrum of host responses should follow exposure to the hypothesized agent along a logical biologic gradient from mild to severe.

6. A measurable host response following exposure to the hypothesized cause should have a *high probability* of appearing [should regularly appear] in those lacking this before exposure (for example, antibody, cancer cells) or should increase in magnitude if present before exposure; this response pattern should occur *infrequently* [should not occur] in persons not so exposed.

7. Experimental reproduction of the disease should occur *more frequently* [*in higher incidence*] in animals or man appropriately exposed to the hypothesized cause than in those not so exposed; this exposure may be deliberate in volunteers, experimentally induced in the laboratory, or demonstrated in controlled regulation of natural exposure.

8. Elimination or modification of the hypothesized cause or of the vector carrying it should *decrease the incidence* of the disease (for example, control of polluted water, removal of tar from cigarettes).

9. Prevention or *modification* of the host's response on exposure to the hypothesized cause should *decrease* or eliminate the disease (for example, immunization, drugs to lower cholesterol, specific lymphocyte transfer factor in cancer).

10. All of the relationships and findings should make biologic and epidemiologic sense.[3]

Several points are worth stressing about these criteria. First, note the use of quasi-statistical concepts such as "significantly higher" and "bell-shaped curve." Second, these notions and others expressed by such phrases as "more commonly," "in higher incidence," "increase," and "decrease," are *comparative* concepts, not absolute such as those found in the expressions "in every case," "must cause," or "eliminate," as in Koch's postulates.

My interpretation of a clinically oriented biomedical concept of causation, then, is that, at least in part, it is now seen as substantially grounded by statistical epidemiological methods. Let us look at some of these methods explicitly and then at the philosophical concept of causation, that is, a prima facie probabilistic notion, which they imply.

EPIDEMIOLOGICAL METHODS
FOR DETERMINING CAUSATION

Generally, if we want to support the claim that "A caused D in person P," we begin by determining that A is *associated with* D in persons *like* P. There can be four reasons why such an association of A with D is found:

1. A can (always, often, sometimes) *cause* D.

2. There may be some other *confounding* factor that causes A and D to "travel together," for example, a *common* cause.

3. The association can be due to *bias*, for example, the ways we *selected* or *measured* the cases.

4. The association can be due to *chance*, for example, a run of good or bad luck or a set of coincidences results in an association.

In order to rule out or diminish the possibility that the suspected cause is actually due either to a confounding cause or to bias, biostatisticians have proposed that we form appropriately selected control groups. To rule out or diminish the effect of chance associations, statistical analysis which estimates the likelihood of runs of coincidences is used.[4]

There are several means of designing studies to test a causal association and control for bias and chance. One appropriate and relatively inexpensive way to test the hypothesis that "A caused D" is to use the case control method. Here, after informed consent is obtained, we identify a small group of individuals with $D(P_D)$ and also select an appropriately similar control group with $D (P_{\sim D})$.[5] We then look back in time and ascertain both groups' exposure to A, and compare results. Because it looks backwards in time this is also called a retrospective study. Because such studies need to rely on faulty memory and often incomplete medical records, the chance for bias is high, and rigorous criteria applied uniformly to both case and control group members are needed.[6] One can then ascertain if there is a statistically significant increase in risk for persons exposed to A: that is, we examine under what circumstances one would find an increase because of pure chance, even though there was in fact no increased risk. We want such a thing to happen (following standard scientific convention) in less than 1 of every 20 studies. This requirement, if satisfied, is written as a *P* value (in this case $P \leqslant .05$). (This is a probability, and it may also be written as a percent and termed a significance level for the study.) Statisticians feel comfortable with this 5 percent figure, in part for historical reasons, but it is by no means sacrosanct.[7]

The increase in risk obtained from such a retrospective case-controlled study is expressed in an odds ratio. In computing such an odds ratio, we divide the odds that a case instance (*a* and *c*) of the disease is exposed by the odds that a control instance (*b* and *d*) is exposed. A tabular summary means of expressing the data is shown in table 6.1.

Table 6.1: Data for Computing the Odds Ratio

	Cases	*Controls*	*Total*
Exposed	*a*	*b*	*a + b*
Nonexposed	*c*	*d*	*c + d*
Total	*a + c*	*b + d*	

It is obvious that the odds that any one case is exposed are
$$\frac{a/(a + c)}{c/(a + c)} = a/c.$$
Similarly, the odds that any control is exposed are
$$\frac{b/(b + d)}{d/(b + d)} = b/d.$$
The odds ratio, then, equals
$$\frac{a/c}{b/d} = ad/bc.$$

Statisticians have shown that this ratio is conceptually and mathematically similar to the relative risk ratio, which would be obtained in the more costly and time-consuming cohort type of study.[8]

A relative risk ratio or odds ratio higher than 1 indicates increased risk of D to the patient from agent A. Basically, relative risk answers the question, How many times more likely are exposed persons to get the disease relative to nonexposed?[9]

It will be helpful to our understanding to illustrate these notions with a few numbers. These are quite close to the data obtained by Herbst and his colleagues in their classic study (1971) of the carcinogenic effects of DES in utero.[10]

Using a tabular summary similar to that in table 6.1, we summarize the data in table 6.2.

Table 6.2: Data for Computing the Odds Ratio for Vaginal Adenocarcinoma

	Cases of Vaginal Adenocarcinoma	Controls (Without Disease)
In utero exposure to DES	7	1
No history of in utero exposure to DES	1	31

The odds ratio for these data yields 7 x 31 ÷ 1 x 1 = 217, a considerable increase in risk! One can perhaps get a better idea of the magnitude of this risk by comparing it with similarly analyzed data for the risk of death from lung cancer associated with cigarette smoking, which yields a relative risk ratio of 13.7.[11] This DES result can itself be tested statistically in accord with the principles mentioned briefly above to determine what the likelihood is that these data would have been obtained if DES were *not* latently carcinogenic. This is accomplished by using an appropriate statistical test, such as the chi-square distribution, which will yield a P value for this study; in Herbst et al.'s work, P was considerably less than .05.

The relative risk ratio, or odds ratio, is but one of several measures of effect used by epidemiologists.[12] One additional measure of effect of particular interest to this inquiry is the concept of attributable risk. Roughly, attributable risk is a measure of the *additional* risk or incidence following exposure over and above that experienced by people who are not exposed.[13] Thus, attributable risk takes into account the background incidence of the disease, say from causes other than the agent A under consideration. The definition of attributable risk is simple:

Attributable Risk = Incidence$_{Exposed}$ - Incidence$_{Not\ Exposed}$.

The concept of incidence used here refers to "the fraction or proportion of a group initially free of the outcome which develops the outcome over a given period of time."[14] The concept of incidence is often distinguished from its sister concept of prevalence, which is "the fraction (proportion) of a group possessing a clinical outcome at a given point in time . . . [which] is measured by a single examination or survey of the group."[15]

Fletcher et al. imply that the above definition of attributable risk cannot be utilized in connection with the easier and less costly case-control type of study discussed above, but it can be employed in a cohort study. In a cohort study we identify a population of individuals free of the disease of interest, some of whom will naturally be exposed over time to the possible disease-causing agent and some of whom will not be exposed. We then follow that group forward in time, periodically gathering data to determine the incidence of disease in the exposed and nonexposed groups. These data will enable us to both determine relative risk ratios and compute attributable risk values. Such a study was initiated for DES daughters after Herbst et al.'s case-control discovery of the carcinogenic properties of DES. A cohort study is obviously more difficult to do and is considerably more expensive, as well as requiring many years to complete, though a *retrospective* cohort group can be identified, in appropriate circumstances.

Though Fletcher et al. raise an interesting question about the legitimacy of applying the attributable risk notion to case-control studies, other epidemiologists such as MacMahon and Pugh and Lilienfeld and Lilienfeld, following the work of Levin and Bertell, do introduce an analogue of attributable risk. Their definition of a population-attributable risk (PAR), or the proportion of a disease in a population attributable to a risk factor, is given by the expression

$$PAR = \frac{a/(a+c) - b/(b+d)}{1 - b/(b+d)}.$$

Using our earlier DES example, this expression would yield a population-attributable risk of

$$\frac{7/8 - 1/32}{1 - 1/32} = 27/31 = 87\%.$$

It must be stressed that the application of this concept is somewhat controversial and depends on the satisfaction of several assumptions: that each group is representative of the respective groups in the population, that the prevalence of the disease is sufficiently low that the prevalence among persons free of the disease is very close to the prevalence of exposure among the total population, and that the odds ratio (given these assumptions) adequately represents the relative risk of the disease among exposed compared with those not exposed.[16] Furthermore, it would be wise to note that these assumptions will not hold for diseases which have synergistic causes operative in the examined populations, such as in mesotheliomas caused by asbestos exposure and cigarette smoking, and in lung cancer in uranium miners who smoke.[17]

As indicated in figure 6.1 from Lilienfeld and Lilienfeld, the retrospective study, or case control, is only one experimental design. The gold standard for determining causation is the randomized controlled clinical trial (RCT), but because of ethical difficulties such a prospective test of an agent considered harmful cannot be done on human beings. In the past such trials were more prevalent: the trial to determine whether retrolental fibroplasia in premature infants was due to high tensions of oxygen being a case in point.[18]

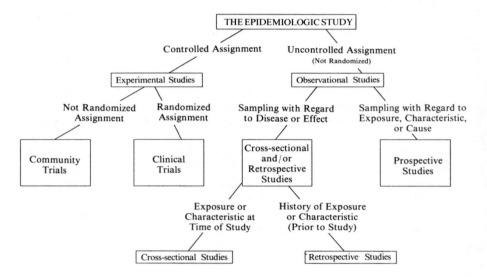

Figure 6.1: The Anatomy of the Epidemiologic Study.

Adapted from: A. M. Lilenfeld and D. E. Lilenfeld, *Foundations of Epidemiology*, 2nd ed. (New York: Oxford Unviersity Press, 1980), p. 192.

PHILOSOPHICAL EXPOSITIONS
OF PROBABILISTIC CAUSALITY

What notion of causation underlies the epidemiological concept of cause elaborated above? A provocative quotation from Lilienfeld and Lilienfeld may help answer this question:

> In medicine and public health it would appear reasonable to adopt a pragmatic concept of causality. *A causal relationship would be recognized*

to exist whenever evidence indicates that the factors form part of the complex of circumstances that increases the probability of occurrence of disease and that a diminution of one or more of these factors decreases the frequency of that disease.[19]

This characterization of epidemiological causation is consistent with a definition proposed ten years earlier by MacMahon and Pugh, who similarly suggested that "a causal association may usefully be defined as an association between categories or events or characteristics in which an alteration in the frequency or quality of one category is followed by a change in the other."[20] In Fletcher et al. we also find a generalization of the notion of causation. They note that "when biomedical scientists study causes of disease, they usually search for the underlying pathogenetic mechanism or final common pathway of disease," and they indicate their agreement with the importance of this approach to causation. They add, however, that:

> . . . The occurrence of disease is also determined by less specific, more remote causes such as genetic, environmental, or behavioral factors, which occur earlier in the chain of events leading to a disease. These are sometimes referred to as "origins" of disease and are more likely to be investigated by epidemiologists. These less specific and more remote *causes of disease are the risk factor* [emphasis added] . . . .[21]

These notions of epidemiological causation appear to be very much like, if not identical to, what philosophers have in the past termed "probabilistic causation." I believe the pioneer in this area is Hans Reichenbach, who characterized the notion of "causal betweenness," used to establish a linear causal sequence and a time order.[22]

An event B is causally between the events A and C if

$$1 > P(C|B) > P(C|A) > P(C) > 0; \qquad (1)$$
$$1 > P(A|B) > P(A|C) > P(A) > 0; \text{ and} \qquad (2)$$
$$P(C|A\&B) = P(C|B), \qquad (3)$$

where $|$ is used to introduce conditional probability. $P(C|B)$, for example, is the probability (P) of C, *given that B is the case.* These relations license the causal chain $A \rightarrow B \rightarrow C$, where $\rightarrow$ denotes probabilistic causation.

Other philosophers of science such as Good and Suppes have developed similar ideas, and still others have provided extensive criticism of such concepts, among them Salmon. Suppes' approach to probabilistic causation is perhaps the most widely known and may be worth a few comments.

Suppes introduces his notion of a probabilistic cause through the idea of a prima facie cause defined in the following way:[23]

The event $B_{t'}$ is a prima facie cause of the event A_t if and only if

$$t' < t \; ; \tag{1}$$

$$P(B_{t'}) > 0; \text{ and} \tag{2}$$

$$P(A_t \mid B_{t'}) > P(A_t), \tag{3}$$

where t denotes time.

Further elaboration of the notion is required, so that "spurious" causes occasioned by some common cause which produces an artifactual association between two variables are eliminated; such extensions of the concept can be found in Suppes' *A Probabilistic Theory of Causality*. Both Reichenbach's and Suppes' proposals encounter problems, however, including that of the improbable alternative causal path (an issue I have examined previously[24]). There are other conceptual difficulties associated with probabilistic causation: for an incisive review, see Salmon and two special issues of *Synthese*,[25] as well as Cartwright and Eells and Sober.

I want to introduce a somewhat different approach to the notion of probabilistic causation which I believe is clearer and ultimately more coherent than Suppes' account. My approach will utilize some helpful suggestions made by Giere, though I depart from his analysis at several critical points, in particular in connection with the application of probabilistic causation to individuals and with his favored propensity interpretation of probability.

There are some useful distinctions in Giere's account which are not explicit in most discussions. First, Giere differentiates between deterministic and stochastic systems, but permits both types to exhibit probabilistic causal relationships. This is important since it distinguishes two different ways in which determinism may fail to hold. This is useful for my account because it licenses a more coherent fit between causation in physiologically characterized biological systems and those we approach from an epidemiological perspective, though it does not exclude stochastic components in physiological processes. In physiology or pathophysiology we are usually dealing with deterministic systems (at least in ideal cases), whereas in epidemiological contexts a more probabilistic or stochastic characterization of causation is evident. Giere also invokes a "propensity" interpretation of probability for stochastic systems and, in particular, maintains that this gives a means of directly attributing probabilistic causality to individuals rather than to populations. In my view, however, the propensity interpretation is neither needed nor desirable in biomedical contexts, though it may have much to recommend it in quantum mechanical situations. I favor a frequency interpretation of probability which I maintain is more natural in epidemiological contexts. A frequency interpretation also permits us to use easily some contributions by Salmon related to a determination of reference classes that ultimately will facilitate reasoning concerning responsibility and compensation. I shall begin by indicating what elements of Giere's approach I find useful.

In Giere's analysis of deterministic systems, a *causal relation* between *C* and *E* is *not necessarily a universal relation.* The entities in Giere's account are individual deterministic systems *which can differ in their constitution,* so that different individuals with the same causal input *C* may or may not exhibit *E*. Furthermore, since *E* may come about from a different cause than *C*, some individuals may exhibit *E* but not have had *C* as a causal input. A good example which Giere often uses is smoking and lung cancer.

For a population of deterministic systems, some number of individuals with input *C* will manifest *E* and some will not. An actual population can be examined to yield a *relative frequency:*

$$\#E/N,$$

where *N* is the number of the individuals in the population and $\#E$ the number of individuals exhibiting effect *E*. This fraction has the properties of a probability (though not a propensity). This is because, for any given individual in the population, a universal law $L(C) = E$ is either true or false, depending on the individual's constitution.

Giere prefers to use counterfactual populations for which outcomes are well-defined. Thus, by hypothesis, two counterfactual populations which are counterfactual counterparts of an actual population of interest are envisaged, and one is provided with causal factor input *C* and the other with input $\sim C$. Each counterfactual population will exhibit some number of effects $\#E$, which will be $\leq$ its *N*. Giere then defines a *positive causal factor* as:[26]

C is a positive factor for *E* in [population] *U* if and only if

$$P_C(E) > P_{\sim C}(E).$$

A reversed inequality will yield a definition for a negative causal factor, and equality will indicate causal irrelevance.

Note that this notion is almost identical to the definition given earlier for a prima facie cause in Suppes' system. What is different is the interpretation in the context of explicitly deterministic systems, and an explicit counterfactual account.

Giere also introduces a *measure of effectiveness* (*Ef*) of *C* for *E* in population *U*, namely:

$$Ef(C,E) = Df P_C(E) - P_{\sim C}(E).$$

This simple definition (*Df*) will prove most useful in the context of our epidemiological examples, since it is equivalent to the definition given earlier of attributable risk, thus tying together again our epidemiological investigation and our philosophical inquiry.

These notions developed in the context of deterministic systems can be extended to stochastic systems, where Giere notes that "the interesting thing about stochastic systems is that we can speak of positive and negative causal factors for *individual systems* and not just for populations."[27]

Giere's counterfactual definition (counterfactual because system S may or may not actually have C or $\sim C$ as input) is

C is a positive causal factor for E in S if and only if

$$Pr_C(E) > Pr_{\sim C}(E),$$

where *Pr* refers to a probability in the sense of a propensity (an inherent objective tendency) of the stochastic individual system.

In a population of stochastic systems, the number of *E*'s is not deterministically by $L(C) = E$, but rather only as a "*distribution of propensities* over possible effect rates."[28] Giere suggests that the mean values of the two distributions μ_C and $\mu_{\sim C}$ can be used as measures of the effect of C in such a population, and, accordingly, for such a population of stochastic systems:

C is a positive causal factor for E in U if and only if

$$\mu_C > \mu_{\sim C}.$$

Similarly, to get a measure of effectiveness we write:

$$Ef(C,E) = Df\ \mu_C - \mu_{\sim C}.$$

I see no reason to adopt a propensity interpretation of probability here. Though there are some conceptual difficulties with the notion, the concept of weight, by which we assign a probability to an individual based on its appropriate reference class should suffice. The determination of the appropriate reference class raises difficulties of its own, but I believe these are soluble by using Salmon's concept of an epistemically and practically homogeneous reference class, a close cousin of Hempel's maximally specific reference class encountered in inductive statistical forms of explanation.[29] From my perspective, specification of appropriate reference classes and populations is exactly what epidemiologists try to do.

I should also add that I see no reason why Giere defends the randomized experimental design as the best way to test a causal hypothesis, since the groups to which he can have access are not in point of fact the counterfactual groups which his approach requires. This, however, is another matter and I shall have to defer comment to another time and place.

In summary, as regards this philosophical section, there are philosophical explications of probabilistic causation available to elucidate further the epidemiologists' notion of causation. What most accounts do not do, but which I believe Giere's does, is allow an identification of the conceptual connections between more traditionally conceived causation and the more probabilistic type of causation found in the writings of the epidemiologist, and also, as I shall argue, in recent law.[30]

CAUSATION IN THE LAW

The concept of causation as used in legal contexts is a critically important one, but it is also a conceptually complex notion about which there is little consensus. The remarkable treatise on the subject written 25 years ago by Hart and Honoré did little to resolve still raging disputes about the proper sense(s) of "legal cause." As a beginning step in clarifying the notion of causation in the law, it must be kept in mind that causal determinations in a legal context are almost uniformly associated with attempts to *fix responsibility*. This notion of responsibility in turn is associated closely with ideas of blame, liability, compensation, and punishment. As the eminent torts scholar Leon Green put it, "in its early tort usage, cause was synonymous with blame, fault, wrongdoing, and culpability." "These are spongy terms," he adds, "each capable of absorbing the meaning of the others, and frequently used interchangeably."[31]

In addition, the specific context such as torts, contracts, and civil or criminal law, will result in somewhat different types of causal questions, as well as different standards of proof (for example, in tort we work with the preponderance of the evidence, or the 51 percent rule, whereas in criminal law we require proof beyond a reasonable doubt). Hart and Honoré point out that sometimes we only want to know whether the causal connection between an act or the omission of an act led to harm; sometimes we want to know the extent of the harm and the extent of the liability; sometimes we want to know both. One must also be sensitive to the variations which arise due to vicarious liability and strict liability. The terminology the law uses varies: "cause-in-fact" seems roughly to mean a necessary condition; "proximate cause" is distinguished from more remote or irrelevant causes. One also finds such expressions as "due to," "owing to," "attributable to," "the consequence of," and the like. In addition, some theorists like to use the term "substantial factor" to describe a cause. All these points indicate the difficulties with achieving a conceptual analysis of the notions of legal cause, and, in truth, these represent but the tip of the iceberg.

In what might be termed a "received view" of legal causation, a sharp distinction is made between cause-in-fact and proximate cause. Unfortunately the former is not necessarily factual, and the latter is not necessarily proximal. Cause-in-fact is generally determined by using the "but for" test: but for the defendant's action, the injury to the plaintiff would not have occurred. Note that this test is expressed in the counterfactual mood.

The but for component of legal causation, however, is not sufficient, and needs to be supplemented with an additional component to limit liability. In science we can, in principle, trace causes backwards ad infinitum, whereas in law we must find some grounds for limiting the attribution of a cause, lest in Prosser's words, it "result in an indefinite liability for all wrongful acts . . . [that] would 'set society on edge and fill the courts with endless litigation.'"[32] Exactly what the similarities and differences between the scientific and the legal concept of cause are, and how to set limits on causal attribution, are difficult questions on which I will speculate later. For now suffice it to note that the required liability-limiting supplement is the notion of "proximate cause." Unfortunately, whereas cause-in-fact or but for causation is viewed as objective and scientific, the notion of "proximate cause" is construed in just the *reverse* way by the received view.

In this received view—which Hart and Honoré also call "the modern approach"—the notion of proximate cause is another word for *policy*. Hart and Honoré provide a quote from a famous case in tort law known as the *Palsgraf* case which they use to summarize the modern view:[33]

> What we do mean by the word "proximate" is that because of convenience, of public policy, of a rough sense of justice, the law arbitrarily declines to trace a series of events beyond a certain point. This is not logic. It is practical politics.

I have dwelt on this received view notion in part to provide a background perspective on the rather different role of causation in the legal context, and also in part to stress the importance of a necessary condition in the legal approach to causation. There is, I believe, much that is valid in the received view approach, though I should point out that most of Hart and Honoré's book is written in opposition to this view. At the same time, I also believe that the concept requires growth in the light of discoveries concerning the complexity of, especially, biomedical causation. Thus I also agree with Hart and Honoré that additional conceptual analysis is a valuable and necessary undertaking. Hart and Honoré, in opposition to what they saw as the *anti*-conceptual thrust of the modern approach, issued an articulate call for more extensive and deeper analysis of causation in the law, with which I find myself resonating.[34]

> It is fatally easy and has become increasingly common to make the transition from the exhilarating discovery that complex words like "cause" cannot be simply defined and have no "one true meaning" to the mistaken conclusion that they have no meaning worth bothering about at all, but are used as a mere disguise for arbitrary decision or judicial policy. This is a blinding error, and legal language and reasoning will never be understood

while it persists. The proper inference from the fact that no common property can be found in cases where causal language is used is that some more complex principle or set of principles may guide, though not dictate its use. The pains of unearthing these, though considerable, seldom go unrewarded.

I have discussed the concept of legal cause in order to give readers a sense of the normative and socially laden character of the causal concept in the legal domain. This discussion also suggests that the notion of legal cause will either go beyond the scientific concept in these normative and policy-oriented directions, or that any complete analysis of the concept will have to embed causation in a context invoking ideas like responsibility.

RECENT DEVELOPMENTS CONCERNING PROBABILISTIC CAUSATION IN TORT LAW

Several legal scholars have noted that mathematically explicit probabilistic and statistical reasoning is quite foreign to the law. David Kaye, a professor of law at Arizona State University, writing in *The American Bar Foundation Research Journal*, states that proof by what he terms "naked statistical evidence" is a "source of bewilderment to the legal profession."[35] Richard Epstein, a noted torts theorist, also has written:

> I do not think that statistical correlations are a kind of causal paradigm to be admitted into the system [of legal reasoning]. Their relevance in my view is confined to matters of proof [such as] [d]id this drug cause this particular illness in this particular case? . . . [W]ithin the law the dominant concern is always with singular causation, with the isolation of decisive conditions from the class of necessary or sufficient conditions. To upgrade therefore the statistical matters into a substantive matter is . . . to admit two inconsistent notions into the system without any clear sense of how they are to be reconciled. To admit it as proof simply means to say that it is, or is more likely than not, that the particular cause had the particular effect, e.g., that this dosage of DES did cause cancer.[36]

In spite of such reluctance to employ explicit probabilistic or statistical reasoning in legal contexts, there have been a few analyses and defenses of statistical reasoning in such contexts. Michael Finkelstein's monograph on *Quantitative Methods in Law: Studies in the Application of Mathematical Probability and Statistics to Legal Problems* is a comprehensive survey of the issues along with references to 1978. Recently there have appeared a few articles defending the use of epidemiological data and epidemiological reasoning methods in the courts, the essays by Mary Ann Mobilia and Annette MacKay Rossignol and Richard E. Hoffman being the most useful.

None of these works, however, deals with the issue of probabilistic apportionment, a key notion for our inquiry for reasons I will indicate below (though Hoffman's suggestions regarding attributable risk can be so interpreted: see my comment on Hoffman in the summary). For our purposes, the inquiry into probabilistic causation and apportionment which the courts have begun to implement (starting about 1980), primarily in the context of DES cases such as *Sindell* and *Collins*, is most important and one on which I shall comment extensively.[37] Also of considerable interest to our analysis is an outline of a paradigm of probabilistic causal reasoning in law being developed by legal scholars such as Mario Rizzo at New York University and David Kaye at Arizona State. This development coincides with the related emergence of an analysis of legal causation using the law and economic perspective pioneered by Guido Calabresi at Yale University and Richard Posner at the University of Chicago, and extended by them and by Stephen Shavell at Harvard University and William Landes at Chicago. Additional papers by Robinson and Rosenberg elaborating a probabilistic risk theory of causation and liability indicate the burgeoning legal interest in this area. It is the task of this section to provide a brief overview of these matters and to indicate further directions such developments might well take.

THE COURTS MOVE TOWARD PROBABILISTIC CAUSALITY

Several court decisions in recent years suggest that the general reluctance of the legal profession to engage in an explicit form of probabilistic reasoning may be yielding to the complex realities of biomedical causation of injuries associated with toxic products. The paradigms in this area tend to be drawn from asbestos and DES cases,[38] but they are applicable to many other substances, ranging from Agent Orange to powerful antipsychotic drugs. In an extensively discussed decision by the California Supreme Court, *Sindell* v. *Abbott Laboratories*, a novel theory of liability was invoked to outflank the problem of proving causation of harm by a specifically identifiable product, DES. On the basis of Herbst et al.'s discovery mentioned above and follow-up studies, it has been demonstrated that clear cell vaginal adenocarcinoma is closely linked to in utero exposure to DES, but that this cancer develops in the daughters of the exposed population 15 to 20 years later. Mothers who took DES, their physicians, and their pharmacists generally do not have the records which would identify the specific drug manufacturer of the DES that was ingested. At common law, failure to identify the manufacturer of an injurious product would usually lead to dismissal, since the legal causation requirement could not be met.

In *Sindell*, the court appealed to two precedents which permitted the joining of a "substantial" number of the manufacturers together as the defendant, and also permitted the burden of proof to be shifted to them. Such a shift would entail that an individual manufacturer would then have the burden of proving that they had not produced the DES which caused the plaintiff's cancer. Compensation costs were to be based on the "market share" of the joined manufacturers, on the grounds that this would best represent the probability that the manufacturer with that market share caused the actual harm.

Not many courts have followed *Sindell*,[39] though this has not stopped other courts from fashioning similar probabilistic schemas for attributing responsibility. An important variant of a probabilistic liability rule was recently articulated by the Wisconsin Supreme Court in *Collins* v. *Eli Lilly*. In *Collins*, the court rejected the *Sindell* market share rule on the grounds that it was too difficult to determine market share due to the lapse of time, poor records, and a shifting market. They proposed instead a "risk contribution" theory of liability which assigns blame to a manufacturer if that manufacturer participated in any activity leading to the marketing of an essentially identical drug.

The *Collins* court wrote that it was motivated by considerations of "justice and fundamental fairness" and appears to have turned to a 1982 law review article written by Glen O. Robinson entitled "Multiple Causation in Tort Law: Reflections on the DES Cases." The Wisconsin court cited the Robinson essay at the critical point in their argument where they assert they "have formulated a method of recovery for plaintiffs in DES cases in Wisconsin" and add "[w]e note that this method of recovery could apply in situations which are factually similar to the DES cases." The court views the Robinson proposal as a "risk contribution" theory, and writes that "although we find Robinson's 'risk contribution' theory sound to the extent it recognizes that all DES drug companies contributed in some measure to the risk of injury, we do not agree that this is a sufficient basis in itself for liability. We still require it be shown that the defendant drug company reasonably could have contributed in some way to the *actual* injury" [emphasis added].[40]

In a key section roughly midway through his lengthy essay, Robinson explicitly considers the relationship between causation, fairness, liability, and compensation. He notes Epstein's (1973) suggestion that causation can be construed both as a necessary and a sufficient condition for the establishment of liability, but disagrees with Epstein, arguing that even the weaker necessary condition thesis is what "created the major problem in the DES cases . . . [in the first place since] there was no proof of a causal link between the actions of any one DES manufacturer and the plaintiff's injuries."[41] Robinson argues that fairness does not require such a link in the criminal context (for there we impose liability for reckless driving and some attempted crimes even if no harm results). Citing philosopher Joel Feinberg[42] and torts scholar Robert Keeton,[43] Robinson maintains that "fairness in civil contexts seems to require only that a defendant's liability be related to his conduct, and that liability, where imposed, be roughly proportional to the seriousness of the *risks* that he has created."[44] Robinson then proposes his thesis in the following terms:

> From the standpoint of fairness, the critical point [for assigning legal liability] is the *creation of a risk* that society deems to be unreasonable, not whether anyone was injured by it.[45]

Robinson applies this principle to the DES cases, arguing that "each defendant made a 'defective' product which created an unreasonable risk of the harm the plaintiff suffered."[46] Robinson sees in *Sindell* and in a generalization of *Summers* (an important precedent for the *Sindell* court) the germ of a new rule which "imposes liability for the creation of a risk and apportions liability according to the magnitude of that risk."[47] In an attempt to determine whether such a rule is feasible, he turns to an examination of multiple causation and probabilistic causation.

Robinson finds he needs to examine the Rizzo and Arnold "probabilistic marginal product" approach as well as to conduct a brief excursion into philosophy of science analyses of the nature of probability and that notion's interaction with concepts of causation. It seems only appropriate that we also turn to these topics though my approach will be rather different from Robinson's.

RIZZO'S (AND ARNOLD'S) THEORY OF PROBABILISTIC CAUSATION

Over the past five years or so, Rizzo has crafted a probabilistic theory of legal causation which he, working with Arnold, has applied to the problem of causal apportionment. Apportionment has traditionally been as foreign to tort law as statistical thinking, though the past 15 years have seen a dramatic reversal of that position. A major statutory movement toward comparative negligence has developed in addition to a rise in joint tortfeasor contribution statutes. We have already encountered the issues of contribution and apportionment above in connection with DES cases, though the issue is both more common and more mundane, and may arise in *any* case in which comparative negligence appears.

Rizzo and Arnold initially rely on a theory of prima facie deterministic causation developed by Epstein in the context of his general analysis of tort law based on principles of strict liability and corrective justice. Epstein's account, which it will not be possible to develop in any detail in this presentation, stipulates that if A causes B harm, then there is a prima facie case that A should compensate B. A causal determination is made in Epstein's theory by deciding that any specific case is a close analogue of *four paradigms* of causal tortious action, such as "A hit B" or "A created a dangerous condition which harms B." Such a prima facie case for compensation may fail, based on a series of admissible defenses and rejoinders made in a legal context.[48] Rizzo and Arnold accept the main features of Epstein's theory, but argue that his causation theory has to be further developed and recast as a relative causation analysis. Rizzo and Arnold write:

> Once two or more wrongful causes of a harm are identified on Epsteinian grounds, it is necessary to determine their relative importance. Where the causes arise simultaneously, this determination is made by hypothesizing a simpler situation in which only one of the causally relevant factors is operative. We appraise the relative importance of the causes by measuring the differential degree of *risk* to which each cause exposes the plaintiff. We employ this *probabilistic analysis because a deterministic analysis is incapable of disentangling the relative importance of causes* [my emphasis]. In those contexts in which each wrongful act is a necessary condition of the harm, the marginal product of each would be the entire damage. If, on the other hand, neither were necessary, then each of their marginal products would be zero. A probabilistic analysis, however, enables us to determine the relative importance of causes by referring to their general harm-producing capacities.[49]

Rizzo's analysis presumes several concepts which appear in the above quotation and which it would be well to elaborate before further analysis of his approach. To do this I turn briefly to another essay of Rizzo's which deals with probabilistic causation and the notion of a marginal product in more explicit terms.

Rizzo introduces his theory of the marginal product in the following manner:

> The theory emphasizes the importance of tracing the relative objective marginal product of wrongful conduct in terms of the probability of that conduct bringing about the harm actually suffered. In less formal language, the theory focusses on the degree of risk to which an instance of wrongful conduct exposes the plaintiff, relative to that of other wrongful conduct or intervening events.
>
> The specific thesis advanced and defended here is: a harm is proximately related to a wrongful act or omission if its *objective marginal product* in probabilistic terms $[= (\beta - \alpha)]$ is higher with respect to that harm than that of any other instance of wrongful conduct, intervening events, or the standard environment $[= \alpha]$. Consequently ... objective or best-informed probability, but not foreseeability, is important to the determination of proximate cause.[50]

This key notion of an objective marginal product can be given a formal definition in terms of conditional probabilities of the type already discussed. Take Z_{t_1} to be the harm resulting at time t_1 from an act A_{t_0} at time t_0, in an environment with other causative factors represented by X_{t_0}. Thus:[51]

If

$$P(Z_{t_1}|A_{t_0}, X_{t_0}) = \beta \text{ and}$$

$$P(Z_{t_1}|{\sim}A_{t_0}, X_{t_0}) = \alpha < \beta,$$

then $(\beta - \alpha)$ is the *objective marginal product* of A_{t_0}, or to put it another way: *the increment in the objective probability of Z_{t_1} caused by Z_{t_1}.*

This use of conditional probability to capture causation is heavily indebted to Suppes' theory of probabilistic causality. In point of fact, the basic concepts utilized to elucidate causal relations in Rizzo's writings involve Suppes' notions of prima facie, spurious, and genuine causes. Without going into details, suffice it to say that cause A_{t_0} in the above expression is a genuine cause, namely, that there is no other common cause which might account for its role in increasing the posterior probability of Z_{t_1}. Rizzo's notions are accordingly similar to what we saw earlier in epidemiology and in the philosophers' approach to probabilistic causality: from the perspective of probabilistic causality, a cause is neither a necessary nor a sufficient condition; rather a cause *raises the probability of its effect.*

Let me now elaborate a bit more on the fine structure of cause in Rizzo's account. Rizzo claims that "deterministic causal analysis is merely a special case of the probabilistic,"[52] and suggests that we can see deterministic causality as a limiting case of probabilistic causation by looking at causation in terms of functional analysis. Briefly, he introduces a "probabilistic production function":

$$P(Q) = F(K,L),$$

which asserts that "inputs K and L produce not a certain output Q, but rather a given probability of a particular output level."[53] Specific values of K and L, say A and X are the specific values, will be *sufficient conditions* for a given *probability level*, but they will not in general be *necessary conditions* since $P(Q)$ may be arrived at by other conditions. As such the event A is what Mackie termed an INUS condition (an insufficient but necessary part of an unnecessary but sufficient complex of conditions), a terribly complex-sounding expression which is nonetheless a very useful notion in analyzing causation.

In what is a clear advance on Suppes' theory of probabilistic causality, Rizzo introduces a definition of a probabilistic INUS condition in the following way:[54]

A is a probabilistic INUS condition of the event Z if and only if:

$$P(AX \cup Y) > 0, \tag{1}$$

$$P(Z|AX) = \beta < 1, \tag{2}$$

$$P(Z|{\sim}[AX \cup Y]) \neq \beta, \tag{3}$$

$$P(Z|A) < \beta, \text{ and} \tag{4}$$

$$P(Z|X) < \beta. \tag{5}$$

Here requirement (1) expresses possibility and requirement (2) asserts that AX is minimally sufficient to produce a given probability level (β) for Z. Requirement (3) says that AX or Y (where Y represents the set of alternative sufficient conditions) is necessary to produce the specified β level of $P(Z)$; (4) and (5) indicate that neither A nor X alone will produce the β level of outcome.

This is as much of Rizzo's technical formalism as we shall need. It indicates the dependence on probabilistic notions of causation, and also a familiarity with recent philosophical analyses of causation. Though prima facie persuasive, it seems that Rizzo's account could profit *conceptually* by being embedded in a non-Suppesian approach to probabilistic causality along the lines of the modification of Giere's analysis sketched above. In addition, I believe that Rizzo's perspective, as well as other legal scholars' approaches to causation using probabilistic concepts, could profit both methodologically and empirically from a closer linkage to *epidemiological* notions which are significantly more *quantitatively* developed rather than relying primarily on *comparative* conditional probabilistic concepts. The epidemiological notions contain, as we have seen earlier, various *measures of effects* which go well beyond such important but less elaborated, and I suspect, less applicable definitions as Rizzo's probabilistic INUS condition.

Rizzo's account is the most technically developed of several contributions in the burgeoning area of risk contribution and probabilistic analyses. It should be noted, however, that Rizzo's approach has not gone uncriticized.

In a recent examination of the Rizzo and Arnold approach to causal apportionment appearing in the *Journal of Legal Studies*, Kaye and Aickin argue that the Rizzo-Arnold analysis is seriously flawed with regard to its mathematical derivation and its justification. Interestingly, however, Kaye and Aickin arrive at essentially the same formulas to describe probabilistic contribution, though they place much less reliance on them. Kaye and Aickin also find that the probabilistic marginal product, an essential concept in Rizzo's analysis, does not lead to any *unique apportionment* in applications, and thus the analysis is seriously incomplete. Though prima facie plausible, Kaye and Aickin's criticisms, I find, do not stand up to a recent rejoinder by Rizzo and Arnold (1986). Kaye and Aickin add further that from the law and economic perspective from which Rizzo writes, it is questionable whether charging for risk creation, or for marginal risk in Rizzo's terms, would create the proper incentives for optimal limits of care on the part of each joint tortfeasor. This is a more speculative issue on which the arguments have not as yet been fully articulated.

Kaye's views are in part motivated by an earlier investigation of his own in which he elegantly demonstrates that a nonprobabilistic apportionment rule, the traditional preponderance of the evidence doctrine, is more efficient from an economic point of view. Kaye is not opposed to probabilistic notions in some restricted circumstances, but his tolerance for statistical concepts is much less than is Rizzo's. Though I will not have the opportunity here to discuss Kaye's arguments, I find them plausible supplements to my own preferred interpretation of the role of probabilistic causation in the law, and will include aspects of Kaye's views in my conclusions.

SUMMARY AND CONCLUSIONS

I have attempted to develop the beginnings of a concept of causation which is robust across the disciplines of medicine, law, and philosophy. I have sketched the manner in which a looser statistical notion of causation has developed in epidemiology departing from the more nineteenth-century deterministic ideas of causation, as we found in Koch's postulates, and have shown how that notion can be applied to a specific case, DES injuries, which has also found its way into the legal arena. I also argued that the epidemiologists' notion of causation is essentially identical to what a number of philosophers have discerned as probabilistic causality, and developed the philosopher Giere's account in preference to the more standard approach of Suppes for reasons of clarity and congruence, though I depart from Giere on several points.

I sketched what is still the received view of legal causation, but agreed with Hart and Honoré that further conceptual analysis, and even further growth in the concept of causation, would be required to make conceptual sense of biomedical causation in a legal context. This led me to turn to an analysis of several recent court decisions which I believe are paving the way for a more extensive use of probabilistic reasoning in legal contexts. I outlined the approach of legal scholar Rizzo to probabilistic causation, noting that it was heavily dependent, conceptually, on Suppes' analysis.

It would take us too far afield to continue the inquiry, but let me offer some tentative hypotheses which will both serve as a summary of this work and as a basis for further research.

First, concentration only on the formal machinery of probabilistic causation with its notions of comparative conditional probabilities is not sufficient to allow application of these notions from law in the medical arena and vice versa; rather, further epidemiologically oriented investigations should be pursued. An especially important feature that is largely missing from probabilistic causal accounts is a set of criteria of causation distinguishing causal connections from coincidences, associations based on subtle biases, and those due to an unidentified common cause. Though some discussion of the grounds for distinguishing spurious from genuine causes does exist in the philosophical and legal literature, it lacks both the sophistication and the quantitative statistical methodology found in epidemiological methodological accounts.

Second, epidemiological notions, especially the concept of attributable risk, are prime candidates for conceptual elucidation and application to legal cases such as DES and radiation injuries. The concept of attributable risk is in point of fact currently being proposed legislatively as a notion which would facilitate fair compensation for radiation-induced injuries. Though I will not analyze these legislative developments, it would be useful to provide a quotation from the *Congressional Record* of March 23, 1983, in which Senator Orrin Hatch introduced his "Radiogenic Cancer Compensation Act." Though the act was not passed by the 98th Congress, it will undoubtedly be reintroduced in the 100th. The Radiogenic Cancer Compensation Act was proposed in part to compensate people who lived downwind from atmospheric nuclear tests and who developed cancer subsequent to the tests. In introducing a mechanism for compensation, Senator Hatch relied on the suggestions of several radiation epidemiologists who urged him to introduce an analogue of the notion of attributable risk, to be termed the "probability of causation." In his summary of the Radiogenic Cancer Compensation Act, printed in the *Congressional Record,* Hatch wrote:

> The idea of the "probability of causation" is a variant of the concept of "attributable risk" which has been a standard concept of epidemiology for at least ten years. The idea is simply to use population data to determine the likelihood that an individual with cancer has an "excess cancer," that is a radiation caused cancer. A cancer victim's "probability of causation" is the probability that he developed his cancer as a result of a prior exposure to a given level of ionizing radiation. The size of this "probability of causation" will vary in accordance with a number of factors such as the age and sex of the person, his cancer, the size of his radiation dose, and the length of time between his exposure and the onset of his disease.[55]

Senator Hatch argues that this approach is the fairest since it is clear that radiation caused some of the cancers, but we cannot determine which specific cancers (or proportion of the cancer) was so caused. In addition, Hatch wishes to provide (reduced) compensation for individuals whose probability of causation is as low as 10 percent. In traditional tort law, such a threshold would be too low, for compensation could only be awarded if, for the appropriate population into which the plaintiff was placed, the attributable risk of injury associated with the alleged injurious product were greater than 50 percent. Regardless of the threshold selected, however, the point remains that the epidemiological notion of attributable risk is a conceptually interesting one to consider in the context of tort compensation. (I am not alone in voicing such a view; recently Hoffman wrote in the *American Journal of Epidemiology* that

"I predict evidence of attributable risk or attributable fraction will be useful in determining the extent of potential losses and, therefore, of future damages [in connection with toxic tort injuries]."[56])

Third, restricting our concerns to tort law, it seems to me that probabilities will best be seen as entering the legal arena in a two-stage process: (1) A decision that a particular plaintiff's injury *more likely than not* has been caused by a specific substance or process. This decision can rely on the construction of appropriate reference groups to whom attributable risk studies assign a probability of more than 50 percent: the groups will be narrow classes of an epistemically and practically homogeneous nature, but the decision will have to be by reference to such *populations* since data available clinically will not be sufficient to *individualize* such a judgment; (2) I also envisage a second stage in which there is a determination of a *proper share* of compensation costs, perhaps to be paid out of a superfund (either quasi-governmental or industrywide) type of mechanism where contributions to the fund are assessed by a national risk-contribution standard appropriately tailored to our knowledge of relevant temporal, geographical, and potential-for-causing-injury factors. The first stage will limit liability to those who were probably injured; the second stage will insure risk-spreading among manufacturers based on a multifactorial probability model—a model which will unfortunately be necessarily freighted with many vague and subjective components. In spite of such defects, however, I maintain it is preferable to the current tort lottery which compensates only some plaintiffs, severely penalizes some manufacturers, and primarily enriches the lawyers.

NOTES

1. Of necessity this essay is limited to a subset of topics that the EVIST project has investigated. For the context of this inquiry, see chapter 1.
2. Taken from Fletcher et al. (1982), p. 188.
3. From Lilienfeld and Lilienfeld (1980), pp. 217-18. The terms in brackets are Evans' original expressions for the similar idea.
4. Based on Fletcher et al. (1982), especially chapter 1. It is important to have some account for distinguishing between "mere statistical correlations" and causal connections for a variety of reasons. As I shall note in a later section, and also in note 48 below, this is one topic which has been largely overlooked by legal scholars interested in probabilistic causation.
5. For a discussion of case control methodology, see Fletcher et al. (1982), pp. 171-84, or any general epidemiology textbook.
6. See Horwitz and Feinstein (1981).
7. See Schaffner (1983b) for a brief discussion and references.
8. MacMahon and Pugh (1970), pp. 270-71; Fletcher et al. (1982), pp. 176-77.

9. Fletcher et al. (1982), p. 102.

10. Herbst et al. (1971) report even stronger data for an association, since their controls indicated zero rather than one case of adenocarcinoma of the vagina. Since this is a simple example, I have slightly altered the data to 1/32 to avoid dealing with division by zero.

11. See Fletcher et al. (1982), p. 102 for an analysis of the data of Doll and Hill (1964).

12. For a useful tabular summary of four measures of effect, see Fletcher et al. (1982), p. 101.

13. Ibid.

14. Ibid., p. 76.

15. Ibid.

16. Levin and Bertell (1978), p. 78; MacMahon and Pugh (1970), pp. 270-75.

17. MacMahon and Pugh (1970), pp. 234-35.

18. See Silverman (1977) on retrolental fibroplasia.

19. Lilienfeld and Lilienfeld (1980), p. 295.

20. MacMahon and Pugh (1970), pp. 17-18.

21. Fletcher et al. (1982), p. 190.

22. Reichenbach (1956), p. 190.

23. Suppes (1970), p.12.

24. Schaffner (1983).

25. See *Synthese*, voume 48, numbers 2 and 3 (1981), especially the articles by Otte and by Suppes and Zanotti.

26. Giere (1968), p. 264.

27. Ibid., p. 265.

28. Ibid., p. 266.

29. Hempel (1965), pp. 399-401 and Salmon (1971), p. 46.

30. Further research into the relation between probabilistic (epidemiological) causation and (usually) deterministic causation in pathophysiology suggests to me that the *key* difference is *not* to be attributed to a distinction between deterministic and stochastic systems. Rather, the principal difference is due to the (often idealized) *uniformity* of the entities constituting the populations under investigation. On this view, which is consistent with the theses discussed in this chapter, probabilistic causation is a *practical* way for examining and drawing conclusions about "averaged" populations. Such inferences *can* be flawed unless *all* relevant individual differences are adequately controlled. I see this as the root of Simpson's paradox discussed by Cartwright (1979) and in more recent literature on probabilistic causation.

31. Green (1962), p. 42.

32. Posser (1971), p. 236.

33. Hart and Honoré (1959), p. 85.

34. Ibid., p. 3.

35. Kaye (1982), pp. 487-88.

36. R. A. Epstein, personal communication, September 28, 1981.

37. See the *Sindell* and *Collins* decisions.

38. But see two workmen's compensation cases: *Bethlehem Steel Company* v. *Industrial Accident Commission* 135 P. 2d 153 (1943), involving kerato-

conjunctivitis; and the *Sacred Heart Medical Center* v. *Washington State Department of Labor* 600 P. 2d 1015 (1979), involving hepatitis B.

39. Different courts have taken differing positions on using *Sindell* as a precedent. See notes 1-3 in Prosser et al. (1982), p. 294. Interestingly, the plaintiff settled out of court for $20,000 [see Epstein et al. (1984), pp. 306-7].

40. *Collins* v. *Eli Lilly*, p. 49, n.10.

41. Robinson (1982), pp. 738-39.

42. Feinberg (1970), p. 213.

43. Keeton (1963), pp. 18-24.

44. Robinson (1982), p. 739.

45. Ibid., p. 739.

46. Ibid., pp. 739-40.

47. Ibid., p. 749.

48. See Epstein (1974) for an elaboration. What I believe is further needed in both the Epstein and the Rizzo-Arnold approaches is an account justifying causal attributions, along the lines of Evans' criteria. Prima facie causal claims can suffice for more ordinary types of causal connection, but in the more complex types of causation which we have been investigating here, a more explicit and statistically informed methodology is required to distinguish causal connections from coincidences, biased assessments, and an association due to a common cause. Use of Epsteinian causation is a suggestive first step, but it requires further elaboration. Referring to the "environment" as do Rizzo and Arnold (1980) will not help answer this question, nor will appeals to Mackie-like INUS conditions [see Kaye and Aickin (1983), p. 194, n.19]. Ruling out "spurious causes" is a reasonable preliminary means of coming to grips with this issue, but it is not sufficient per se and could profit from epidemiological methodology.

49. Rizzo and Arnold (1980), p. 1408.

50. Ibid., pp. 1007-8.

51. Ibid., p. 1016.

52. Rizzo (1981), p. 1009.

53. Ibid., p. 1011.

54. Ibid., pp. 1013-14.

55. *Congressional Record* (1983), p. S3922.

56. Hoffman (1984), p. 201.

BIBLIOGRAPHY

Calabresi, G. 1975. "Concerning Cause and the Law of Torts . . ." *University of Chicago Law Review* 69:43.

Cartwright, N. 1979. "Causal Laws and Effective Strategies." *Nous* 13 (November):419-37.

Collins v. *Eli Lilly*. 1984. 342 N.W. 2d 37 (Wis.), p. 45.

Congressional Record. 1983. 98th Cong., 1st sess. Vol. 129, no. 39, 24 March, pp. S3918-26.

Doll, R., and A. B. Hill. 1950. "Smoking and Carcinoma of the Lung: Preliminary Report." *British Medical Journal* 2:739-48.

Eells, E., and E. Sober. 1983. "Probabilistic Causality and the Question of Transitivity." *Philosophy of Science* 50:35-57.

Epstein, R. A. 1973. "A Theory of Strict Liability." *Journal of Legal Studies* 2:151.

_____. 1974. "Defenses and Subsequent Pleas in a Theory of Strict Liability." *nal of Legal Studies* 3:165.

_____. 1979. "Causation and Corrective Justice: A Reply to Two Critics." *Journal of Legal Studies* 8:477-504.

_____. 1980a. *Modern Products Liability Law.* Westport, CT: Quorum Books.

_____. 1980b. *A Theory of Strict Liability.* San Francisco: Cato. [Reprints of "A Theory of Strict Liability" and "Defenses and Subsequent Pleas in a Theory of Strict Liability."]

Epstein, R., C. O. Gregory, and H. Kalvin. 1984. *Cases and Materials on Torts.* Boston: Little, Brown.

Evans, A. S. 1976. "Causation and Disease: The Henle-Koch Postulates Revisited." *Yale Journal of Biology and Medicine* 49:175-95.

Feinberg, J. 1970. *Doing and Deserving.* Princeton: Princeton University Press.

Finkelstein, M. 1978. *Quantitative Methods in Law: Studies in the Application of Mathematical Probability and Statistics to Legal Problems.* New York: Free Press.

Fletcher, R. H., S. W. Fletcher, and E. H. Wagner. 1982. *Clinical Epidemiology—the Essentials.* Baltimore: Williams and Wilkins.

Giere, R. 1980. "Causal Systems and Statistical Hypotheses." In *Applications of Inductive Logic,* ed. L. J. Cohen and M. B. Hesse. Oxford: Oxford University Press, pp. 251-70.

Green, L. 1962. "Duties, Risks, Causation Doctrines." *Texas Law Review* 41:42-72.

Hart, H. L. A., and A. M. Honoré. 1959. *Causation in the Law.* Oxford: Oxford University Press.

Hempel, C. G. 1965. *Aspects of Scientific Explanation.* New York: Free Press.

Herbst, A. L., H. Ulfelder, and D. C. Poskanzer. 1971. "Adenocarcinoma of the Vagina: Association of Maternal Stilbestrol Therapy with Tumor Appearance in Young Women." *New England Journal of Medicine* 284:878-81.

Hoffman, R. E. 1984. "The Use of Epidemiologic Data in the Courts." *American Journal of Epidemiology* 120:190-202.

Horwitz, I., and A. Feinstein. 1981. "The Application of Therapeutic Trial Principles to Improve the Design of Epidemiological Research." *Journal of Chronic Diseases* 34:575-83.

Kaye, D. 1982. "The Limits of the Preponderance of the Evidence Standard: Justifiably Naked Statistical Evidence and Multiple Causation." *American Bar Foundation Research Journal* 2:487-515.

Kaye, D., and M. Aickin. 1983. "A Comment on Causal Apportionment." *Journal of Legal Studies* 13(1984):191-208.

Keeton, R. 1963. *Legal Cause in the Law of Torts.* Columbus: Ohio State University Press.

Landes, W., and R. Posner. 1980. "Joint and Multiple Tortfeasors: An Economic Analysis." *Journal of Legal Studies* 9:517.

—————. 1983. "Causation in Tort Law: An Economic Approach." *Journal of Legal Studies* 12:109-34.

Levin, M. L., and R. Bertell. 1978. "Re: Simple Estimation of Population-Attributable Risk from Case-Control Studies." *American Journal of Epidemiology* 108:78-79.

Lilienfeld, A. M., and D. E. Lilienfeld. 1980. *Foundations of Epidemiology,* 2d. ed. New York: Oxford University Press.

Mackie, J. 1974. *The Cement of the Universe.* Oxford: Oxford University Press.

MacMahon, B., and T. F. Pugh. 1970. *Epidemiology: Principles and Method.* Boston: Little, Brown.

Mobilia, M. A., and A. M. Rossignol. 1983. "The Role of Epidemiology in Determining Causation in Toxic Shock Syndrome." *Jurimetrics* Fall:78-86.

Otte, R. 1981. "A Critique of Suppes' Theory of Probabilistic Causality." *Synthese* 48:167-89.

Posner, R. A. 1977. *Economic Analysis of Law,* 2d ed. Boston: Little, Brown.

Posner, R., and W. Landes. 1983. "Causation in Tort Law: An Economic Approach." *Journal of Legal Studies* 12:109-34.

Prosser, W. L. 1971. *Handbook of the Law of Torts.* St. Paul, MN: West Publishing.

Prosser, W. L., J. W. Wade, and V. E. Schwartz. 1982. In *Torts: Cases and Materials,* 7th ed. Mineola, NY: Foundation Press, pp. 364-70.

Reichenbach, H. 1956. *The Direction of Time.* Berkeley: University of California Press.

Rizzo, M. 1981. "The Imputation Theory of Proximate Cause: An Economic Framework." *Georgia Law Review* 15:1007-38.

Rizzo, M., and F. Arnold. 1980. "Causal Apportionment in the Law of Torts: An Economic Theory." *Columbia Law Review* 80:1399.

—————. 1986. "Causal Apportionment: Reply to the Critics." *The Journal of Legal Studies* 15:219-26.

Robinson, G. O. 1982. "Multiple Causation in Tort Law: Reflections on the DES Cases." *Virginia Law Review* 68:713-69.

Rosenberg, D. 1984. "The Causal Connection in Mass Exposure Cases: A 'Public Law' Vision of the Tort System." *Harvard Law Review* 97:851-929.

Salmon, W. C. 1971. *Statistical Explanation and Statistical Relevance.* Pittsburgh: University of Pittsburgh Press.

—————. 1980. "Probabilistic Causality." *Pacific Philosophical Quarterly* 61:59-74.

Schaffner, K. 1980. "Theory Structure in the Biomedical Sciences." *Journal of Medicine and Philosophy* 5:57-97.

—————. 1981. "Causation and Responsibility in Medicine, Science, and the Law." In *The Law-Medicine Relation,* ed. S. Spicker, J. Healey, and H. T. Engelhardt. Dordrecht: Reidel.

—————. 1983a. "Explanation and Causation in the Biomedical Sciences." In *Mind and Medicine,* ed. L. L. Laudan. Berkeley: University of California Press, pp. 75-124.

_____. 1983b. "Clinical Trials: The Validation of Theory and Therapy." In *Physics, Philosophy and Psychoanalysis*, eds. R. S. Cohen and L. Laudan. Dordrecht: Reidel.

Shavell, S. 1980. "An Analysis of Causation and the Scope of Liability in the Law of Torts." *Journal of Legal Studies* 9:463-92.

Silverman, W. A. 1977. "The Lesson of Retrolental Fibroplasia." *Scientific American* 236(June 1977):100-107.

Sindell v. *Abbott Laboratories*. 1980. 26 Cal. 3d 588, 163 Cal. Rptr. 132, 607 P. 2d 924.

Suppes, P. 1970. *A Probabilistic Theory of Causality*. Amsterdam: North-Holland.

Suppes, P., and M. Zanotti. 1981. "When Are Probabilistic Explanations Possible?" *Synthese* 48:191-99.

7

Moral and Legal Responsibility

Kurt Baier

In thinking about the moral and legal concepts of responsibility, it appears that the same concept applies in both, and that this concept can be elucidated without exploring the several different conceptions found in the literature. In the first section of this chapter, I will examine this unitary concept and throw light on some of the normative problems which are our special concern. In the second part, I will explore various normative principles that might be considered in settling a case under discussion here, namely, *Sindell* v. *Abbott Laboratories.*

THE CONCEPT OF RESPONSIBILITY

ASCRIBING RESPONSIBILITY

Ascribing responsibility is part of a much broader social practice whose overall aim is to minimize the mutual infliction of harm, loss, or damage, to maximize desirable mutual help in attaining personal ends, and, when necessary, to provide adequate redress. Achieving these aims depends on causal knowledge. We must know what sorts of events bring about or prevent what sorts of harm; we must know how to intervene suitably in the natural course of events so as to prevent such harm or avoid bringing it about; and we must know how suitably to allocate this task of intervening. Thus, a society may require some people to, say, build dams to prevent floods, or it may at least officially designate as flood-prone those low-lying regions likely to be flooded, or perhaps forbid developers to build in such areas, or else make public funds available to help owners rebuild after a flood. Alternatively, society may altogether forbid certain forms of behavior known to endanger others or, alternatively, to allow such behavior, but impose various duties on those who engage in it, for example, duties of special care or duties of compensation. The means employed by society to attain the aims of this social enterprise could therefore be described as requiring people to do what tends to make others better off or prevent their being worse off, and forbidding them to engage in behavior which tends to make others worse off.

Three distinctions should be drawn immediately. The first is between harms that are acts of nature, such as a brain tumor or death by lightning, and those that are due to human action or inaction—and so could have been avoided—such as the deaths of President John F. Kennedy or Kitty Genovese.

The second distinction is between those types of human behavior and their effects which society tries to prevent from occurring, such as murder, assault, or fraud, and those in which society ensures compensation to the victims, as in the case of automobile or industrial accidents. In the first case, society forbids such behavior and attaches punitive sanctions to it. In the second case, society sets up social arrangements that ensure adequate redress for the innocent victims. Often both types of social response are appropriate, as when a drunk driver loses control of his car and does extensive damage to a shop window.

The third distinction is between those interactions for which society empowers the parties to engage in activities that are generally forbidden because they involve harm, and those interactions for which society does not so empower the parties, thus setting limits to the legal principle *volenti non fit injuria*. We may perhaps agree that contracts in which people undertake, for pay, to engage in gladitorial combat to the death of one, ought to be invalid and the behavior punishable.[1]

This broadly conceived social enterprise of which ascription of responsibility is part rests on the common sense idea of intervening in the natural course of events. It may be difficult to give a clear account of how to isolate that natural course of events and of what constitutes an intervention, but I assume that these problems can be solved.[2]

Now the point of ascribing responsibility is to single out entities, whether events, states of affairs, doings, material objects, or persons, that satisfy two criteria: one, being directly and unproblematically under someone's control; and, two, being capable of playing a significant role in the deflection of events from their natural course, and in a direction society finds desirable.

THING- AND AGENT-RESPONSIBILITY

We ascribe responsibility in two senses of the term: "thing-responsibility" and "agent-responsibility." When we claim that the failed brakes—as opposed to the giant pothole, the tree across the road, or the carelessness of the driver—were responsible for the accident, we ascribe thing-responsibility. In ascribing thing-responsibility, the central idea is to single out the decisive factor that *must actually be operative* when an undesirable event is being prevented or a desirable one produced. This factor may be singled out because it is the most easily controlled (the brakes were responsible for the accident) or perhaps because it is abnormal (the unusually good rainfall was responsible for the bumper crop). Even when the factor identified as responsible is not itself controllable, knowledge of its responsibility may be of some, albeit limited, practical use, since it may prevent us from wasting our efforts on controllable factors which are not efficacious, or may warn us that there is nothing we can do (for example, we cannot prevent the multimillion dollar devastation caused by a tornado). However, when one causal factor is an artifact with a function it has failed to perform, that factor is an especially suitable candidate for thing-responsibility.

The rationale of ascribing responsibility is thus ultimately forward-looking, to improve the future; but the actual ascribing of thing-responsibility is backward-looking. We identify the "culprit" only after the mishap has occurred, but of course the general purpose of identifying such a culprit is to prevent future damage. The brakes and the storm *were* (not *are*)[3] responsible for the particular harm suffered. The harm is done and cannot now be undone; but if we know what was responsible this time, we can take steps to prevent it next time. We can repair the brakes, and though we can as yet do nothing about storms, we can build houses or ships or windbreaks that can withstand them. Ascribing thing-responsibility is thus similar to identifying cause.[4]

Ascribing agent-responsibility differs in several important ways. Although it is also backward-looking, it is not merely so; the consequences of the identification of the culprit are much more complex. The main reason for these differences is that agents, especially human agents, are extremely complex entities, particularly as far as their response mechanisms are concerned. Unlike things, human beings cannot only be blamed, they can be found *blameworthy*; not only have faults, but be *at fault*; and not only be due for repair, but be *culpable* and deserving of *condemnation* or *punishment* or liable to payment of *damages*.[5]

Why? Because normal human beings are moral agents. This means, for one thing, that what they do to their environment is done for a variety of reasons. Hence agents can modify one another's responses without necessarily having to tinker with their response mechanisms. Different persons can, by threats, inducements, cajoling, persuasion, and arguments, be made to respond to the same situation in quite different ways. It is only when that capacity to respond is impaired that we need to treat them as abnormal and so in need of "cure," that is, in need of treatment that will restore their response mechanism to good working order. Only when we must give up hope even of this, is there any question of treating human beings by means of the implantation of electrodes in their brain, prefrontal lobotomy, chemical treatment, and the like.

But having such a faculty of choice (will) is not all there is to moral agency. Moral agents must also be capable of understanding guidelines for action, of being able to act on them, and of understanding that they ought to do so. They must understand that they have certain obligatory tasks, are subject to certain requirements, and must discharge them. Small children, who have not yet acquired this ability, and the insane, who have lost it, may be capable of performing intentional actions but not of understanding why they are required to have certain intentions and not others. Hence they are not, as we say, responsible for their actions, not even for what they do intentionally. Ascribing responsibility in this sense of capacity-responsibility[6] is ascribing responsibility not for a particular past event or state of affairs but for a certain basic ability presupposed by all such particular ascriptions.

Agent-responsibility thus differs in two important respects from thing-responsibility. Agent-responsibility has a forward-looking aspect to which its backward-looking aspect is closely tied. The brakes become thing-responsible for the accident (in the backward-looking and only sense) simply by virtue of being the significant causal factor. The driver becomes agent-responsible only if he has failed in the forward-looking aspect of agent-responsibility. Simply being the cause is not sufficient nor even necessary. A company's decision to close a plant may cause harm to many people, but that does not make the company agent-responsible (in a backward-looking sense) unless its closing of the plant was a failure in, or breach of, the forward-looking aspect of its agent-responsibility; unless, in other words, the company had a duty which the plant closure has breached. The fact that plant closure causes harm is not sufficient to establish such a duty. Parents are responsible for their children, employers for their employees. This means that they are agent-responsible, in a forward-looking sense, for the state of the world that is free of harm caused by these children or employees, and agent-responsible, in a backward-looking sense, for harm the children or employees do cause. In these cases of vicarious responsibility, those who are responsible for the harm are not those who have caused it.

DUTIES AND TASK-RESPONSIBILITIES

The forward-looking aspect of agent-responsibility consists in a social requirement, whether customary, legal, or moral. It may be a duty, an obligation, or a responsibility in the forward-looking sense which I call a "task-responsibility." Such social requirements may be designed in various ways, and two must be distinguished here. First, that one must not lie specifies an action without requiring that it be performed for a particular end or purpose. Second, that when one is well-placed to do so, one should try to rescue others in peril, does specify the end, that is, the event or state of affairs to be brought about, prevented, or maintained, without requiring that it be attained by particular means. A task-responsibility is a social requirement of the second form. A ship's captain is task-responsible for the safety of the passengers, a ship's doctor for their health. They are under a social requirement to see to it that the passengers are safe and well. Their task is not merely to do, or refrain from doing, various actions on a list. Rather, their task is to do, or refrain from doing, whatever is necessary to attain that end of safety and health, and they must continually bear in mind what is necessary for that end. Thus, the social requirement which constitutes the forward-looking aspect of someone's agent-responsibility is often a (task-) responsibility for some event or state of affairs; but not always, for sometimes it may be a duty or an obligation to do something specific, such as telling the truth or filling in a form.

ANSWERABILITY, ACCOUNTABILITY, CULPABILITY, LIABILITY

If I fail in a social requirement, whether a task-responsibility or not, I ipso facto become responsible in a backward-looking sense, namely, answerability. If I am task-responsible for X, then I am answerable for not-X. Answerability is the logical consequence not necessarily of a failure in a task-responsibility, but of a failure to discharge a social requirement of any sort. If there is a social (for example, legal or customary) requirement to submit a tax return by April 15, then I am answerable for *not* submitting one by that date. If the ship's doctor has a task-responsibility for the health of the passengers, then he is answerable for any illness that any passenger contracts on the ship.[7]

Answerability presumptively implies liability, but that presumption can be rebutted by an exculpatory explanation of the failure to discharge the requirement. Exculpatory explanation is either a justification, as when a killing is in self-defense, or it is an excuse,[8] as when it is done under duress.

Of course, there are cases in which this presumption cannot be rebutted. We then speak of strict liability. Later we shall look briefly into the question of whether some or all ascriptions of strict liability are morally objectionable.

The most important notion in the backward-looking aspect of agent-responsibility is liability, which does most of the important practical work for the social practice I have sketched. Sometimes when we claim, for example, that Jones is responsible, say, for the damage caused his neighbors by his children, we mean that he is liable for that damage. This can, however, mean two importantly different things. One is liability to punishment, the other is liability to or in damages. The two types of liability serve different purposes.

Punitive sanctions are applied in those cases in which a social requirement or prohibition has been imposed in order to ensure or prevent the conduct in question, and the culprit has shown by his conduct that he lacks the appropriate motivation. He has no justification or excuse; it is not the case that even the person with the best or at least minimally acceptable motivation would have failed in just the same way. There is, therefore, some reason to remotivate such a person, and for this purpose to apply the punitive sanctions, not, however, without interposing the culpability safeguards.

These safeguards have the following rationale. Children are taught their social tasks and as far as possible motivated to shoulder them. We also threaten punitive social sanctions to motivate those adults whose socialization has not taken well enough to elicit conduct in conformity with social requirements. That still leaves those who are not appropriately motivated even by the threat of punitive sanctions. It is only upon this last group that we are justified in imposing punitive social sanctions, because we may hope that it will remotivate (reform or rehabilitate) them, that it will influence others who, in the absence of a credible threat of these sanctions, would not comply, and that by inflicting these sanctions we shall at least temporarily incapacitate culprits from committing further breaches of the social requirements. But the actual imposition of these punitive sanctions is allowable only under culpability safeguards. One of these safeguards is that the violator have no exculpatory explanation of his behavior. We think of the punitive sanctions as applicable only to those whose motivation is at fault, but that necessarily would not be the case if they had an exculpatory explanation, an explanation which shows that their motivation was not at fault. Hence strict criminal liability is morally objectionable.

We also do not allow the imposition of punitive sanctions on those whose rational response mechanism is not yet fully developed, as in children, or is out of order, as with the insane.[9] In the latter case, we treat human beings in somewhat the way we treat things. We try to repair their rational response mechanism in various manipulative ways, by drugs and the like, so that if this works, the person can again be treated as befits a fully rational and moral agent. If we fail in that, we feel justified in dealing with such a person manipulatively, to ensure that he does not harm others or himself.

The other kind of liability, liability in damages, is imposed for the solution of a very different problem. In these cases, the social requirement does not necessarily aim at preventing people from behaving in certain specified ways. On the contrary, the conduct may be permitted or even encouraged, perhaps under certain safeguards (such as the requirement of due care), but then the agent is required to compensate those who suffer harm in the course of such permissible but dangerous activities, for example, blasting or running nuclear power stations or selling socially wanted but dangerous medication, such as the whooping cough (pertussis) vaccine. It should be noted that in these cases we are not embarrassed, as we are in criminal cases, by the distinction between successful and unsuccessful attempts at murder. In the criminal case it seems we ought to punish the unsuccessful as much as the successful attempts, for what counts is the motivation and the intention based on it, not the good or bad luck, the skill or clumsiness in execution. The person attempting murder wants to cause death and so needs to be remotivated; the wrecker does not want to cause harm, for he is engaged in a socially useful and approved but dangerous activity whose harmful side effects he may do his utmost to avoid.[10] Thus, it seems fair to permit the activity but if, as is usually the case, he profits from it, to impose on him the duty of covering the losses that others suffer as a result. In such cases, difficult moral questions arise about the importance of the dangerous activity and the fairness of exposing some to dangers for the sake of the benefits derived by others.

The concept of responsibility, which includes the notion of liability in damages, thus strongly suggests or implies that a person should be able to recover from the person who is culpably answerable for that damage (that is, should be held liable for that damage) if he has culpably failed in a social requirement. However, if what I said in the preceding paragraph is sound, we should not accept the normative principle that he should necessarily be able to recover *only* in these cases—that strict liability in damages is always morally objectionable. For in the cases considered, the person who caused the damage had the choice of not engaging in that profitable but dangerous activity.[11]

CAUSAL RESPONSIBILITY AND CAUSATION

Some writers distinguish yet another sense of responsibility, which they call "causal responsibility." They use this term in somewhat the same way as I have used the expression "thing-responsibility," but they also use it interchangeably with "cause."[12] I have avoided this term altogether because it tends to blur the differences between two different types of social activity, one concerned with making a favorable difference to the future course of events, the other with explaining the past. Historically speaking, the distinction between these two activities has emerged only slowly, and even now the affinity of responsibility with the former, of cause with the latter is not firmly established.[13] However, the distinction is discernible in ordinary usage and, in my opinion, deserves to be developed and sharpened. When we observe the distinction, we affix responsibility to intervene in the natural course of events so as to deflect it in a desired direction by modifying people's motivation or rectifying the outcome of their behavior; we then single out something by which we can influence the future. By contrast, we pick out the cause when something calls for an explanation of why it has happened. We ascribe responsibility when intervention in the natural course of events is warranted either to prevent an undesirable occurrence or to make up for it. That which calls for causal explanation is an event in relation to which we want to identify some other past event tied to the explanandum by a reliable connection. Causal explanations only incidentally identify what was thing-responsible. Although the tornado may be said to be the cause of, and so responsible for, the damage to the town, the two claims have different content. That it is the cause purports to explain how and why it happened—we now think we understand and so are no longer puzzled or perplexed; that it was responsible tells us that this (and not something else) is the factor we must worry about if we wish to prevent such losses in the future, either by building stronger houses or building elsewhere or taking out more insurance.

Of course, the further we move from the primary use of responsibility (that is, agent-responsibility), the closer the connection between responsibility and cause. An uncontrollable event, such as a snowstorm, or thing, such as a comet, is *necessarily* responsible for the harm it causes, and is the cause of the harm it is responsible for. It is therefore easy to overlook the differences between these claims, and the expression "causal responsibility" tends to obscure them further.

However, the differences are significant in the primary cases. The person who hires the assassin, who instigates a murder, is (ultimately) responsible for the death of that person, although he did not do the killing and in that sense has not caused the death (though we may also want to claim that he is the ultimate cause of that death).[14] The person who is (vicariously) responsible for the damage his children or employees inflict has not caused that damage nor need he be in any sense even their ultimate cause, or in any other way causally involved.

That one can be agent-responsible without having caused the occurrence can easily be overlooked because agent-responsibility gives rise to a new quasi-causal relationship, namely, a duty-breaching failure to use one's power to prevent. To see this, we must attend to two further distinctions. The first is between *having* causal power over an event and *exercising* that power. We may think of some parts of the universe as systems which in the normal course are headed for some predictable event (for example, a pregnant woman's body heading for the birth of her baby, a drowning person's heading for death within a roughly predictable time) or as systems that in the normal course maintain themselves in a certain state (for example, a person's maintaining himself at a stable temperature, in a state of good health, or full consciousness). In such cases, some people may have and either exercise or fail to exercise causal power over some events in the system; the woman, for instance, may have an abortion or take DES to prevent a miscarriage. They can exercise that (supposed) causal power in two importantly different ways: they can bring about an event or state which would not come about in the normal course, or they can prevent one that would otherwise occur. Killing is an exercise of the first kind (strictly speaking, one cannot kill someone at the very time at which that person dies from natural causes, that is, independent of intervention), saving someone's life is of the second kind (one cannot at a given time save a life unless it would at that time come to an end from natural causes). A person has causal power over event E if and only if he has both positive and negative causal power over E. He has positive causal power over E if and only if, when E would not come about from natural causes (that is, would not come about but for someone's intervention), he can bring E about by suitably intervening. He has negative causal power over E if and only if, when E would come about from natural causes, he can prevent E by suitably intervening. A person or his behavior has caused E if and only if he has exercised his positive causal power over E. We can say that he or his behavior has caused not-E if he has exercised his negative causal power over E. Neither using one's negative causal power over E nor failing to use that power is causing E.

The second distinction is between being the cause of a death and death being a consequence. When A has a duty to save B's life or has a responsibility for B's life, then that situation can give rise to a special quasi-causal connection. For in such a case, in which A has causal power over B's life (whether to bring about B's [premature] death or to prevent [delay] B's death), A is required not to use his causal power to bring about B's death; A may use his power only to prevent B's death should B's life be in danger. Because of A's responsibility, his *not* using his causal power to save B's life would be a violation of his duty. Hence what A does, his behavior in these circumstances, can be described as such a violation, one that consists of his *not* using his causal power to save B's life. In such cases we can say that B's death *was a consequence of* what A did, that is, of his doing nothing to save B. But obviously A did not kill B or cause B's death; nor was A the cause of B's death. Rather, B's death is the (logical or internal) consequence of *A's letting B die*, but this is so only if A was under a requirement to save B. Of course, it is not plausible to maintain that everyone is under such a requirement: this is the important truth in the widespread belief that killing is worse than letting die, for everyone is, other things being equal, under a requirement not to kill or to cause anyone's death.

The upshot is that such a nonintervention (not saving) cannot be the cause of something (death). What can be said is merely that an event E (death) is the causal consequence of such a nonintervention by someone, provided that (1) intervention would have prevented E; (2) one was required to intervene; and (3) one was able to. Not intervening was not the cause of E, because it was a nonuse of causal powers to prevent E, not their use to bring it about.[15]

Failure to draw these two distinctions can have important normative consequences. Thus, theorists with libertarian sympathies, who accept something like the everyday interpretation of "causing" and "being the cause of," which I have just given, and relying on the normative principle SL_1, that that one should be held liable for all and only the harm one has caused, are led to the conclusion that one cannot be responsible—and so should never be held legally liable—for anything that one has not caused, for example, the death of a drowning man one has failed to rescue.

Now, principle SL_1 is plausible, but should not be thought to hold for all situations. We should consider the desirability, from the point of view of all concerned, of making it a conventionally recognized duty. Thus, it does not seem desirable to impose on rescuers strict liability for harm done to rescuees. For such an arrangement—required by SL_1—is likely to deter voluntary would-be rescuers. It seems, on the contrary, more desirable to make rescuers liable only for culpably inflicted harm, and, indeed, to impose on the rescuee a duty to compensate the rescuer.[16] In a well-known article, Antony M. Honoré[17] has indicated ways in which the law can encourage such rescuing behavior, without imposing a duty to rescue, by imposing on the rescuee a duty to compensate the rescuer.

At the other end of the normative spectrum, Marxists and others who also accept principle SL_1 but cannot accept the libertarian normative conclusions derived from it, feel they cannot escape it except by giving a different interpretation to causation. They therefore maintain that the person who does not rescue the drowning man, though he could do so by throwing a rope, causes or is the cause of his death and is therefore liable for it. They are especially concerned to refute the view that a person's behavior can be a causal antecedent of an event only if that behavior is a failure of the duty to prevent that event. For to admit that would preclude them from showing that they had such a duty on the ground that it is such a causal antecedent. In an article defending this interpretation of causation, John Harris[18] tries to show that the drowning man's "death *results from our failure,* whether we have a duty to save him or not. (We might have a duty to kill this particular man and discharge it by failing to save him.) It is not the existence of the duty that makes the death of the [drowning man] *a consequence of our failure* to save him, rather it is the fact that unless we save him he will die that makes it our duty to save him" [emphasis added].

If my distinctions are sound, it is true both that the existence of my duty to save the drowning man makes his death a consequence of my failure to save him, and that the fact that unless someone saves him and the additional facts that I am in the best position to save him and that saving him does not impose an unreasonable burden on me, is regarded (in my view, rightly) as a sufficient ground for conventionally recognizing this (at least in our custom, but perhaps also in law) as a duty on me. But, as we have seen, none of this means that failing to rescue the drowning man is causing his death, or that it could not be my duty to save him *unless* failing to rescue him was causing his death, or that the reason why his death is a consequence of my failure to rescue him must be that it was the cause of his death, rather than that its being such a consequence follows from the fact that I had a duty to rescue him.

MORAL AND LEGAL RESPONSIBILITY

I can now draw the distinction it is my main task to elucidate. Plainly there are no legal or moral thing-responsibilities; brakes cannot be morally or legally responsible, only agents can. As far as such agent-responsibility is concerned, there are two main distinctions, one based on the ground, the other on the sanction involved.

Take first the distinction based on ground. Moral responsibilities are those based on moral grounds; legal responsibilities are those based on legal grounds. However, the two types of grounds are not always as analogous as they seem nor are they mutually exclusive. A legal ground is always one that originates in the relevant legal system—the context will usually make clear which that is; for example, in the case of my legal responsibility for my tax return, the ground is that my income is above a certain tax-free level, and the relevant legal system is that of the United States. By contrast, "moral task-responsibility" often means something that implies nothing about the origin or pedigree of the ground—it may be legal or customary in my society or it may not be conventionally recognized in my or any society at all. Huckleberry Finn notoriously senses moral grounds which his in-group, and he himself as a well-indoctrinated member, does not officially recognize. What makes a ground a moral one in this sense is not a special mode of conventional recognition but rather its appropriateness or soundness from the moral point of view. The claim that a responsibility is a moral one in this sense is analogous to the claim that the ground of the validity of an argument is a logical one. It is based on a certain test passing which attests to a certain merit in the argument. Thus, if an argument conforms to *modus ponens*, it passes this test and has this merit. If a certain type of utilitarianism states the truth about morality (as most logic textbooks do about the validity of arguments), then a certain ground, say, that my income is above $10,000, is a moral one if and only if its adoption maximizes utility. Other moral theories offer other criteria of what makes a moral ground. That my task responsibility for my tax return is a moral one (in this sense of moral) implies that it is licensed or required from that point of view, whether or not it is conventionally recognized. Claiming that it is a moral task-responsibility implies that one would suitably change one's view that it is, if one discovered that it is not so approved from that point of view. Such moral claims are, therefore, analogous in this important respect to factual assertions: they, too, imply that one's views are tied to the evidence available, quite independently of what is generally thought or recognized in one's society.

One can, of course, make claims about moral grounds, and about what is based on them, from what has come to be known as "an external point of view,"[19] that is, one that distances itself from the commitments implied in one's remark. Thus, when we speak of the morality of the Navajo, or even "our own" morality, in the sense of our society's public morality, we do not imply that we, the speakers, accept what that morality says. It makes no sense to claim "I have a moral task responsibility for my tax return, but I do not believe it,"[20] because such a remark is made from the internal point of view. By contrast, it is perfectly good sense to maintain that, according to our public morality, one has such a responsibility but that one does not believe one (really) has it, because this is said from an external point of view.

To sum up: legal and moral responsibilities are distinguished by the different grounds on which they are based. But whereas legal grounds are always those anchored in some particular legal order, moral grounds are often those appropriate from the moral point of view. This should make clear why one and the same responsibility may be both moral and legal, and indeed why many should be both. This is typically so in the case of task-responsibilities, but we also distinguish in this way between moral or legal answerability—which is the failure in a moral or legal requirement—and moral or legal culpability— which is such a failure in the absence of an explanation that is exculpatory, either from the moral point of view or on the basis of exculpatory grounds actually recognized in the relevant legal order.

By contrast, in the case of liability and accountability, the distinction between the legal and the moral is usually based not on the ground, but on the sanction. Legal liability sometimes means not, or not merely, liability on legal grounds, but liability *to legal sanctions*; the same is true for moral liability. Legal sanctions include, as we have noted, a range of coercive and other social pressures designed to ensure an adequate degree of conformity with the social requirements. The term "moral sanctions" applies to things such as the expression of approval and disapproval, commendation and condemnation, the passing of favorable and unfavorable moral judgment on others, or even the pangs of conscience and the like. It implies that people want to be or, at least thought of by others to be, morally upright persons, hence that the mere passing of favorable or unfavorable moral judgment on their conduct or character would have some appropriate influence.

What is true of liability is to some extent also true of accountability. As we noted, accountability is similar to answerability, but has closer ties with liability. Moral (or legal) answerability follows logically from one's failure to discharge a moral (or legal) requirement. Moral accountability is accountability to a specific person for a specific thing which is based on sound moral ground, whether conventionally recognized or not. Legal accountability by contrast is accountability to a specific person for a specific thing which is based on a ground actually recognized in the law of some legal system.

If this is right, then there is not, as the legal positivist tradition has held, an exact parallel between what John Austin called "positive law" and "positive morality."[21] Rather, we should distinguish between, on the one hand, the conventionally established practices and institutions that make up a society's custom and law, each characterized by its peculiar ways of generating and enforcing the society's requirements, and on the other hand, a moral point of view from which these actually existing, conventionally established practices and institutions can be critically examined and improved. The positive morality of a society is not, then, a third parallel part of the conventionally accepted social order with yet a third, peculiarly moral, way of generating and enforcing the society's requirements. There are no specifically moral sanctions and no specifically moral rules. Rather, the positive morality of a society consists of the society's publicly accepted *beliefs* about which of the conventionally accepted social requirements, whether customary or legal, are or are not justifiable from that moral point of view, and about which hitherto unrecognized ones should be recognized. Of course, as we have already noted, insofar as people wish to be morally upright persons, in passing moral judgments on one another they will exert relevant pressures on one another to comply with the social requirements. Hence the passing of such judgments can be construed as the imposition of the peculiarly moral sanctions.

However, if we construe them in this way, we must note an important difference between such moral and other types of sanctions. Whereas the imposition of moral sanctions consists simply in passing moral judgments on people, for example, claiming that they have failed to discharge certain morally justified social requirements, the imposition of the peculiar sanctions of custom and law consists in exerting on people specific social pressures, such as ostracism or imprisonment, whenever they are judged to have failed to discharge a requirement of custom or law. Thus, in the sense in which there are sanctions peculiar to custom and law, there are no sanctions peculiar to morality. For moral sanctions are not social sanctions over and above moral judgments, but are the public passing of those moral judgments themselves.[22] These judgments function as moral sanctions only to the extent that people want to be moral, or at least be regarded as such. By contrast, the sanctions of law and custom are not the analogous effects of legal judgments or judgments of what is customary: they are threats of the imposition of deprivations whose motivating effects can be relied on even in the case of people who do not want to be law- or custom-abiding. It follows that so-called positive morality is not a peculiar system of directives parallel to law or custom but, rather, a widely held belief that all or the bulk of these directives satisfy a certain criterion, are acceptable from a certain point of view—the moral one. It seems to me, therefore, that the legal positivist construal of the relation between law and morality is a philosophical mistake, and in my judgment a deep one.

NORMATIVE PRINCIPLES
FOR ASCRIBING AGENT-RESPONSIBILITY

This completes the summary of the analytic part of my paper, in which I tried to elucidate what we claim when we ascribe responsibility. I turn now to the second part, in which I survey a variety of normative principles society might adopt to guide us in our ascriptions of responsibility and especially liability. We should, however, bear in mind that the concept of responsibility itself contains such normative principles, for example, that no one can be answerable except through failing in a social requirement, whether a duty or a task-responsibility, and that no one can be liable for something unless answerable and so task-responsible for it. As we shall see, the concept of agent-responsibility also strongly suggests, if it does not imply, certain other normative principles for handling certain practical problems.

The most general formulation of the problem we encounter in the domain of human interaction is, What should be done if someone suffers harm, loss, or damage? The simplest, most general solution seems to be to let the damage lie where it falls unless there are good reasons for shifting it to someone else. The concept of responsibility strongly suggests that the only good reason for shifting responsibilities is that the harm suffered by someone is (1) something (for example, a death) which someone else was under a social requirement to prevent or not to bring about and which was the consequence of that person's failure to discharge that social requirement, or (2) something which was the consequence of someone's failure to discharge a duty to do or not to do something specific, for example, to drive within the speed limit or not to pollute the air. This is true regardless of whether we allow only liability for fault or also strict liability. For even in the latter case it is only if someone has failed to discharge a requirement not to cause someone harm or to prevent it that the loss someone suffers may be shifted to another person, namely, the one who has caused it.

We may expect the structure of a concept to be such that it does not commit us to any normative principles for its use, so that nothing whatever follows about the justifiability of any claim we make with the word "responsibility," simply from the meaning of the word itself. However, this does not seem to be true for this concept, for it appears to rule out the so-called deep-pocket policy which allows shifting (the cost of) the damage to some other person even though he has not violated any justifiable social requirement. For the concept of responsibility implies that a loss should be shifted to another only if that other is liable to pay compensation, but that implies answerability and so failure in a social requirement. The deep-pocket policy therefore violates not only a normative principle firmly embedded in our individualistic ideology, namely, that nobody should be made to lighten the blows of fortune suffered by another—that such transfers should be entirely voluntary—but a principle implied by the very concept of responsibility itself. Since we think of liability as presupposing answerability, we tend to reject the deep-pocket policy as contrary to the very idea of responsibility. It should be clear, however, that this normative principle need not be acceptable to every moral theorist. A utilitarian, for instance, can think of such transfers as required by the principle of diminishing utility, since utility tends to be increased when goods are transferred from deep to shallow pockets.

There are in any case other plausible ways of looking at the possibilities. It is by no means obvious that the best way to cope with losses suffered as a result of interaction between people is either to forbid such interactions altogether or forbid them in the absence of the potential victim's consent or else to allow them but then impose the duty to compensate the victim, when there is one, out of the pocket of the person who caused the damage. Two weaknesses of this arrangement implied by responsibility are obvious. One is that the individuals who have caused the damage may not have sufficient resources to pay for it. The other is that the requirement to pay damages may not adequately motivate people, especially those who have nothing to lose, to refrain from such dangerous activities or to take adequate care. This is particularly true in the case of the manufacture and sale of unsafe products. In these cases, if the manufacturer, who will not normally be the one actually causing the damage, is made answerable or strictly liable for the damage caused by use of the product, it may induce the manufacturer to produce safer products to decrease liability, and the victim will be more likely to receive adequate compensation because manufacturers tend to have the deeper pockets. Thus, there seems to be no a priori reason to think that, in order to minimize the incidence of damage, society must aim to deter or shift the loss to those most likely to *cause* the damage. Another effective policy might be to induce those in the best position to *prevent* the damage, either to do so or else pay for their failures. This seems especially appropriate in those types of interaction which are socially desirable but, though profitable to most, dangerous to some. It seems only fair that those who derive great benefit from these interactions should be called upon to ensure that in conducting these activities they exercise reasonable care to prevent harm and that where harm occurs despite such precautions they compensate the victim.

SINDELL V. ABBOTT LABORATORIES

The relevant facts of this case can be briefly summarized. To avoid miscarriage, some women, including Judith Sindell's mother, took the drug DES, which was manufactured by a number of firms, including Abbott Laboratories. Judith Sindell and other so-called DES daughters have suffered a variety of serious and costly impairments of their health. There seems to be no reasonable doubt that these impairments were caused by their mothers' taking DES during pregnancy. However, it is no longer possible to determine which of the roughly 200 firms that manufactured DES actually produced the particular DES those mothers took.

The manufacturers did not themselves perform tests for effectiveness and safety, though they advertised the drug as such. In fact, the drugs were not effective in preventing miscarriage and were not safe, and it seems the manufacturers could have known this.

MORAL RESPONSIBILITY

Thus although there seems no doubt that the cause of Sindell's health impairment was a DES drug, and that such a drug was (thing-) responsible for it, it is not possible to ascertain who caused it; and therefore it seems impossible to say who, if indeed anyone, is (agent-) responsible. Does this mean, then, that, morally speaking, Sindell and the other women in the same position ought to bear the cost of these health impairments themselves? If my account of moral responsibility is correct, then that will depend on the answers to the following three questions:

1. Is the health impairment the consequence of someone's failure to discharge a task-responsibility?

2. Is it the consequence of someone's failure to discharge a duty?

3. Is there any other reason why all or part of the cost incurred in the health impairment should be shifted to someone other than the persons who suffered it?

Did anyone have such a moral task-responsibility? Presumably the physicians of these women had such a responsibility for their health. However, it would seem plausible to say that these physicians did not fail in that responsibility by prescribing DES. After all, they were in no position to challenge or test the manufacturers' assurances of safety and effectiveness. In their position, they simply had no reason to doubt the manufacturers' claims, and no choice but to rely on them.

Do the manufacturers, then, have such a task-responsibility? Plainly, it could not be one analogous to that of the physicians, for manufacturers stand in no special relationship to any particular patient, as physicians do, but they can hardly be burdened with responsibility for the health of everyone. Nor does it seem reasonable to hold them task-responsible for a state of affairs in which there always is an adequate supply of safe and effective drugs for this purpose.

We can perhaps make a case for such a task-responsibility where there is a special public interest, as with infectious diseases. Thus, it is undesirable for manufacturers to stop or threaten to stop production of whooping cough vaccine when they find mandatory testing and safety requirements too burdensome, because the whole community, not only those immediately threatened by the disease, has an interest in protection from the disease.

It does not, then, seem plausible to say that the health impairments were (or were the result of) a failure of the manufacturers to discharge their task-responsibility for a state of affairs directly or indirectly involving the absence of these impairments. Nor does it seem likely that these impairments were (or were the result of) anyone else's failure in such a task-responsibility, for who could have such a responsibility?

Is the health impairment, then, the consequence of someone's failure to discharge a duty? It may, for instance, be thought that manufacturers, like everyone else, have a duty not to harm others and that Judith Sindell's health impairments are a case of some manufacturer's harming her and other women in the same position. But this would be a mistake. For what the manufacturer did, namely, producing and selling these drugs, is quite unlike the typical case of harm, such as killing or blasting, in which the victims are entirely passive, mere targets that may or may not be hit as a (logically internal) result or consequence of what the agent does. A purchaser of a product is not passive, but must do something to effect a purchase, and can quite easily avoid the relevant harm by simply not buying. Judith Sindell's mother's behavior was a causally contributory factor of the medical mishap that befell Judith. The interaction was consensual. In a sense, Judith's mother herself brought the harm on Judith, for she must be assumed to have known that taking a drug by and large involves a health risk. No doubt for this reason, the legal principle which for a long time governed this sort of interaction was caveat emptor. However, for various reasons, among them the purchaser's inability under modern conditions to ascertain whether a product is safe and effective and, because of the standardization of contracts, to shop around for comparable products with better warranties, the law has imposed on manufacturers, especially in the field of food and drugs, more or less strict product liability.[23] It seems to me these recent changes accurately reflect the considered judgment of our public morality. This is all the more so when the manufacturers in their publicity assure the public that their drug is safe and effective.

We can construe these legal and moral changes as the imposition of certain new duties on the manufacturer—roughly the duty to manufacture and sell only products that can be safely used by anyone—and the harm suffered by the user as a consequence of the product's use. In this case, although it would be wrong or misleading to say that the manufacturer inflicted the harm on or caused it to the purchaser, it would seem fair to say that the harm occurred as a *consequence* of the manufacturer's failing to discharge a duty, namely, the duty not to sell hazardous products.

In *Sindell*, it seems clear that all the manufacturers of DES failed to discharge that duty, hence that the harm Sindell and other women suffered was a consequence of that failing. Since we do not know which manufacturer's drug caused Sindell's illness, the question therefore is whether all, some, or none of the manufacturers, any of whose drugs may have been the cause of these health impairments, should be held liable for that harm.

The answer to this question can be found by detailing all the desiderata we wish to achieve by such liability arrangements and to work out which of these arrangements achieves them best. The most obvious desiderata in this case seem to be the following.

The availability of adequate quantities of drugs that are as effective, safe, and inexpensive as possible. One way of ensuring such availability would be to set up a tax-supported government-run research and testing facility, whose results would be made available to private manufacturers. Another would be to let the manufacturers themselves finance their own research and testing facilities and pass the cost on to the consumer. A third would be to combine this latter arrangement with setting up a government facility, such as the FDA, which would perform its own tests for effectiveness and safety of the products developed in private laboratories. And there may be others.

The maximal prevention of the disease in question and the minimal incidence of harmful side effects. This would be achieved by providing the strongest motivation inclining manufacturers to produce adequate quantities of effective and safe drugs, and also inclining those threatened by the disease to use the drugs.

Adequate compensation for those suffering harmful side effects of the use of the drug. This is desirable for its own sake, but also as a way of encouraging people to use the drug to combat the disease. It is also especially important since it may be desirable to have such drugs available as soon as possible, that is, in some cases even before testing has shown the drug to be safe. Where the deleterious side effects may well be long-range, as in DES, it could be particularly desirable to put the drug on the market before such long-range effects have been ascertained. It is then especially desirable that people who take the drug are not used simply as guinea pigs, hence that the harm they suffer be adequately compensated, since they are suffering it also in the interest of later users.

The minimal cost of the arrangement to be chosen. We must bear in mind the administrative and other costs of imposing either strict liability or fault liability on one of the parties involved or on the public at large. As we know from recent discussion of no-fault automobile accident insurance, making liability depend on fault may be administratively very costly because determining fault is usually a difficult and time-consuming endeavor.

The fairness of any arrangement designed to achieve these ends. When we choose between letting the damage lie where it falls and shifting it to some other person or persons, we should give preference to the fairest ruling.[24]

Consider the simplest liability arrangement:

P_1, every damage should lie where it falls.

Plainly this principle involves no administrative errors and costs at all and is therefore attractive on that score. It is not clear, without empirical investigation, whether such an arrangement would also keep the incidence of harmful side effects of drug use at a minimum. Even if it had that effect, it might have it only because people, fearing such side effects, would tend not to use the drug. But that would tend to increase the incidence of those illnesses the drug is designed to combat. It also may have another possibly undesirable effect, namely, that the harmful side effects of using the drug will affect people in rather unequal ways, since those who will have to bear those effects will not always be those best equipped to cover the costs. There would also seem to be another undesirable aspect of this arrangement: it will not be rational for people to assume that products on the market are effective and safe. Unless persuaded by manufacturers' dishonest advertising that their products are effective and safe—which would be morally objectionable—people might tend not to use these products and manufacturers not to produce them, and this would tend to make everyone worse off. It would seem to be best for all concerned if it were rational for the general public to believe that the products on the market are effective and safe. But it would seem that the arrangement based on principle P_1 might well not have this desirable effect.

Let us then consider another principle:

> P_2, any damage should lie where it falls, except where some other individual (1) has failed to discharge his moral requirement either to prevent that damage to that other or to refrain from doing something specific which caused that damage or as a consequence of which that damage occurred and (2) lacks an exculpatory explanation for this failure.

This principle would impose on the manufacturer a fault liability for the harm its product has caused to a user. By such an arrangement the manufacturer would pay compensation for the harm done, unless the manufacturer can show it is not at fault, that all reasonable care in testing and in manufacture, as well as in advertising, was exercised.

This fault liability arrangement would seem to have several advantages over the first. It would in all probability increase the general confidence in the products on the market and would increase their use, thereby enabling people to better attain various ends. It would, surely, encourage the manufacturers to improve the effectiveness and safety of their products, thus reducing the harmful side effects of the use of their products and, because of limitation of liability by fault, it would not discourage manufacturers from putting their products on the market.

However, this arrangement has at least one serious drawback, the high administrative cost of determining fault, which, from certain relevant angles is, as we shall see, pure waste.

This drawback can be lessened by adopting strict liability, that is, by dropping the second clause of P_2. This arrangement thus rests on the following principle:

> P_3, any damage should lie where it falls, except where some other individual has failed to discharge his moral requirement to prevent that damage to that other or to refrain from doing something which caused that damage, or as a consequence of which that damage occurred.

Because the manufacturer usually has a deep pocket, the user of its products need not worry about failing to recover financially. The manufacturer has various ways of protecting itself: it can make safer products and pass the cost on to the consumer; it can take out insurance to cover the costs of paying compensation; or it can stop manufacturing the product. As in the case of the whooping cough vaccine, it is undesirable that the manufacturer stop manufacture; there is likely to be a guaranteed market for the product and so any additional costs could be covered by a price increase.

It may be thought unfair to burden the manufacturer with the costs of compensation even when all reasonable precautions to ensure the safety of the product have been taken. This seems especially plausible if we construe liability in damages on the model of liability to punishment. For since punishment aims to remotivate the wrongdoer and since, in strict criminal liability, the criminal is punished even when an exculpatory explanation of the crime exists (that is, when there is no reason for remotivation), strict criminal liability is indeed objectionable. But this point does not apply to liability in damages. For damages are extracted not in order to remotivate the person liable, but to relieve the harm sufferer. Thus, strict liability in damages is not necessarily objectionable. There may well be types of interaction—and selling technologically complex and potentially hazardous products seems to be one of these—in which the manufacturer ought to bear the cost of damages suffered by the bona fide user, even though the manufacturer has not failed to observe a reasonable standard of care. The main reason for such strict liability would seem to be that it is desirable for people to feel confident that they can buy and use such products without risking serious harm. The best way to achieve this is to ensure that customers can rely on receiving compensation if they do suffer harm, and perhaps the best way to assure that is to make the manufacturer strictly liable.

Strict liability still has two serious drawbacks. One is that there is still not complete assurance of recovery, since even manufacturers may not have adequate resources. The other is that people are told, at least by implication, not to do things which cannot be separated from activities they are permitted to engage in. The driver is told not to inflict harm on other drivers and is made to pay for such harm, although he cannot be sure that he will not inflict harm when driving. The drug manufacturer is told not to put drugs on the market whose use might harm the user, but he cannot ensure that without giving up the activity of manufacturing.

We can avoid these drawbacks by another liability arrangement for desirable but dangerous interactions—though "liability" is here perhaps a misleading term since we think of liability as coming out of answerability and since this arrangement drops the answerability requirement. We need to make two changes. One is that a person can become liable for something although he has not violated any moral requirement. The second is to require potential harmdoers to pool their resources (through insurance) and make all of them economically liable for the harm that any one of them inflicts. If it best assures recoverability for the harmed, the insurance should be compulsory; those who cannot afford to pay must be carried by taxation or by other insurers or be forbidden to engage in the activity. This shifts the burden from those who suffer uncompensated harm to those with a deep pocket or to the community as a whole. Imposing the burden on the pharmaceutical industry is probably not unfair, since the greater depth of their pocket is probably due to sales to those who stand to be harmed. In the case of driving cars, the problems can perhaps be avoided by forbidding driving without third-party insurance.

The principle to be used for these cases thus introduces two novelties. One is that it applies only to cases of certain sorts of harm, namely, harm suffered by some people as a result or as a causal consequence of others engaging in socially desirable but dangerous activities. It does not apply to cases in which people suffer harm through socially undesirable activities, such as deliberate harm. The other novelty is that it presupposes the existence of social arrangements which enable or require those engaging in such activities to buy insurance which would pay for the damage their activities may cause, and that the cost of this insurance can be passed on to the consumer. However, the causal condition would be retained. A person who suffered harm through the use of a product could recover only if he could show whose product caused the harm. The principle would therefore read as follows:

> P_4, to cover the cost of damage through socially desirable but dangerous activities, those engaging in them should or must take out liability insurance; the damage caused by their activity is to be borne, through their insurance company, by those of whose activity the harm was an effect or consequence.

It may be thought that under this arrangement liability in damages will not effectively deter those whose actions cause harm and so this will lead to an increase in the incidence of harm and the cost of compensating for it. But this need not be so. In the first place, this arrangement retains the causal requirement—that is only those can recover whose damage is *a consequence of* the relevant activities of the harmdoers. If I suffer harm in the course of driving, I cannot recover from another unless the harm is a consequence of that person's driving. If I suffer harm when taking a drug, I cannot recover unless it is a consequence of taking a drug manufactured by someone in the relevant class of harmdoers, that is, drug manufacturers. Hence the insurance premium could be made to vary at least roughly with potential harm, calculated on the basis of harm actually inflicted, and so will be a deterrent, though possibly a weak one. At the same time, a person whose behavior falls below a certain level of care—whose harm-causing behavior is culpable—should perhaps be held liable to punishment in addition to being liable in damages.

The above arrangement still has certain shortcomings. The most obvious is the frequently great administrative cost and difficulty of proving the causal link, and, where this cannot be proved, as in *Sindell*, the inability of the harmed to recover. This can be remedied by a further modification of the arrangement, namely, by dropping the causal link. The principle governing this arrangement should therefore read:

> P_5, to cover the costs of any harm through socially desirable but dangerous activities, all those engaging in them can or must take out liability insurance from one insurance company, and the damage caused by these activities is to be borne by that insurance company, irrespective of whose activity caused it.

Under this arrangement everyone can recover for harms caused in a certain way, irrespective of who is actually responsible. It is then a matter of social policy how much a person can recover and what classes of people must take out insurance and how large a premium they must pay to the fund that pays for such losses or harms. This treats the accidental harmful consequences of desirable interaction on a par with illnesses whose treatment and cure are covered by health insurance. The benefits may or may not be directly related to the premiums; they may, for instance, include all or a portion of the losses, while the premiums could be a percentage of income, as in social security payments, or proportional to market share, and so on. Carelessness and worse might then have to be deterred by culpability-based liability to punishment.[25]

One could go further still in that direction and adopt something like the Marxian principle, From each according to his ability; to each according to his need:

> P_6, to cover the costs of any harm, damage, or loss one may suffer, everyone must pay social liability insurance, and everyone receives compensation up to a certain level from this insurance for any harm, damage, or loss suffered, irrespective of causal origin.

Under this arrangement, recovery does not depend on who or what caused the harm. This obliterates any differentiation between harms that are blows of nature and harms that are caused by human action, and compensation is not necessarily limited to harms of a certain sort. This arrangement would have to rely, for deterrence of criminal, reckless, and careless conduct, on the criminal sanction alone.

These different liability arrangements yield different answers to the question of whether Sindell should be able to recover. Under the first arrangement, P_1, she plainly would not. Under P_5 and P_6, she would because the main obstacle, namely, the knowledge of whose product actually caused her illness, is irrelevant. However, at present we clearly do not have anything like these arrangements. It seems that the disadvantages of P_1 speak strongly against it. Perhaps P_5 would be a good arrangement for the production and sale of dangerous drugs. However, even if it is, we cannot very well judge *Sindell* under this arrangement, since it was not the accepted arrangement at the time. Morally speaking, it seems that we must go by the rules of the arrangement actually in operation unless that arrangement is so bad that it should be ignored or overridden, and that seems not to be so.

That leaves P_2, P_3, and P_4. Let us, then, consider which of these is currently in operation and acceptable. I think we would not find any of them morally objectionable, and all three have been in operation in various contexts at various times. In cases of product liability the law has for some time favored P_3, strict liability. However, in *Sindell*, it would seem to make little difference whether we apply strict or fault liability (P_2), since the manufacturers would seem unable to provide an exculpatory explanation of having marketed an ineffective and hazardous drug, having advertised it as effective and safe, and having been negligent about testing the drug before or even while putting it on the market. Whichever arrangement we apply, it seems the companies behaved in ways that call for remotivation under all three models. However, all three models retain the causal conditions and so *Sindell* raises two difficult questions: (1) Who has the burden of proof concerning the causal condition? and (2) Can the causal condition be met even when the burden of proof cannot be discharged?

All three relevant principles (P_2, P_3, and P_4) fall under two more general principles, namely that the damage should lie where it falls unless there is adequate reason to shift it, and as long as that reason conforms to the causal condition, that is, the requirement that the damage be the result, effect, or causal consequence of something done by specifiable others. Only P_5 and P_6 reject the causal condition, and only P_1 rejects the very possibility of shifting the damage from where it falls. As long as these two more general principles are socially accepted, it seems fair to put the burden of proof for the satisfaction of the causal condition on the person who has suffered the harm. For otherwise, anyone who suffered harm could shift it to anyone unable to prove that he did *not* cause it. For this reason it seems that in *Sindell*, the objection by the dissenting minority of judges to the majority's departure from traditional tort doctrine about the burden of proof would be sound from the moral as well as the legal point of view.

Can the causal condition be clinched one way or the other without either side's discharging its burden of proof? Here is a possible way. All 200 or so manufacturers failed equally to discharge the social requirement of not marketing an unsafe product. We may assume that most of the damage occurred as a consequence of this failure since, if the existing tests had been more carefully evaluated or more tests made, the product would either have been more effective and safe, or it would have been advertised as ineffective and hazardous, or it would not have been put on the market. If it were known, with regard to all the harm done, *whose* product caused *which* harm, and if each harm causer were held liable exactly for all the harm it had caused, then although all harm would be repaired, the magnitude of each harmdoer's liability would be a matter of luck, depending on which drug user happened to be caused harm and which drug user escaped harm. This allocation of liability would not meet the desideratum that those whose behavior called equally for remotivating sanctions should have the same remotivating sanctions applied to them. But it would appear that in this case the best and fairest way to allocate liability would be on the basis of culpability, hence on all manufacturers without exception (because all manufacturers had been equally willing to take the impermissible risk of selling a drug that should have been known to be ineffective and unsafe and to advertise it as effective and safe). This would be so even if the causal ancestry of all the harm were fully known, but plainly even more so where the causal ancestry is not known, especially since shifting the burden of disproof to the manufacturer is unfair, as already stated; allocating the burden of proof to the plaintiff has the undesirable result that some innocent victims cannot recover. If this is correct, then it would seem fairest to allocate liability to each manufacturer in proportion to market share, since that most fairly represents its share of the total burden. It would seem to follow that the majority decision in *Sindell* to allocate liability to manufacturers on the basis of their market share is in accordance with our considered moral judgments, though the moral reasoning differs from the legal.

NOTES

1. Compare Irving Kristol, "Pornography, Obscenity, and the Case for Censorship," *New York Times Magazine,* March 28, 1971, reprinted in *Philosophy of Law,* ed. Joel Feinberg and Hyman Gross. (Encino, CA: Dickenson, 1975), pp. 165-71, especially 165-66.
2. The world appears to us to consist of a number of more or less independent self-contained systems (such as the solar system, the earth, the human body, the economic system) and a variety of events, including above all deliberate human actions, which fall outside these systems and interfere with the expectable changes within these systems. In a recent article, Erhard Scheibe puts it this way, "The creation of the concept of such a *closed system,* as it is called technically, together with the fact that such systems are readily found in physical reality, was fundamental for the

establishment of modern physics. Physical laws are concerned with what occurs in them, and what these laws bind together are not events or things which relate as causes and effects, but quantities, properties and states of the particular systems. However, it often happens that the closed character of a system is significantly violated *from without*, that is, from beyond the boundary separating it from its surroundings, and that what occurs within it more or less suddenly starts to go awry in a manner that can no longer be made intelligible in terms of the conditions that have gone into the concept of the system itself. These are the cases in which the occurrence of an event can no longer be understood or even formulated if the closedness of the system is maintained and for which relative to the system—which had previously been considered closed—the notion of cause is introduced." ["Remarks on the Concept of Cause," trans. David J. Marshall, Jr., in *Contemporary German Philosophy*, Vol. 4, ed. Darrel E. Christensen (University Park: Pennsylvania State University Press, 1984), p. 239].

3. See H. L. A. Hart, *Punishment and Responsibility* (Oxford: Oxford University Press, 1968), p. 215.

4. Compare, for example, R. G. Collingwood, *An Essay on Metaphysics* (Oxford: Clarendon Press, 1940), especially pp. 285-87 and 296-311, and D. Gasking, "Causation and Recipes," *Mind* 6(1955):479-87. For the long and difficult process of disentangling causality from responsibility and other normative terms, see Hans Kelsen, *Society and Nature* (London: Kegan Paul, 1946).

5. For an excellent discussion of the notion of fault, see "Sua Culpa," a chapter in Joel Feinberg's *Doing and Deserving* (Princeton, NJ: Princeton University Press, 1970), pp. 187-211.

6. I can find no colloquial term for this basic sense of agent-responsibility. Hart called it capacity-responsibility (*Punishment*, pp. 227-30). Herbert Fingarette has called it response-ability (Herbert Fingarette and Ann Fingarette Hasse, *Mental Disability and Criminal Responsibility* [Berkeley: University of California Press, 1979], p. 208), but these are rather clumsy neologisms. German has a good word to mark the sense (*Zurechnungsfähigkeit*, that is, capacity to have something charged to one's account, to have it debited or credited to one), but the closest English equivalents, "imputability" (Hans Kelsen, "Causality and Imputation," in *What is Justice? Justice, Law, and Politics in the Mirror of Science*, ed. Hans Kelsen [Berkeley: University of California Press, 1971], pp. 324-49, especially p. 327) and "accountability" (which I used to favor), mean something rather different, so I shall stick to Hart's capacity-responsibility.

7. We may want to distinguish answerability from accountability, being socially required to give an account to some specified person of how one has discharged a given social requirement. One can be answerable for something without being answerable to some specific person, but one cannot be accountable without being accountable to someone. One becomes answerable if and only if one has failed in a social requirement, but one must give someone an exculpatory explanation only if there is a

specific person to whom one is answerable. By contrast, one becomes accountable if the task of accounting to someone for how one has discharged a social requirement has been imposed on one on top of discharging that social requirement, and if one must do so irrespective of whether or not one has so discharged it. Thus one may be answerable without being accountable (since one may not have the task of giving an account of one's performance to a particular person) and one may be accountable without being answerable (since one may have duly discharged all social requirements). Thus, it has been said, not implausibly, that corporations will not discharge their social responsibilities (that is, their task-responsibilities for certain social states of affairs, such as an unpolluted environment) until they are made *accountable to society.*

8. For the distinction between justification and excuse, see, for example, J. L. Austin, "A Plea for Excuses," in *Proceedings of the Aristotelian Society, 1956-7.* Reprinted in *J. L. Austin, Philosophical Papers*, ed. J. O. Urmson and A. J. Warnock (Oxford: Oxford University Press, 1961), pp. 123-52.

9. For a relevant discussion of the meaning of rationality in this sense, see Herbert Fingarette and Ann Fingarette Hasse, *Mental Disability,* chapter 14.

10. Negligence lies between these cases. The negligent person is not set on causing harm, but he is at fault. He is too much concerned about his own project to consider the risks to others. He needs to be remotivated, and having to pay damages may be sufficient to do it.

11. See Richard A. Wasserstrom, "Strict Liability in the Criminal Law," *Stanford Law Review* 12(1960):731. Reprinted in *Philosophical Issues in Law*, ed. Kenneth Kipnis (Englewood Cliffs, NJ: Prentice-Hall, 1977), pp. 28-41. There has been a great deal of disagreement among jurisprudentialists about the relationship between strict liability and fault liability. Some would agree with what I have just said and would regard the two types of liability as mutually exclusive. Those who follow this line tend to interpret the change in tort law in the 1850s as a move from strict to fault liability [for example, O. Holmes, *The Common Law* (1881); James Barr Ames, "Law and Morals," *Harvard Law Review* 22(1908):97-113]. Others see this change and the relation between strict liability and fault liability (or negligence) quite differently. They see the change in the 1850s as a change from a reciprocity model to a reasonable man model. In this view, strict liability is compatible with excuses.

The reciprocity model assumes that everyone has an equal right to security from risk. Where the risks people inflict on one another are reciprocal, as in driving a car, losses lie where they fall, except where people drive carelessly or recklessly, in which case the risks are not reciprocal. Thus, on this model, the underlying condition of liability is unexcused, nonreciprocal risk taking. By contrast, the model of reasonableness assumes that (1) no one is liable for anything that results from such reasonable behavior and (2) the reasonable person acts so as to maximize expectable utility, that is, he takes precautions whose cost is equal to the expectable losses his action will cause. (For an excellent discussion of these issues, see George P. Fletcher, "Fairness and Utility in Tort Theory," *Harvard Law Review* (1972), reprinted in *Law, Economics, and Philosophy*, ed. Mark Kuperberg and Charles Beitz (Totowa, NJ: Rowman and Allanheld, 1983), pp. 248-84.

12. See, for example, H. L. A. Hart, *Punishment*, p. 214: "That he caused the disaster may be expressed by saying that he was responsible for it."

13. For a good discussion of a closely related difference—that between "cause" and "his fault"—see Joel Feinberg, "Sua Culpa," especially pp. 200-7.

14. For hints about a plausible distinction between "causing" and "being the cause," see, for example, Joel Feinberg, "Causing Voluntary Actions," in *Doing and Deserving*, pp. 152-86, especially pp. 160-86.

15. But surely, it may be said, nonoccurrences can be causes: the sailor's not getting any vitamin C is the cause of his scurvy. True, but only because this nonoccurrence can be construed as analogous to an intervention to bring about the scurvy rather than as a nonprevention of it. What makes a killing an intervention is not that it was a doing rather than a not-doing, but rather that death would not have occurred at that time if the event (the shot) involved in the killing had not occurred and if the death did occur only because of that event. In other words, the nonoccurence of something can be the cause of something else only if it was an intervention, that is, a deflection from the normal course of events, hence only where there is a normal course of events. In the case of the sailor's scurvy, we can construe the situation as one in which there is a normal course of events, namely, the sailor's choosing a diet which contains a sufficient quantity of vitamin C to maintain health (including the absence of scurvy). The normal course of events thus is one in which the sailor has a health-maintaining (and thus scurvy-preventing) diet. His being forced to live on a diet of polished rice thus is an interference with that normal course of events, which by removing the scurvy-preventing vitamin C causes the scurvy. The difference between the two cases is therefore this: in the case of the sailor, what happens (his not getting sufficient vitamin C to prevent scurvy and to maintain health) is an interference with or deflection from the normal course of events, hence it is a cause of the scurvy. In the case of the patient who dies as a consequence of the doctor's failure to administer the appropriate vaccination, the nonoccurrence of the vaccination, far from being an intervention in the normal course of events, is a nonintervention in the normal course of events; hence it cannot be said to be the cause of that death, although the death can be its consequence.

16. See, for example, Antony M. Honoré, "Law, Morals, and Rescue," in *The Good Samaritan and the Law,* ed. James M. Ratcliffe (New York: Doubleday, 1966). Reprinted in *Philosophical Issues in Law*, pp. 105-17.

17. Antony M. Honoré, "Law, Morals, Rescue."

18. John Harris, "The Marxist Conception of Violence," *Philosophy and Public Affairs* 3(1974):192-220. Reprinted in *Philosophical Issues in Law*, pp. 136-58.

19. See H. L. A. Hart, *The Concept of Law* (Oxford: Clarendon Press, 1961), chapter V, section 2, especially pp. 86 on.

20. G. E. Moore, "A Reply to My Critics," in *The Library of Living Philosophy*, vol. IV, *The Philosophy of G. E. Moore*, ed. Paul Arthur Schilpp (Evanston, IL: Northwestern University, 1942), pp. 542 on.

21. John Austin, *The Province of Jurisprudence Determined,* ed. H. L. A. Hart (London: Weidenfeld and Nicholson, 1954).

22. This is easily overlooked if one thinks of moral approval, commendation, and so on on the hurrah-boo model and fails to realize that moral disapproval (or approval) of someone is expressed by moral judgments, such as that what he did was wrong (or right).

23. See, for instance, *Henningsen v. Bloomfield Motors Inc.*, and the discussion following it, in William L. Prosser, John W. Wade, and Victor E. Schwartz, *Cases and Materials on Torts*, 6th ed. (Mineola, NY: The Foundation Press, 1976), pp. 748-55.

24. In *The Cost of Accidents* (New Haven: Yale University Press, 1971), Guido Calabresi distinguishes several classes of persons who might be required to shoulder the costs of accidents (p. 22). I have left out some, for example, the broad categories of people who are likely to be victims, which would not be a plausible solution to *Sindell* and similar cases.

25. There is, of course, a glaring difference between the cases of driving and of selling dangerous drugs, which seems to make arrangement E acceptable for the former but not the latter case. The difference is that, in the former case, the same people (namely, all the drivers) are both potential harmdoers and sufferers, hence it seems only fair to ask all of them to take out insurance. In the case of selling drugs, this is not so. After all, the drugs are produced for the benefit of the consumers, but it is the producers who are asked to pay the insurance. Nevertheless, the difference alone does not seem to be decisive. The manufacturer seems to be better placed to buy insurance than the drug buyer: he can pass the cost on to the consumer, and he can get out of the business if it is not profitable. By contrast, the consumer cannot test the product before buying; he normally cannot, and should not have to, take out insurance to cover against health impairment; and he should be able to assume at least that the advertising is truthful, if not that the drugs are safe.

8

A Broader View of Medical Responsibility

James M. Gustafson

The purpose of this text is to examine the resolution of conflict between the mandate to pursue and apply new medical knowledge *and* what is due to persons who suffer bad outcomes as a result of innovative medicine. As the introductory essay stated, the purpose is to examine issues concerning causation, responsibility, liability, and compensation for "bad outcomes."

The chapters by Schaffner, Gray, and Baier properly pertain to the purpose. They examine what Baier calls the backward dimension of the general area of responsibility. Thus they address ways in which answers can be given to the questions Who did it? or What did it? and focus on bad, rather than good, outcomes.

I am not by profession a historian or philosopher of science, a historian of law, or a moral philosopher, and thus have limited competence to engage in technical critiques of these chapters. Indeed, I have nothing to add to the analyses presented with reference to the backward dimension of responsibility.

Thus I have chosen to write an oblique response to these works, for two reasons. First, it might cast in broader relief the ways in which focus of attention on the backward dimension limits, and perhaps even stipulates, how one thinks morally about medical innovation. The focus on who did it requires a certain vocabulary, a certain set of concepts, and a certain use of those concepts. If, by contrast, one attempts to focus on what Baier calls the forward dimensions of responsibility, or task-responsibility, the frame of reference for thinking about responsibility is enlarged and altered significantly.

The second reason I have chosen to write an oblique response stems from my own intellectual history and interests. To acknowledge this is not to admit that those interests are arbitrary. In some theological literature, the idea of responsibility is not used only in the backward dimension. Another possibility is the capacity to be responsive; responsiveness is context-dependent and involves both the resources required relative to the context and a discernment of what is fitting in relation to it. I think all physicians can understand this; clinical judgments are responsive in this sense. A second way, related to responsiveness, the idea is used in some theological literature is this: responsibility requires that agents and institutions develop the necessary conditions to achieve certain ends; they must have the *ability* to respond. Their accountability, then, is judged not merely in terms of backward causal analysis for outcomes, but also in terms of their fulfillment or non-fulfillment of the ends or purposes proper to them.

These usages of the idea of responsibility have equivalents or similarities in philosophical literature; they are not the exclusive property of theologians. For example, Hans Jonas' *The Imperative of Responsibility: In Search of an Ethics for the Technological Age* has affinities with what I shall briefly develop. One of his theses can be put oversimply in the following way: in the light of certain ends, for example, keeping the planet habitable for human beings, restraints upon certain kinds of action are required. One moves from a future dimension to the present and counsels actions or restraints upon action. Thus, responsibility is set in a context somewhat different from that of the previous chapters.

I take my cue for this oblique response from an essay that my mentor and former colleague H. Richard Niebuhr wrote in 1946. A simple descriptive statement is important. He wrote that "The idea of responsibility . . . has its place in the context of social relations. . . . To be responsible is to be able and required to give account to someone for something." The second sentence obviously includes the backward dimension, and requires the kinds of specifications and analyses that have been presented.

The scope of responsibility, however, depends upon the answers to the questions, To whom? and For what? How the medical profession answers the questions of to whom it is responsible and for what it is responsible sets the context in which thinking about the general issue will occur. If the answers include forward dimensions, as the mandate to medicine in this project clearly affirms, then there is a relocation of the issue. It becomes more inclusive than the limited purpose of the essays to which I am responding, though it includes accountability for the outcomes of actions of agents, in our case the medical profession. Its moral responsibility (to use the term "moral" in a sense not all persons would accept) is bound to its *role* or task-responsibility, that is, its effectiveness in fulfilling chosen and justified purposes. Its moral responsibility is not limited to its causal accountability for bad outcomes.

I shall play freely for a few moments with To whom? and For what? in order to illustrate the difference this can make in construing the issue.

The basic line of this book answers the question For what? in terms of bad outcomes; To whom? is primarily the victim of the bad outcome; *and* the previous writers have also involved the issues of what other persons, institutions, and things can be held accountable. The most nearly similar process in the religious traditions takes place in the analysis of sin and sins; the refined discussion of Roman Catholic moral theologians and Jewish Halahkists are equivalent in degree of precision to those of moral philosophers and lawyers.

As a forward-looking procedure let me suggest a contrast. In the division of labor in society the medical profession is responsible *for* the health of persons and the public. The medical profession has an end, a *telos*; or it has ends, *teloi*. The choice of ends is critical to the morality of medicine. Let us prescind from the issues of the definition of health since my purpose is more general. The prima facie justification for every medical innovation is that it will provide better means to fulfill the purposes, the ends, of the profession. *If* the medical profession is responsible for prolonging the lives of persons with diseased hearts, one way in which it exercises its social role responsibility is to develop implantable artificial hearts. It would be remiss in its responsibilities as a profession if it did not develop the technology to extend the life span in these cases. *If* women patients have symptoms that can, on the basis of contemporary knowledge, be treated by a substance called DES, then physicians have a responsibility to use the substance to achieve what is deemed to be in the best interest of the patient. The prevention of lung disease is a legitimate end of medicine, and thus the profession has a responsibility to the public to support regulations which will reduce its incidence insofar as it is reasonably the outcome of certain environmental factors.

The expansion of the answer to the question For what? can get out of hand unless some other qualifications are considered. If malnutrition and starvation in Africa are the outcomes of civil wars, imprudent uses of land resources, unwise economic policies on the part of national governments, excessively high birth rates, and alteration in meteorological conditions, it is clear that the medical profession is not responsible to do something about all these factors. If the ends of medicine are defined in such general terms as the prevention of disease and death, and the "causes" of death are malnutrition which makes persons susceptible to diseases and starvation, the medical profession is only one of many professions, its institutions only one of many institutions, that have the power—that is, the causal capacity—to make a difference in outcome.

This illustrates my general point. If one begins the discussion of responsibility in medical research and care not with the causal responsibility for bad outcomes of innovation, but rather with the ends or purposes of medicine, one has a different construal of the moral issues because innovation is described and interpreted in a different and larger context. The pursuit of the issue of responsibility leads to a different set of questions than those which have shaped the agenda of the Schaffner, Gray, and Baier chapters. The main questions become: what ends ought medicine to choose that are more precise than "health" in general? What conditions are necessary for the medical profession to fulfill its responsibilities for the preservation of health? The chapters to which this is an oblique response are set in a different context; they remain, but *might* be qualified by this different context. To reiterate in terms of Baier's distinction, what conditions are necessary for the medical profession to exercise its forward dimension of responsibility? And, since medicine is necessarily interrelated with other institutions to fulfill those responsibilities, it is important to delineate more precisely what special capacities (and thus roles) medicine has relative to other institutions.

The To whom? question of responsibility becomes different as well; it is not limited to the individuals who have experienced bad outcomes of innovation. I do not like the generality and abstraction of the term "society" as it gets bandied about, since what it refers to is never clear, but for the sake of brevity I must use it here. In the division of functions medicine is responsible to society for certain ends, just as educational institutions, the legal profession, and others are. By reconstruing the To whom? (as with the reconstrual of For what?), the matter of medical innovation is set in a different context, and this *might* qualify the way in which at least the moral issues involved are interpreted and understood. It will enlarge the morally relevant features of medical innovation.

From this I suggest a descriptive statement, too simply to be sure, as a premise that leads to another way of talking about the moral responsibility of medicine relative to innovations. Medicine is responsible *to* society *for* preservation of health (or, for provision of health care). This descriptive statement, then, necessarily requires an enlargement of the context in which responsibility is considered in comparison with the limited purpose of this work, as quoted above, and a different set of factors becomes morally relevant.

In order to fulfill its responsibility in this forward dimension, medicine must meet certain conditions. Some conditions are distinctively and primarily the responsibility of the medical profession; others have to be met by other institutions and resources because of the interdependence of medicine with other aspects of society.

I would suggest that a basic area of responsibility of medical institutions and professions be to develop the *knowledge conditions* necessary to meet its ends. Because specialization of research and knowledge is required, no other institutions in society have the capacity to provide those conditions. By knowledge conditions I refer to various areas of research, basic and applied, and to the skills and capacities for judgment that come through clinical training and practice. Since the knowledge conditions are always developing, there is no avoiding the risks that are involved in experimentation and innovation. Continual innovation is simply a matter of fact in contemporary medicine. In terms of this project, one issue seems to be the degree or extent of moral and legal responsibility to which medicine can be held for knowledge conditions which can never provide absolute certitude of outcomes. One could argue, I think, that the forward dimension of responsibility of medicine requires conditions other than just the resources for the development of knowledge. Many of these conditions are within the capacity of medical institutions to provide.

Economic and social conditions have to be met. Resources are needed for research and for clinical application of innovations. This is not the place to outline the obvious, but only to indicate the importance of the provision of these resources. These conditions might include the provisions for compensation of the risk takers, that is, those who submit to experimental therapies with the knowledge of the probabilities of benefit and harm.

Legal conditions have to be met. In light of the different construal of the medical profession's responsibility that I have drawn, it is arguable, at least, that the fear of liability for bad outcomes *might* impede the development of certain necessary knowledge conditions. I have no specific proposal to make, but my remarks about the responsibility of medicine to sustain health for both present and future patients and for the sake of individuals and society might induce some thinking about how, legally, research and innovation could take place so that the risk factors can better be taken into account.

Moral conditions have to be met. If the perspective I have suggested is to be entertained seriously, the ways in which medical ethics are now conventionally developed might require some alteration. The dominant feature of current medical ethics fits the dominant model of this book: moral responsibility is related primarily (if not solely) to causal accountability for actions of particular agents on particular subjects. The proscription, do no harm, is dominant. The descriptive context tends to be limited to the contractual relation between the physician engaged in innovative medicine and the particular subject patients. If, however, medicine is responsible to society for health and health care, different criteria of judgment about morality might follow. Medicine might be held morally irresponsible if it did not fulfill its social role to provide the best possible health care. It would be blameworthy if it did not pursue the conditions necessary to fulfill its purposes. Concepts from ethical traditions which judged the morality of actions in light of the securing of beneficial outcomes, or in the light of the provision for the elusive common good of a community might well gain prominence.

Responsibility is a relational term, and as Baier indicates it has forward as well as backward dimensions. How any person or group answers the questions of responsibility to whom and for what will set the scope of the context in which moral and even legal issues are discussed. My oversimple proposal is that, if we describe medicine as being responsible to society for health and health care, we would likely enlarge the agenda of the Schaffner, Gray, and Baier chapters.

9

The Morals and Technique
of Medical Innovation

Richard A. Epstein

Medical innovation is here with us to stay. So too are its ethical and technical issues. No one would take the line that all innovation should cease because some innovation has unfortunate side effects. No one would take the line that all medical resources should be devoted to innovative research. The routine treatment of routine cases often reflects the successful innovation of prior generations. Low-cost care that provides quick and certain relief provides the welcome payoff of the sound investments of a previous generation.

It is therefore possible to rule out these two extremes quickly. Having said that the hard work has only begun, what should the sound middle position be? To use an analogy, we are quite confident that the optimal level of taxation is neither 0 nor 100 percent. The range of possible rates and tax structures that satisfy these dual constraints defines the problem, not the solution. A similar problem exists with medical innovation. The decision to go forward with medical research in a bounded way also defines a problem, not a solution.

Working with medical innovation brings us back to the point of departure for all serious social inquiry: scarcity. It is a commonplace observation that there are more good things in the world than there are resources to obtain them. Paul Meier has stressed rightly that inconsistent legitimate desires are the ordinary stuff of human relationships. What is unrealistic is the thought that they can all be satisfied simultaneously—a conclusion which the constraint of scarcity necessarily precludes.[1] The effects of scarcity reveal themselves with a vengeance in the area of medical innovation. We should all like a world in which every patient is treated only with drugs and therapies that have already been subject to complete and thorough experimental tests. We also desire a world in which no one has to participate as guinea pig in any experimental program that exposes him or her to enormous risk. It is not possible to have a world in which every person has the benefits of previous testing done on others. Someone must take some risk at some time.

In one sense we must learn to aim low, but hit the target. The best we can hope for is a set of institutions, practices, and rules that minimizes the sum of the relevant risks: some drugs and therapies may not be tested enough, which creates the major danger that they will cause widespread harm when placed into general use. Others may be tested too long, which creates the risk that beneficial therapies are kept off the market because of lingering, principled— and erroneous—doubts about their effectiveness. To use the metaphor of the veil of ignorance, one relevant inquiry can be stated as follows: if a person did not know whether he was to be the guinea pig or the ordinary patient, what set of procedures would he desire, assuming he knows the probabilities and payoffs of being in each position?

The question of designing the right regime to minimize the competing risks is not made any easier by the fact that, to control relevant risks, scarce resources must be drawn off from other activities. Nor does it help that there are enormous deficits of information that have to be confronted at every stage of the process—deficits individual consumers have about the drugs in question, and deficits producers have about the preferences of their consumers. It sorely oversimplifies the problem to assume that the only ignorance worth talking about is that of consumers. Ignorance runs in both directions. To give but one example, producers often need to know the trade-offs consumers desire between efficacy of treatment and risk of side effects. Any system of information control must be directed to making sure that the persons who should rightly make the decision—be they technical or moral—have the relevant information on which to act. All this must take place in a world in which the creation or transfer of information comes at a very high cost.[2]

In view of the relevant constraints, it seems that the dominant unresolved questions are not moral, but technical. What set of legal and social institutions should be used to optimize the flow of useful innovations and to distribute the gains of these innovations to various members of the public at large, both as taxpayers and as users of the system? In formulating this question, I am comforted by Kurt Baier, who in chapter 7 identifies first the appropriate moral constraints and then the possible systems of legal control consistent with them. The moral constraints are both powerful and important. I know of no one who would advocate that it is a good thing for people to be coerced or deceived into participating in innovative research. The experiments of the Nazis are so clearly out of bounds that they do not require discussion; the Tuskegee study of syphilis is less so, but is nonetheless clearly indefensible.[3]

No one should forget the importance of these powerful constraints, but the territory of permissible options that they leave is very substantial indeed. Baier notes five separate approaches to the question of medical innovation that range from a simple rule of no compensation to participants, to a rule of negligence liability (with or without personal excusing conditions), to a rule of strict liability for maloccurrences caused by the procedures, to a rule for comprehensive insurance protection for any maloccurrences arising in the course of treatment. Each scheme is subject to many variations: what are the burdens of proof; what persons or institutions should be held responsible; what portion of payments should come from general revenues; what should be the interaction between private rights of action (if any) and direct public controls?

If all these are consistent with our moral intuitions, then the only hard questions are technical. What set of arrangements gets the right choices made by the right persons at the right price?[4] The task is still how to minimize the relevant risks. Given the complexity of the problem, the risks may be minimized while remaining extremely substantial. Any system worth proposing will have its horror stories. But it is a great mistake to look at the system strictly from the point of view of its chief losers after the fact, as is the temptation in many circles today with respect to the pertussis vaccine. It may well be that any alternative system would have different (or simply more) persons who would have lost to the same or greater degree, such as those struck down by the disease. The question therefore is one which must address a far harder task—the *magnitude*, not the *existence*, of unfortunate outcomes.

Just how does one conduct the appropriate cost-benefit analysis within the broad constraints identified? One could argue that any such analysis is wholly inappropriate in organizing social institutions. Costs and benefits have an inescapably subjective dimension about them, which makes them extremely hard to measure in the absence of organized markets. In addition, it is necessary to aggregate preferences across separate individuals, which raises vexing problems of the interpersonal comparisons of utility and of collective action. All these objections have their intellectual force, but the haunting practical problem remains. Someone has to use some technique to decide which programs should be put in place and which should not. If the noninstrumental moral arguments carry us only a short part of the journey, then instrumental arguments necessarily take on greater weight once the force of moral argument is exhausted. As that is the case, then the familiar objections take on reduced power. They become difficulties to be minimized; they are no longer impassible roadblocks that prevent further inquiry from taking place.

The proper effort therefore seeks to do the cost-benefit analysis in a way that tends to minimize the problems at hand. It may be, for example, that key decisions on whether to proceed are left to persons whose subjective preferences are likely to be substantial. In one sense this points to the increased role of individual patients in the process, but it speaks as much to their obligations as to their rights. Thus, they may have the right to decide whether to participate in various programs, but they may also be under a duty to inquire about the particular risks that they regard as most troublesome about the entire operation. It is doubtful that the entire burden of initiation would fall on one side or another. But after the general risks and benefits of treatment are identified, it is not inappropriate to ask any individual participant to voice whatever unanswered concerns remain.

In addition, the use of cost-benefit analysis does not entail the adoption of any practice which requires the legal system to make a formal cost-benefit determination of its own, should a certain practice be called into question or an outcome go awry. Thus a principled utilitarian should be opposed to a legal rule that simply states, "Decide each case in ways that maximize social utility." The indeterminacy of such a rule and the possibility of abuse in its application make this form of utilitarianism profoundly anti-utilitarian. Instead the proper procedure in many cases is to make institutional cost-benefit analysis at the *wholesale* level. The object of forming a rule is to have a general guide for concrete action, and that enterprise remains worthwhile even if it is known that the rule must necessarily have a positive error rate. Case-by-case determinations have error rates as well, and such determinations are more expensive to undertake. Unless there is good reason to believe that individual determination of matters of principle are both cheap and reliable, then the inquiry is best not made. Individual trials or administrative hearings should be left to the task of finding out the relevant facts that determine the application of general rules, itself an inquiry of no mean difficulty.

With medical innovation these insights translate into a position that tends to give greater weight to medical custom and less weight to arguments (after the fact) that the custom itself misstates the relevant risks.[5] In drug cases (such as the swine flu episode referred to by Stephen Toulmin),[6] it points to the use of administrative procedures to establish authoritative warnings before the start of a liability program: warnings that no court or jury can thereafter declare inadequate in a tort action for actual or punitive damages. Both situations involve numerous similar instances that have to be resolved by a common rule. Consequently there are enormous economies of scale in having a single determination that lets people know where they stand before they commit themselves to action. To be sure, there are always risks in concentrating decision-making power in the hands of a single person. With customary care those risks are countered by the simple fact that the practice of a single person never establishes a general custom. Within the institutional setting appropriate to a product's mass use, those risks can be reduced by taking testimony from independent experts before making a determination, and by establishing procedures to change the wording or format of the warning or license on the basis of new information, as it is acquired by field experience and systematic scientific research.

There is a more general point lurking here. The last thing a sound utilitarian wants is a formula that flaunts its utilitarianism. The animating concerns of individual and social utility should be used to devise rules of general application that have beneficial consequences. I believe that the recent advances in many quarters have provided useful tools for this inquiry. I include on the list a greater understanding of imperfect information, of the conflicts of interest between contracting parties, of game and bargaining theory, and of complex organizations. The difficulty of the inquiry that remains should not lead to a conclusion of general skepticism or despair. It is not the case that any tax system is as good as any other (flat tax is best). It is not the case that any system of legal, administrative, and social sanction works as well as any other. Generally speaking I think that in recent times we have moved in the wrong direction because we have been misled into overestimating our ability to fine tune the legal and social control of medical innovation. Fine tuning does not work. Clear and simple general rules offer a great chance of solving the host of technical problems that remain once the moral questions have been settled.

NOTES

1. Paul Meier, chapter 4.
2. The study of imperfect information is a booming business in modern economics. The seminal paper is George J. Stigler, "The Economics of Information," in *The Organization of Industry*, ed. George J. Stigler (Homewood, IL: Irwin, 1968), p. 171.
3. See Meier, chapter 4, and James H. Jones, *Bad Blood: The Tuskegee Syphilis Experiment* (New York: Free Press, 1981).
4. I speak about these issues in my principal contribution to this volume, chapter 11.
5. I address the question at greater length in "Medical Malpractice, Imperfect Information and the Structure of the Firm," *Law and Contemporary Problems*, forthcoming.
6. Stephen Toulmin, chapter 2. See also E. W. Kitch, "Vaccines and Product Liability," *Regulation* (May-June 1985):11-18 for a damning critique of the current legal position.

Section 3

Legal Frameworks for Providing Compensation to the Injured

10

Different Compensation Approaches to Bad Outcomes from Standard Treatment, Innovative Treatment, and Research

Alexander Morgan Capron

The subject of this book invites consideration of a wide range of fundamental questions about the relationship of modern medicine to society and particularly to the legal system. Although directing special attention to the harms that sometimes result from medical innovation in its various guises, the questions provoked herein raise in turn questions about noninnovative (standard) medical practices. Nor does inquiry come to a natural stop there; it spreads outward to questions about the consequences of nonmedical activities and generally about the means that should be used to balance the harms caused to certain people by an activity against the benefits it brings to them and to others. Indeed, is the fact of activity important in evaluating the legally (or ethically) appropriate outcome? When—and how—ought society to intervene to alter what would otherwise be the distribution of harms and benefits? Should it matter whether the harms are labelled an "injury" (typically resulting from some human activity) rather than an "illness" (the causes of which may be more obscure)? Should an attempt be made to treat all cases similarly, and if so, by what measure of "likeness"—the type or degree of injury? The cause of injury? The need (or other characteristics) of the "victim"?

Needless to say, no attempt is made to answer all these questions in this essay. Instead, the objectives are to examine the manner in which compensation is provided to persons injured by several types of activities carried on by physicians and to explore distinctions among these activities that might explain the different means of compensation employed. The conclusion is that the distinctions sometimes suggested are not persuasive, except for a distinction between interventions intended to benefit only the patients-subjects involved and those that have broader purposes. The essay closes with suggestions about improving methods of compensation.

PRELIMINARY DIVISIONS

The current use of the negligence system as the major means for deciding which "bad outcomes" from medical intervention will be redressed beyond the payment of medical bills (and to what degree) is scrutinized elsewhere in this volume; here that system will be assumed, despite the critical attacks it has sustained of late.[1] Based on that assumption, the issue is whether innovative medical interventions, including formal research projects, have certain distinctive features that would argue in favor of treating their bad outcomes outside the negligence framework.

ILLUSTRATIVE CASES

In order to begin to explore these distinctions, it may be useful to consider the following cases.

Case 1

Last month, Imogene Infant, a healthy two-month-old, received her first DPT (diphtheria-pertussis-tetanus) vaccination; she rapidly developed a fever from acute disseminated encephalitis, which caused permanent brain damage. The vaccine used was manufactured according to standards approved by the Food and Drug Administration and was accompanied by appropriate warnings. Because it was made from inactivated whole cells of the *pertussis* bacterium, it contains both toxins and antigens, which induce an immune response. Her pediatrician routinely recommends a course of five vaccinations for all her patients, despite the risks (3.2 cases of brain damage, 575 cases of "collapse," and 1,600 very high fevers per million patients). The shots are compulsory for admittance to school under state law.

Case 2

Adam Adenoid, a married father of three children (ages 25, 21, and 16), was employed as a stockbroker. Last December he was found to have thyroid cancer, which was discovered through a thyroid scan performed by his regular physician after Mr. A complained of feeling lethargic and unusually sensitive to cold. As a child, Mr. A had suffered from tonsillar enlargement and repeated colds, some quite severe and disabling. In 1944, at the age of eight, he underwent tonsillar irradiation, a widely used procedure that was selected by his pediatrician both because of its popularity at the local hospital and because the physician believed that Mr.

A's frequent infections made him a poor candidate for a tonsillectomy. The physician (who was fresh out of his residency in 1944 and is still in active practice) stopped using radiation on enlarged tonsils in 1954, when studies were published demonstrating the association between irradiation and subsequent development of thyroid cancer. Mr. A died last week during surgery to remove the carcinoma.

Case 3

Gary Gladstone, a 56-year-old patient of Dr. Skeptic, was found to have asymptomatic gallstones during a routine physical four years ago. Although aware that most physicians favor removal of the gallbladder in these circumstances, Dr. S did not recommend this procedure to Mr. G because he does not believe that elective surgery has been shown to lengthen life expectancy significantly. Last week, after increasing pain and severe indigestion, Mr. G died during emergency surgery to remove his gallbladder.

Case 4

Twin sisters, Mrs. Mary Miscarriage and Mrs. Florence Fecund, were attended during their first pregnancies in the fall of 1949 by Dr. Curious, a member of the obstetrics department at University Hospital. Both women miscarried during the second month. One year later, when each again became pregnant, they returned to the same physician. Aware that a synthetic estrogen, diethylstilbestrol (DES), was being widely used as an antimiscarriage drug, but sharing the skepticism of some of his academic colleagues about its efficacy, Dr. C decided to enter the sisters into a randomized, double-blind clinical trial of DES. As it turned out, Mrs. M received the placebo and miscarried again in the second month; the resulting strain on her marriage led to divorce, and she has remained unmarried and childless. She is, however, a doting aunt to her sister's four daughters, who include First Fecund (born in June 1951) and Fourth Fecund (born in 1959); thus, she was very distressed to learn last month that both First and Fourth (who themselves are now married and attempting to begin families) have serious problems with their reproductive systems, including clear cell adenocarcinoma. Although Dr. C attended Mrs. F during all her pregnancies, he ceased administering DES after the first one, based upon the demonstration of its ineffectiveness as a means of preventing miscarriages. (Neither of Mrs. F's other two daughters has clear cell carcimona or other reproductive problems.)

Case 5

Sam Studious, a 25-year-old engineering graduate student, responded last week to a poster seeking "Healthy Volunteers, 21-30 Years of Age" who were willing to participate in a "Two-Day Study of Exercise Stress" at the University's physiology laboratory for $250. The procedures and risks were explained to Mr. S, and he agreed to participate. Yesterday, during the positioning of a catheter to monitor his cardiac output during part of the test, Mr. S experienced cardiac arrest (a very rare complication in healthy subjects); by the time he was revived, he had suffered irreversible brain damage and will probably never regain cognitive functioning.

ECONOMIC EFFICIENCY?

These five cases are presented for illustrative purposes, though it is apparent that many further details would be needed for a full exploration of the complexities they raise. The one thing that seems certain is that the cases will be regarded as complex by the present legal system(s) and will not be disposed of by any simple legal rule. For example, it seems doubtful that the outcomes here could (or should) be predicated on having the legal system attempt to discern which allocation of the costs of bad outcomes would be most economically efficient. To cite only one difficulty, the barriers to information exchange are so tremendous, particularly along the frontiers of biomedical innovation, as to make any notion of a medical marketplace, much less a transaction cost-free Coasean world, totally unrealistic.

Prior examinations of this subject have reached similar conclusions. Although some have suggested, for example, that requiring persons engaged in a medical activity such as clinical research to carry non-fault insurance would provide an ideal means for internalizing its costs and checking "overly dangerous" conduct,[2] others have concluded that a compensation mechanism would not be the best way to control the research enterprise and allocate injuries appropriately between the present and the future.[3]

Furthermore, the relative imbalance of knowledge and power between the professional and institutional participants in health care, on the one hand, and patients and their families, on the other, and the symbolic and existential qualities implicated in many health care interventions (for example, suffering, illness, and death—and indeed, evil, sin, and injustice) are frequently the unspoken subtext of evaluations of moral responsibility (and legal liability) for bad outcomes. An inquiry that ignored these factors and looked only to "rational calculations" would prove unable to explain the rules that have governed past cases and would provide an unworkable basis for the resolution of future cases, because it would offer no avenue for the expression of these moral intuitions.

CATEGORIZING THE CASES

Since economic arguments seem unlikely to provide an adequate basis for constructing legal rules in this field, other means will be needed to sort out the complexities illustrated by the foregoing hypothetical cases. Several categories of medical intervention that are frequently employed provide a helpful beginning point.

Standard treatment—practices "designed solely to enhance the well-being of an individual patient"[4] through diagnosis, preventive treatment, or therapy;

Innovative treatment—a deviation from standard practice, the efficacy or safety of which has not yet been validated;[5]

Clinical research—an activity designed to produce generalizable knowledge through the application of procedures of potential diagnostic or therapeutic value to those involved as patients-subjects;[6]

Nontherapeutic research—an activity designed to produce generalizable knowledge through the application of procedures without the intention of directly benefiting those involved as subjects.

While each reader will have his or her own views about the correct way to apply these terms to our hypothetical cases, they might be categorized as follows:

Case 1: Standard treatment, because DPT vaccination has been shown to be very effective in providing immunity, with many fewer adverse consequences than when children are not vaccinated;

Case 2: Standard (or innovative?) treatment, because irradiation was widely used but not adequately tested;

Case 3: Innovative treatment (or nontreatment), because even the omission of an accepted (though perhaps nonvalidated) treatment amounts to an innovation;

Case 4: Clinical research, because randomized, double-blind trials are the paradigm of clinical research;[7]

Case 5: Nontherapeutic research, because there was no intention to benefit Mr. S.

POSSIBLE GROUNDS FOR DISTINCTION

With these initial descriptions in mind, what factors might determine the liability or compensation status among such an array of bad medical outcomes?

INNOVATIVENESS?

Concerns are sometimes expressed that the existence of the tort system is having a depressing effect on medical innovation;[8] if that were true, one would expect that the likelihood of the injured person (or his or her survivors, in the case of death) collecting damages would increase as one moved down our list of cases, from standard treatment to research. Yet, if one assumes no problems of "informed consent" in any of these cases, none of the potential plaintiffs stands a good chance of collecting: case 1 might succeed if strict products liability is found applicable to the facts; cases 2 and 3 might be awarded damages by sympathetic juries, unconvinced of the statistical wisdom of the choices made; in case 4, some of the potential plantiffs' claims contradict others'; and case 5 seems dubious.

Thus, while it may once have been the courts' view that a physician "experiments (that is, innovates) at his peril,"[9] the innovative nature *vel non* of a medical intervention is no longer an adequate basis for predicting whether damages would be awarded to an injured party. Instead, recognizing the need to achieve an appropriate balance between the acquisition of new knowledge and the protection of personal safety and well-being, various means (from requiring a process of obtaining subjects' informed consent to providing prior review of the design of research protocols by scientific peers and others outside the research process) have been put into place since the Nuremberg trials and the renewed interest of the federal government in this subject two decades later, spurred by revelations of unethical experimentation.[10]

Are there, then, other factors that might serve to sort out the cases—such as the balance between risks and benefits, or the identity of the intended beneficiaries?

RISKS AND BENEFITS?

It is commonplace to view research as risky, and risk *is* "inherent in medical research, no matter how conscientious the investigator and careful the research."[11] Nevertheless, the degree of risk alone can neither explain present liability rules for bad medical outcomes nor provide the criterion on which such rules should be constructed.

Probability and Severity

First, "risk" is a complex concept that encompasses both the likelihood of harm and its severity. Because of the extensiveness and complexity of many medical interventions and the variation in individual physical response, the types of harm that result from such interventions will often vary widely from mild and temporary pain to death or permanent and total incapacitation. Thus, when a procedure is described as "not very risky," it will typically be associated only with minor harms or a very low probability of severe injuries, or both; the same harms, however, might be regarded by many people as constituting a "high risk." (The difficulty that people have with statistical risks is well known, as is the confounding effect of very low probabilities in people's attempts to evaluate severe harms such as death.) The 3.2 per million chance of permanent brain damage from DPT vaccine illustrates this phenomenon.

Balancing the Chances
of Good and Bad Outcomes

Perhaps of even greater importance, the concept of risk by itself is relevant only to a subjective (and after-the-fact) evaluation, not to the setting of liability rules. Rather than risk alone, the reference point for decision making will be the relative balance of likely good versus likely bad outcomes from an intervention. Seen in this way, it is apparent that some forms of standard treatment carry risks of far greater probability and severity than the risk of almost all research, because the needs of some grievously ill patients justify "desperate appliances."[12]

Barriers to Quantification

Even in cases not at the outer extremes of risk and benefit, the notion of balancing these two categories ought not to suggest that any very precise measurement is possible. The problems that frustrate all such attempts at quantitative decision making are only too apparent in the health care arena. First, data on outcome are very weak, with respected sources giving a wide variation in the expected results of even very common procedures.[13]

Second, the benefits and harms may be of such different sorts as to make comparison difficult or meaningless. In case 3, the choice of whether to do elective gallbladder removal earlier or emergency removal later balances similar factors (time without pain or limitation versus surgical injuries) on both sides of the equation; yet this is frequently not the case. Were it an inflamed prostate that was the possible candidate for surgery, the choice would be between relieving discomfort and the risk of further complications, on the one hand, or the likelihood of loss of potency and the risk of surgical complications, on the other. Similarly, in case 4, had DES been effective in preventing miscarriage and had the risk of cancer been known, the choice would have been between avoidance of fetal loss versus later problems in the reproductive systems (involving infertility, pain, suffering, and even death) of the daughters.

Latent Harms

The DES example also serves as a reminder that in the biomedical sphere, the notion of risk is further complicated by delays in the manifestation of some harms. This problem may be one of the reasons why illness is treated differently (and usually less generously) by compensation programs than is injury, which can typically be identified with a direct cause.[14]

The latency complication can, of course, occur in any health care intervention: standard treatment, innovative treatment, or research (as well as from environmental or occupational exposures). It is, however, the *one* type of risk that might with good reason be thought to occur more frequently in innovation or research than in standard treatment since, by definition, standard treatment has been validated (that is, its outcomes—for good and ill—have been documented in a sufficient number of cases to predict the results it will produce when used). Yet too much ought not to be made of this possible distinction because, even among those standard practices that have achieved this hallowed status through research verification rather than through unquestioned custom, very few have been used long enough to rule out latent defects. Moreover, even in the field of drugs (which undergo the most systematic form of evaluation of any biomedical procedure), the lack of a comprehensive system of postmarketing surveillance in this country means that complications which manifest themselves slowly (as well as those occurring very infrequently) usually go undetected unless they are bizarre, since they are unlikely to be turned up by the standard experimental protocols.

Subjectivity in the "Standard"

A final problem in any attempt to base compensation decisions on quantification of risk is the inherent subjectivity of such measurements. (This difficulty comes as no surprise to utilitarians, of course; indeed, it lies behind the younger Mill's effort to construct a justification for individual liberty.) Again, standard treatment might seem to suffer less from this problem than its more experimental cousins, since one sense of the word "standard" would designate those treatments that have been shown, by objective measures of reasonableness, to provide a favorable balance of benefits over harms. Yet the conventional use of the term "standard" in the medical (litigation) context is merely that of a practice that is accepted by at least some recognized school of professional opinion—a source of judgment which, while perhaps informed, is obviously subjective.

In sum, while it is possible to draw distinctions among the categories of medical interventions (as illustrated by the hypothetical cases) based on the varied ways they are characterized by risk (or a balance of risk versus benefit), none is very precise and collectively they cut in several directions. In particular, "risk" provides no clear ground for placing standard practices into a class distinct from various innovative methods.

INFORMATION AND CONSENT?

Though riskiness does not provide a bright line for dividing cases of injury appropriate for compensation outside the tort system from those in which compensating patients or subjects would seem unnecessary, information about risk might still have an important role to play in dealing with the bad outcomes of biomedical activities. In the initial description and evaluation of the five hypothetical cases, it was assumed that the patients-subjects were provided all information that would be material to their decisions and voluntarily agreed to the course of action undertaken. This assumption reflected ethical principles that have been translated into parallel sets of legal rules (for "informed consent") in the therapeutic and investigatory settings.

These rules not only impose obligations on biomedical professionals in intervening with patients-subjects, they also provide an ethical and legal basis for denying compensation should injuries occur, in that the patients-subjects have voluntarily accepted the intervention. In moral terms, informed consent is sometimes taken to obviate claims of reparative or compensatory justice;[15] in legal terms, consent may be seen as a waiver of the right to recover or even as a denial of the existence of a compensable wrong (*volenti non fit injuria*).

On this view, consent *vel non* provides one means of separating cases in which compensation should be provided from those in which it need not. The view faces substantial objections both of principle (such as concern that the rule emphasizes mere disclosure of risk instead of real choice among alternatives, and doubts about the willingness or ability of physicians to engage in the necessary discussion with their patients[16]) and of technical implementation (such as questions about the effect of the legal basis—negligence, battery, or some hybrid—on the relationship, if any, that must be shown to exist between the information omitted and the harm that occurs[17]).

More important for the present discussion, however, is that the consent requirement does not provide a basis for distinguishing among the categories of biomedical intervention under discussion, unless a systematic difference were demonstrated between therapeutic and research settings in the informed or voluntary nature of the consents given. Several such differences deserve examination.

First, it is often assumed that research subjects are more vulnerable to being drawn into participating in a procedure against their wishes than are patients. In actual fact, research subjects (at least outside institutions) are more likely to give voluntary, informed consent partially because of the elaborate means that have been established for prior review of research risks and of the adequacy of consent documents (which are never examined by outsiders in the typical physician-patient encounter) and partially because of the freer position of research subjects to decline compared with patients in need of medical assistance. Perhaps the most problematic case of informed consent would thus be the innovative treatment category, where the degree of risk is relatively greater and any expectations that a patient would have independent, prior knowledge about the procedure would be relatively weaker than for standard treatment. Further, a patient's need for treatment (perhaps even a desperate need, which has driven the physician to attempt a novel cure) and the patient's existing dependency on the physician may render the patient less able to withhold consent for the innovation than a volunteer subject in comparable research.

A second possible difference between innovation or research and standard therapeutic practices lies in the quality of the information on which the patient or subject (as well as the physician or investigator) must base his or her decision. As discussed in the preceding section, too much is sometimes made about the degree of precision that attaches to data about the risks and benefits of standard therapies; often the quality and predictive value of such data will not significantly exceed that of innovative or research interventions, which (more often than not) are novel only in one small respect, and are otherwise made up of standard steps and procedures. For example, the factors that accounted for the risk (and the actual harm) in cases 1 and 5 (the *pertussis* toxins and the catheterization) are both known on the basis of experience. This precision probably exceeds that of the risk information pertinent to the decision making about either the standard treatment given in case 2 (tonsillar irradiation) or the clinical research involved in case 4 (DES for miscarriage).

Nonetheless, biomedical scientists and practitioners, like patients and subjects, are probably not wrong to assume that, generally and on average, research involves a greater degree of uncertainty in outcome, for good or ill. Is this uncertainty such that it would be appropriate to distinguish injuries arising in standard treatment from those in an innovative or research setting on the ground that the latter are instances of absence of informed consent? While the conclusion that informed consent is lacking may be justified as to any particular innovative therapy or research intervention (just as to any instance of standard treatment), the uncertainties in those settings are not so different from the uncertainties that are inherent in medicine[18] as to offer a reliable basis for framing liability and compensation rules.

BENEFICIARIES OF THE INTERVENTION

If these doubts are justified about the possible grounds for drawing distinctions among categories of biomedical interventions for purposes of framing legal rules, is there anything to the visceral reaction that, between instances of "experimentation," case 5 is more deserving of remedial financial attention than case 4 (just as, among instances of "standard treatment," case 1 seems more deserving than case 2)?[19] Even after deciding that possible differences in novelty, risk, or consent do not alone provide grounds for different legal rules, do they (perhaps together with some other factor) justify the conclusion that, when harm occurs to people in research, the obligation on those carrying out the intervention to "make them whole" is greater than it is for physicians providing standard medical care? In other words, given the somewhat greater uncertainty of outcome and the risk that subjects may obtain "mere knowledge of the harm" without "true appreciation of the nature and extent of the risk,"[20] is there any further significant difference among the categories of intervention that would argue for a non-fault form of compensation for some injuries, even if most medical bad outcomes are left to the tort system?

The central distinction with moral weight is one often associated with the concept of fairness: in the words of John Rawls, "a duty of fair play" binds a person who has accepted the benefits of an arrangement "not to take advantage of the free benefits by not cooperating."[21] In the case of biomedical research, the obligation to redress subjects' injuries would thus rest with the investigator, the sponsor of the research, and society at large (since the object of research is to produce generalizable knowledge, an archetypical public good).

How might this notion of compensatory justice[22] be applied to the categories of interest here? One approach would draw a simple distinction between benefiting oneself and benefiting others. Accordingly, a grid of the sort in table 10.1 could be constructed.

As this table suggests, biomedical professionals ought not to undertake interventions that offer no prospect of benefiting either an individual patient or society (science). Some interventions (nontherapeutic research) aim to benefit society, but their success offers no benefit to the

Table 10.1: Distinctions Among Cases by Intended
Beneficiary

	Benefit to Individual	No Benefit to Individual
Direct benefit to society	4, 3(?), 1(?)	5, 1(?)
No direct benefit to society	2, 3(?), 1(?)	

subjects involved; conversely, the application of standard treatment to an individual patient will not benefit society through the provision of new knowledge (though the avoidance of illness or disability among its members provides an indirect benefit to the collectivity). Clinical research straddles the two categories because it has as its objective benefiting both the patients-subjects and scientific knowledge. The status of innovative treatments (like case 3) is less clear. In theory, they belong with standard therapy, since they are not systematic enough to provide predictable, generalizable knowledge, but some may be performed in a fashion that is careful enough to yield more than anecdotal data, so that, when combined with historical control cases, for example, useful information can be derived.

Finally, case 1 (vaccination) is the most difficult to classify. As an approved procedure that will benefit the patient by conferring immunity against a dread disease, it would seem to benefit the individual rather than society. Yet a program of vaccination is of great value to society, both in avoiding preventable disabilities among those who are immunized and in providing general protection for everyone (even those with faulty immunizations) by restricting the spread of pathogens (and in some cases, as with smallpox, eliminating them entirely). Indeed, once *most* people are vaccinated, it can then be argued that an individual exposes him- or herself to *unnecessary* risk by being vaccinated and is at that point only providing a benefit to society (the realization of which imbalance may explain the necessity of enacting mandatory vaccination laws). In any case, this sense of being a victim for the benefit of others lay behind the earlier distinction (on the visceral level) between case 1 and case 2, though both are matters of standard, accepted "treatment."

What ethical and legal conclusions can be drawn from the distinction between interventions that aim to benefit those who participate (among others) and those that aim only to benefit the larger society? First, such distinction might be denied on the ground that—provided informed consent has been obtained—a subject who chooses to participate in an experiment designed to benefit others has thereby signified that such participation (including the taking of the necessary risks) is of benefit to himself or herself as an individual. While this strict version of autonomy is morally coherent (and legally enforceable), the danger remains that what appears to be an altruistic act is nothing more than the subject being cooperative with the investigator. This danger is particularly pronounced when the subjects are, in the words of the 1975 Declaration of Helsinki, "patients for whom the experimental design is not related to the patient's illness." Moreover, while an investigator might be morally justified in holding a subject to the consequences of his consent if non-negligent harms occur, it would seem fairer (in the Rawlsian sense) for society not to ask the subject to expose him- or herself to the peril of an injury in socially beneficial research for which compensation would be unavailable without proof of negligence.

PRACTICAL CONCLUSIONS

For more than a quarter century, commentators have suggested that, since "society is more than the ultimate beneficiary of research" but "through governmental action" is also "the initiator of most research,"[23] the government should underwrite an insurance program that would provide liability without fault. The creation of such a program would seem, however, to require some proof of need—that is, that a sufficient number of injured subjects is actually going without compensation—to justify taking on the administrative costs of a formal system. That proof does not yet exist.[24] Instead, the partial and informal data now available suggest that subjects who are injured without negligence (whose numbers, though unknown, are apparently small) are typically provided with necessary medical care (though not lost income or other expenses) even though tort law does not now require compensation for those who have consented to participate unless they can prove the investigators have been negligent.

If a study of the incidence and severity of research injuries (and the effects of providing non-fault compensation for them) revealed that a formal program were needed, how might it be organized? One approach would be to identify the particular unmet needs and provide special compensation for them. This is, in effect, what the Swedes do with a special add-on to their existing programs; the add-on provides medical care for all and special coverage for medically created injuries.[25] Another approach would be to require each institution conducting research to arrange its own non-fault coverage; though doubts have been raised about the willingness of insurance companies to write such coverage, interest in experimenting with such policies has been expressed, and several research institutions already include research subjects in their workers' compensation policy.[26]

The adoption of any form of non-fault compensation scheme for injured research subjects would pose several problems. First, while the existence of the compensation plan might encourage the participation of subjects,[27] the opportunity to obtain compensation creates a moral hazard and might bias the selection of subjects—just as the present failure to promise to redress research injuries may create a bias by discouraging certain subjects from participating.

A second and related problem is that the existence of a compensation fund may lead sympathetic physicians-investigators to certify patients-subjects who suffer "bad outcomes" as qualified for compensation, without particular regard for whether the intervention caused the bad outcome. This is one manifestation of the objection about causation that is often raised against non-fault schemes in the medical sphere, namely, that dealing with the human body (rather than something more mechanical and predictable) creates special difficulties of proof: the often unpredictable outcomes may result not only from medical interventions but also from diseases and disorders. Limiting a compensation program to injuries that arise in nontherapeutic research[28] would lessen if not totally eliminate this problem, because subjects would be healthy volunteers, or at least their initial condition would be unconnected with the intervention under investigation. With this limitation, a non-fault program would not be at risk of compensating for many "bad outcomes" that in reality are just the inevitable process of disease (as in case 4) or the inherent problems of the treatment chosen by the patient in preference to allowing the disease to run its course unchecked. One indication of the troubles that arise if clinical research, or innovation, is included in the compensation plan can be seen in case 3. When nontreatment is the course chosen and the treatment is of doubtful efficacy, which outcomes deserve what amount of redress?

One final issue—which goes to the heart of this book—would remain even with a compensation program limited to nontherapeutic research. By what logic would a program (or programs) designed especially for injured research subjects be justified? If the justification were on the fairness grounds suggested above, then the logic would carry over to a program for vaccine injuries as well. But that logic would not necessarily extend to the sorts of innovative (that is, newly accepted) treatments that have been discussed in other chapters, nor to the nonvalidated treatments that have been classed in this chapter—as in general parlance—as innovative in the sense that they are potential substitutions (or replacements) of existing, standard practices. While activities of physicians (and others) that fall into this category are doubtless often justified on scientific grounds (and have, in any event, accounted for a great deal of the development of medicine historically), the analysis presented in this essay leads to the conclusion that injuries resulting from such innovative activities ought not to be included in a non-fault compensation program. Yet the limitations of the underlying justification must be admitted, for in the minds of many people the notion of "unfairness" on which it rests is too narrow. Given the many unexplained causes of much human illness and disability, it seems unfair for those so burdened to suffer without some relief, at least from the heavy burdens of medical bills and lost income. Yet this interpretation is too broad, for it would convert a plan to compensate for certain bad medical outcomes into a comprehensive social welfare program.

NOTES

1. The malpractice system has been criticized as slow and inefficient, wasteful in administration (in the costs of collecting premiums from physicians, the proportion of total funds absorbed by attorneys, and so on), unfair (in rewarding some cases too richly while leaving most injured parties without funds), and unpredictable, hence not an effective deterrent to unsafe practices or unskilled practitioners.

2. See, for example, Delford L. Stickel, "Organ Transplantation in Medical and Legal Perspectives," *Law and Contemporary Problems* 32(1967):597, 609, note 32; see also Irving Ladimer, "Clinical Research Insurance," *Journal of Chronic Diseases* 16(1963):1229, 1233, arguing that the cost of protecting research subjects from bearing the burden of injuries should be regarded as "a proper charge to the business of doing research."

3. Guido Calabresi, Dean of Yale Law School, suggests that having to compensate injured subjects would stimulate better analysis of the risks and benefits of a research proposal, but he concluded that requiring prior committee review (of which more later) offered a more likely means of calibrating and controlling the risks of the activity. See Calabresi's "Reflections on Medical Experimentation in Humans," in *Experimentation with Human Subjects,* ed. P. Freund (New York: George Braziller, 1970), pp. 395, 398-399.

4. This concept, from the National Commission for the Protection of Human Subjects of Biomedical and Behavioral Research's Belmont report (1978), is elaborated by Robert J. Levine in *Ethics and Regulation of Clinical Research* (Baltimore: Urban G. Schwarzenberg, 1981), p. 2. Levine, professor of medicine at Yale Medical School, a special consultant to the commission, and an influential writer on the subject of human research, argues for the use of the word "practice" in place of "treatment," since not all actions are for therapeutic reasons (for example, a diagnostic test); the term "standard treatment" (or "accepted treatment") is commonly used, however, and will be employed here to include preventive and diagnostic measures.

5. While many commentators use the term "innovative treatment" or "innovative therapy," Levine argues that, since more than novelty is involved, the class is better described as "nonvalidated practices":

A practice might be nonvalidated because it is new; i.e., it has not been tested sufficiently often or sufficiently well to permit a satisfactory prediction of its safety or efficacy in a patient population. An equally common way for a practice to merit the designation "nonvalidated" is that in the course of its use in the practice of medicine there arises some legitimate cause to question previously held assumptions about its safety or efficacy [Levine, *Ethics and Regulation*, p. 3].

6. The 1975 revision of the World Medical Association's Declaration of Helsinki uses the term "clinical research" for what had earlier been termed "medical research combined with professional care." Many commentators, including the National Commission for the Protection of Human Subjects of Biomedical and Behavioral Research in its early work [see, for example, *Report and Recommendations: Research on the Fetus 73-75,* DHEW publ. no. (OS) 76-127 (Washington, D.C.: Government Printing Office, 1975)], use the term "therapeutic research" as a shorthand description. Levine has objected vehemently to it, pointing especially to the risk that the term "therapeutic" will cause those who review such research to take too lenient a view and fail to focus on those aspects of the research not intended to benefit patients-subjects. His objections (which are not logically persuasive) have been largely unavailing, and the term is still widely used, particularly (by those who are nonetheless aware of its pitfalls) as convenient shorthand to distinguish it from "nontherapeutic research."

7. Surgical experiments, such as those now being conducted with the permanent artificial heart, provide more familiar examples of therapeutic research, combining as they do the intention of benefiting a patient with the intention of using the procedure to provide generalizable knowledge. It is the latter feature that distinguishes such activities from innovative practices.

Levine has recently reiterated his argument that randomized clinical trials cannot be thought of as therapeutic for the subjects who receive the placebo. [Robert J. Levine, "The Use of Placebos in Randomized Clinical Trials," *IRB* 7(March-April 1985):1.] In fact, as the DES experiment demonstrates, the person in the placebo branch is often better off than the person receiving the active treatment. When there is another method of treatment available, it is advisable (for both scientific and ethical reasons) to use that with the control group, rather than using an inert placebo.

8. Though sounded loudly today by those who claim that the threat of legal liability is paralyzing physicians' use of their judgment in responding to individual patients' particularities and destroying the incentives of drug and device manufacturers to develop new products, this concern is not of recent coinage:

> Much was said on the argument, as to the right of a surgeon to exercise his own judgment as to the mode of treatment he will adopt in the case of a wound, or of a disease which he is called upon to treat; that neither the rules prescribed by writers, nor those acted upon by other physicians or surgeons, can apply to every case, and hence latitude must be allowed for the application of remedies which the attending physician or surgeon

has found to be beneficial. If this is not allowed, the argument is, that all progress in the practice of surgery or physic must cease, and the afflicted lose altogether the benefits of experience and of remedies that science furnishes for the alleviation of human suffering [*Carpenter* v. *Blake*, 60 Barb. 488 (N.Y. Sup. Ct. 1871), *rev'd on other grounds*, 50 N.Y. 696 (1872)].
The court found "this danger . . . more apparent than real," and held the physician who departs from a long-established "system of treatment" to "take the risk of establishing, by his success, the propriety and safety of his experiment" [ibid., pp. 523, 524].

9. *Jackson* v. *Burnham*, 20 Colo. 532, 39 Pac. 577 (1895): "[W]hen a particular mode of treatment is upheld by a consensus of opinion among members of the profession, it should be followed by the ordinary practitioner; and, if a physician sees fit to experiment with some other mode, he should do so at his peril." See also *Slater* v. *Baker and Stapleton, C.B.*, 95 Eng. Rep. 860 (1767): because it was "the first experiment made with this new instrument," defendants' action was "rash" and hence "ignorant," and they were thus negligent, however skillful they may have been, for having acted "ignorantly and unskillfully, contrary to the known rule and usage of surgeons."

10. See, for example, Henry K. Beecher, "Ethics and Clinical Resarch," *New England Journal of Medicine* 274(1966):1354.

11. President's Commission for the Study of Ethical Problems in Medicine and Biomedical and Behavioral Research, vol. 1, *Compensating for Research Injuries* (Washington, D.C: Government Printing Office, 1982), p. 9.

12. See especially, *Hamlet*, act IV, scene 3: "Diseases desperate grown/ By desperate appliance are relieved,/ Or not at all."

13. See Harvey and Levine, "Risk of Injury Associated with Twenty Invasive Procedures Used in Human Experimentation and Assessment of Reliability of Risk Estimates," in President's Commission, vol. 2, *Appendices*, p. 73.

14. One recent empirical study of victims of accidents and illness in England and Wales by a research group at the Centre for Socio-Legal Studies at Oxford concludes that, although "illness causes much more incapacity than accident, both in terms of numbers of people affected, and the length and severity of consequences . . . compensation under the damages system is virtually confined to [certain types of] accident cases [and] . . . benefits under the industrial injuries scheme are concentrated almost entirely on accident cases." Donald Harris; Mavis Maclean; Hazel Genn; Sally Lloyd-Bostock; Paul Fenn; Peter Corfield; Yvonne Brittan, *Compensation and Support for Illness and Injury* (Oxford: Clarendon Press, 1984), pp. 325-27.

15. See, for example, James Childress, "Compensating Injured Research Subjects: I. The Moral Argument," *Hastings Center Report* 6 (December 1976):21, 24.

16. See, for example, Jay Katz, *The Silent World of Doctor and Patient* (New York: Free Press, 1984); President's Commission for the Study of Ethical Problems in Medicine and Biomedical and Behavioral Research, *Making Health Care Decisions* (Washington, D.C.: Government Printing Office,

1983); Mark Siegler, "Searching for Moral Certainty in Medicine: A Proposal for a New Model of the Doctor-Patient Encounter," *Bulletin of the New York Academy of Medicine* 57(1981):56.

17. See, for example, A. M. Capron, "Informed Consent in Catastrophic Disease Research and Treatment," *University of Pennsylvania Law Review* 123(1974):340.

18. Though often unacknowledged, see Katz, *The Silent World*, pp. 165-206.

19. Explicit attention has not previously been drawn to one feature of the hypotheticals which was raised as a possible factor in the opening paragraph of this chapter, namely, the relevance, if any, of the need (or other characteristics) of the "victim." Plainly, the preexisting circumstances of a victim, like the extent of the injury, affect the measurement of damages: injuring a married "breadwinner" (case 2) typically has greater impact than injuring a single youth (cases 1 and 5), just as an injury that results in a need for permanent medical and nursing care (cases 1 and 5) usually results in a larger damage award than does an injury that results in a quick death (case 2). But the characteristics of the victims (particularly if most of the victims of an intervention share salient characteristics) can also affect the determination of liability itself and not solely the measure of damages. The blameless babies affected by the immediately comprehensible and very pathetic injuries caused by thalidomide are one example (contrast with the diversity of the victims affected by the less easily understood Guillan-Barre syndrome from swine flu vaccine).

20. D. P. Dietrich, "Legal Implications of Psychological Research with Human Subjects," *Duke Law Journal* 1960:265-72.

21. John Rawls, "Legal Obligation and the Duty of Fair Play," in *Law and Philosophy*, S. Hook, ed. (New York: New York University Press, 1964), pp. 9, 10.

22. Unlike retributive justice, compensatory justice need not rest on a finding of fault or blame on the part of the person called upon to make redress.

23. Dietrich, "Legal Implications," p. 273.

24. See President's Commission, vol. 1, *Compensation*, pp. 2-4, 101-12.

25. See Harry Boström, "On the Compensation of Research Subjects in Sweden," in President's Commission, vol. 2, *Appendices*, p. 309.

26. See, for example, John D. Arnold, "Incidence of Injury During Clinical Pharmacology Research and Indemnification of Injured Subjects at the Quincy Research Center," in President's Commission, vol. 2, *Appendices*, p. 275; Thomas S. Chittenden, "Compensation for Injured Research Subjects: Funding Mechanisms," in President's Commission, vol. 2, *Appendices*, p. 423.

27. And thus overcome any problems of "insufficient" research activity that *may* now result from fewer people being willing to participate in research than would optimize the benefits to society from research.

28. And for injuries in therapeutic research or innovative practice that are caused by procedures (such as tests) *added solely* for the purpose of providing generalizable data rather than for the benefit of the individual patient-subject.

11

Legal Liability
for Medical Innovation

Richard A. Epstein

Many of the major issues of health care today revolve about two familiar questions to students of tort and regulation. What are the proper institutional arrangements to minimize the level of risk associated with the delivery of products and services, and what level of compensation, if any, should be provided to those persons who are injured when the remaining risks materialize in losses? These questions are especially difficult in cases of medical innovation, where both risks and rewards are frequently great. The enormous complexity of issues is revealed by the range of institutional responses. Deterrence and compensation can be approached under the tort law, specifically through suits for medical malpractice and products liability. They can be handled by various forms of direct legislative and administrative overview, from Food and Drug Administration control over drugs to institutional review boards in local hospitals and medical centers. They also can be handled by private contracts amongst the various parties.

Each system of controls works in a different way. The tort remedies tend to operate by indirection: there is no direct supervision over the behavior of the various parties, who (it is hoped) nonetheless are induced to perform properly by the threat of damage actions. The administrative controls, adopted in part out of the fear that some defendants may prove insolvent or some harms (death, serious disabilities) will prove irreparable, represent direct public controls that deploy a mixture of fines, inspections, licensing, and approvals to prevent most losses from occurring. The private contractual element is designed to preserve for patients and consumers some measure of autonomy and choice, at least within the constraints of tort and direct regulation.

The hardest problems arise over the mix of remedies. I will start with the tort approach to these questions, specifically medical malpractice and products liability, and then consider how regulation complements or substitutes for it. Although I refer to the issue from time to time, I do not stress an argument that I have made elsewhere, which is that contractual solutions for all the flaws are better than the regulatory and tort alternatives that are so much in vogue today.[1] Instead, I want to address the various methods for the public control of medical innovation, and indeed medical practice generally. That inquiry begins with a discussion of the connections between medical malpractice and products liability law; thereafter, it addresses the integration of tort remedies with direct public control.

One central theme is that more need not be merrier. Throughout this essay I want to stress the importance of the coordination between the tort and the regulatory sides of the issue, and to emphasize the great benefits that follow from the adoption of clear rules to handle complex problems. Much of what I have to say is a plea for a return to safe harbors, whether by custom or by statute, for new therapies or products introduced into the marketplace. The sheer number of concrete situations influenced by possible private actions makes it imperative that there be some known and observable standard to guide parties who must act under the applicable legal rules. The present system tends to offer injured persons repeated bites at the apple, wherein it is commonplace to examine medical or manufacturing practices under different standards, first in administrative and then in judicial settings. In my view the duplication of supervision is the source of conflict, cost, and contradiction, all of which should be controlled to help medical innovation, indeed medical treatment, proceed on rational lines.

This essay is organized as follows. The first section argues that the rules of product liability and medical malpractice should be understood as an integrated whole: that is, they are best understood if their interactions with each other are taken into account. The second section then examines the way in which these rules should be applied to three distinct contexts: routine cases and known risks, experimental treatment, and routine treatment that reveals an unknowable risk. In each case the key objective of the liability system is to insure the proper transmission of information. Where the information to be transmitted is standardized in form, an official, uniform determination of its adequacy should be made before it is disseminated, not afterwards. As in so many areas of law, the greatest mistake in the current liability rules is their excess of ambition. Certain major risks can be controlled at low price, but in the effort to endow the system with a certainty that it cannot possess, the limited, but vital, gains that are possible are systematically undone. The best again becomes the enemy of the good.

THE COMMON LAW OF MEDICAL MALPRACTICE AND PRODUCTS LIABILITY

The two bodies of tort law most relevant to questions of medical innovation are medical malpractice and products liability. The conventional understanding places them in separate domains. For physicians, liability is said to depend upon negligence, with its usual elements of duty, breach, cause, and damage. Liability for products is said to be strict, where proof of negligence is irrelevant once the causal connection between the product defect, however defined, and the plaintiff's injury is established. The difference in liability rules is then reflected in two critical but subsidiary points. Where negligence is the test of liability, custom becomes at least probative and in medical contexts is often regarded as dispositive in determining the standard of care.[2] Where negligence is irrelevant, then customary practice tends to become irrelevant as well. Where negligence is the test of liability, res ipsa loquitur, "the thing speaks for itself," may assist in drawing the inference of negligence from proved facts.[3] Where it is not, then the principle is said to be as irrelevant as the negligence that res ipsa could help establish.

These traditional views of the subject tend to mislead. The similarities between medical malpractice and products liability are far more pronounced than the usual accounts might otherwise allow. The critical point often depends not upon the status of the defendant, that is, not upon whether the defendant provides medical products or medical services, but upon the nature of the enterprise in which that defendant is engaged and the types of risks that must be confronted. That the same pattern of liability rules should emerge in both areas should not be surprising. Most medical treatments involve coordinated interaction between the providers of goods and services. As the goods and services work in combination, so too should the liability rules that govern them.[4] The ideal system is one which makes the choice between different inputs to health care turn upon the benefits that they provide. Where products are subject to more stringent standards than medical services, there is a risk that treatment will be substituted for products, even when the latter is more suited to the task.[5]

Consider the traditional distinction between liability for bad services and liability for bad products. By hornbook law, liability for products is strict and that for services is not. Yet in particular instances the alleged disparity could only be a source of difficulty. Thus in some of the early hepatitis questions, the issue was the appropriate standard for holding a blood bank liable when a transfusion caused hepatitis in the recipient. Those cases which took the line that blood was a product were willing to apply strict liability principles. Yet if the provision of blood had been found to be a service, negligence rules would apply. The obvious point is that the sale of blood contains both types of inputs, so the proper question is, What regime of liability will tend to increase the net benefits from using blood, which is known to carry a certain risk? For reasons that shall be developed later, the strict liability system tends to work awkwardly in this context, and the negligence standard (at least as properly defined) is preferable. But the structural point is that there is little reason to have one standard of liability for the blood bank that sells the product and another for the hospital or physician (as providers of services) that uses it. The distinction between products and services can be viable in some contexts, but the determinants of liability should be functional, not formal. As a general matter, close substitutes should be subject to identical regimes of liability in order to avoid skewing the choices between them. Indeed, in this area, where contracting is possible, the question should not be decided collectively at all, for private markets will work to create the desired parallelism in liability rules.

FROM ROUTINE TO INNOVATIVE RISKS

The need for a systematic approach to liability across separate systems is pervasive and applies whenever products and services are used in mixed proportions. With medical malpractice it is important to contrast, at the poles, the liabilities of physicians for routine practice with the liabilities of physicians who are engaged in developing experimental or innovative techniques for diagnosis and treatment. The intermediate case, of great importance and difficulty, is where a standard practice turns out to have a systematic defect that was unknown (and perhaps unknowable) at the time of its general adoption. The same classification is at work in the law of products liability. At the extremes, the rules governing the production of standard drugs are quite different from those governing the testing and development of new drugs. Similarly, the intermediate case is one where a standard drug turns out to have a uniform, undisclosed risk that is revealed only years later.

The simple distinction between medical malpractice and products liability, therefore, must give way to more complex inquiry, which asks how both products liability and medical malpractice law respond to the three dominant kinds of cases. It is useful to examine both dimensions of the problem simultaneously, in order to show how the doctrinal differences between products liability and medical malpractice can be harmonized once the institutional profiles of these three different situations are understood. In particular, the pitfalls for innovative treatments and therapies are by

definition greater than those for routine treatments and therapies. The rates
of return for innovative treatment may be very high, but so are the risks.
Long-term latent risks of routine practices and products are, if anything,
more difficult to control, precisely because of the apparent success of the
standard practice. Once a treatment has passed from the innovative to the
routine without identification of its major adverse effects, the probability of
any loss occurring may be very low. Yet should anything be amiss, the
danger of widespread disaster becomes far greater, for even the prompt
removal of the dangerous drug or discontinuation of the dangerous
treatment still leaves large numbers of people at risk. Finally, routine
treatments with known risks are investments that have known returns and
known risks, whether we speak of medical malpractice or products liability.

The question, What is the proper way to deal with medical innovation?
reduces itself to the treatment of these three cases. I shall begin with the
treatment of routine risks in routine cases and then move on to both the
experimental and latent defect settings.

ROUTINE AND KNOWN RISKS

Correction or Warning

As might be expected, the liability rules for routine cases are not without
controversy, although they are in principle the easiest to articulate. The
sources of risk are generally understood, and, while they may be great,
efforts can be made to counter them. Sometimes the appropriate defense is
to eliminate the peril in its entirety; therefore compensation after the fact
need not be examined in the vast majority of cases, where the precautions
are successful. Where correction is possible before the fact, and where its
benefits exceed its costs, someone will normally try to do it, no matter how
the law sets the original liability.[6] The innovator need not be any party who
might have to bear the loss in the absence of innovation. Thus if the medical
loss were left with patients, they would pay handsomely for any test that
reduced that risk. Similarly, if liability were imposed upon either a blood
bank or a hospital, independent firms would still have the incentive to
develop cost-effective tests. The new liability only means that blood banks
and hospitals, as well as patients (who rarely receive perfect compensation
for injury), would all be willing to pay the innovator a price greater than the
costs of production, but less than the loss averted. It is for just this reason
that drug companies introduce new products whether or not they are at risk
for liability. The hepatitis B vaccine, for example, was developed *after* the
vast majority of states made it clear that liability for the supply of bad blood
depended upon proof of negligence and could not be maintained on a strict
liability theory. The same principles apply to new advances in medicine,

most of which are developed by persons who have no personal risk of liability.

In other cases, however, correction of the peril is simply impossible, or at least too costly. In the extreme, the effort to remove the risks of a certain treatment can rob that treatment of its promised benefits. Many lifesaving drugs have very serious, known side effects: it is worth bearing the debilitating side effects of steroids in order to control some life-threatening condition. Yet here, too, it should be possible to avoid the question of damages by *warning* of the side effects that follow from the use of this treatment or product. In principle there is the question of whether the warning should be directed to the physician or to the patient. Where the information is technical, there is good reason to warn the physician, who can in turn (as is now required under the doctrines of informed consent) make the information intelligible to the patient and relate it to the concrete particulars of individual cases. In other circumstances, package inserts for patients may be appropriate, if only as supplements to warnings to physicians. Once informed about side effects, the patient (who best knows his own preferences) can compare risks and benefits of treatment, allowing for the uncertainties of the case.

More controversially, I believe that one can go further, for so long as there is notice to the patient that further information is needed, it becomes possible for him to make independent inquiries (through a second opinion, for example) on how to treat the known risks and hazards. The key point, therefore, is to assure that relevant information is transferred, not necessarily that the defendant will do the transferring. In some cases that burden will be assumed in order to avoid the need to refer to third parties, but in other cases the independent judgment may well prove essential to the job. Indeed, it may well be that this system is far better than one which demands that generic warnings (especially in products cases) be complete, for second opinions allow the individuation of risk in a way that any collective determination of standardized warnings does not.

No matter how one phrases the duty-to-warn question, the transfer of information to the proper party should be the limit of the relevant duty for both the drug company and the physician. Once all the benefits and costs of any action rest upon the same individual, there is no danger that one person (say the physician) will externalize costs while preserving benefits. The normal conflict of interest between private contracting parties is therefore eliminated, either by transferring a safe product or by providing accurate information as to why and how the product is dangerous, or even by providing information about the need to inquire further about certain material risk. Information transfer is the key; accordingly, the patient's decision should not be reviewable afresh in the public arena by some social cost-benefit calculation. Legal intervention has placed it in the hands of the parties with every incentive to get it right.

In doctrinal terms this argument leads to the adoption of a position which says that the patient assumes the risks once the relevant information about the risks is received.[7] It contrasts with the view that liability should turn in any way on the *reasonableness* of the private evaluation, corresponding to the principle of contributory negligence, which accordingly should be kept out of the discussion. No one should claim that every person always does his sums correctly under conditions of uncertainty and stress. But it is proper to claim that the inevitable errors of calculation made by individual patients should not be the source of extensive liabilities for either physicians or manufacturers who have properly supplied the relevant information.

The Choice of Liability Rule

Fitness of goods and services. The next question is what the rules of liability should be to ensure a safe course of action is taken or proper information supplied. With correctable risks, I think that the appropriate standard of liability is strict in both medical malpractice and product liability: indeed, I believe further that this solution would be adopted consensually even if not required by law. But strict liability for what? For the requisite standard of treatment or for the wholesomeness of the drug, *not* for the cure or recovery of the patient. In essence, therefore, the defendant becomes an insurer, but only of his own product or conduct, *not* of the health of the patient.

Within the framework of medical malpractice, this result is reached in essence under the negligence rubric, when the custom of the profession becomes the standard of care. The traditional formulation understates the strictness of the rule by treating medical custom as one deposit of a uniform standard of reasonable care. But while the scope of the strictness may be narrow, within that domain it is remorseless. There is, of course, more than one permissible approach to a given problem, and it is possible to depart consciously from a known but fallible procedure in the effort to find a superior alternative. Yet putting these complications to one side, the physician who deviates from the permissible set by inadvertence does so at his peril. He can surely defend himself on the ground that the deviation in question was not causally connected with the losses in question,[8] an issue of great difficulty when the inferior treatment only works to increase the probability of loss.[9]

There is a precise parallel with respect to the production of drugs. Under the law of products liability there has emerged a threefold classification of defects: production or formula defects, warning defects, and design defects. Where a drug is manufactured that does not meet its own formula specifications, then the construction defect is established. It is no defense to say that all reasonable care was taken in order to produce the safe product. As before, the finding of liability does not follow from the finding of defect because of the lurking causal difficulties that remain. But with liability clear, cases of this sort are rarely tried today once the factual matters are resolved.

In both medical and product contexts there is good sense to the strictness of the liability. The control of risk lies exclusively within the hands of the defendant, as it is unlikely that any unusual conduct by an individual plaintiff or by any third party can change the magnitude of the risk.[10] The questions of product misuse or patient misbehavior are of very minor importance and are best handled by affirmative defenses, which should apply when a consumer knows (say because of discoloration or smell) that a given drug is indeed defective.[11] These rare cases aside, a simple rule which says to the defendant, Bear the losses that you have caused, will serve to induce the appropriate level of care, with a minimum of administrative costs and without creating any unwanted distortions in the patient's behavior.[12] Creating the liability also works to the benefit of both the physician or manufacturer, as the case may be, and the patient, because it induces individuals to accept the services or goods in question even when they cannot fully understand what the services are or how the drug is manufactured. The rules of liability state with sufficient clarity what outcomes should follow if an accident occurs. They give a neutral road map that allows disputes to be resolved in accordance with known and reliable standards when and if they occur, so that an investigation into standards does not have to be undertaken upon receipt of the drugs or treatment, when the probability of any failure or defect is too low to warrant it.[13]

The pattern of mutual benefit suggests that such a rule would be adopted by contract where these are permitted by law (as they now are not) and that they should be kept, at least as "off the rack" provisions to minimize the cost of contracting when it is allowed in these areas. One persuasive piece of evidence of the desirability of the powerful, but limited, domain of strict liability comes from the various proposals for reform in both medical malpractice and products liability. During the ebbs and flows of the past ten years, both physicians and manufacturers have worked to restrict the scope of liability rules, but none of their proposed reforms has ever been directed toward either of the stringent liability rules at issue here.

Most efforts by physicians to revise the rules of liability in medical malpractice cases have been to return custom to its dominant position, and not to invent a position in which no liability attaches to well-understood forms of malpractice.[14] Nor should we expect otherwise, for within limits it is in the interest of physicians to be able to warrant their services in order to induce individual consumers to sign on with them. There are enormous imperfections in information in medical markets, none of which is necessarily eliminated by direct regulation.

The same point is true for drugs. It would be nothing short of calamitous for drug companies, which are often not in privity of contract with their users, to be forced to try to duplicate by contract the express warranties that the tort law now commands. In the swine flu fiasco, the entire dispute among the drug companies, their insurers, and the government was the question of the adequacy of warnings. But throughout the dispute, the companies were willing to take full responsibility for production errors, that is, for vials of vaccine that did not meet government standards. Again, the warranty on balance costs the company less than it benefits consumers. The question of liability standards, then, is pretty much solved in this easy case. To be sure, many difficult matters of fact will arise in individual cases, but these fact-dense issues (Who took what drug when?) have little precedential value and do not raise any institutional concerns.

Warnings. The question of warnings is, however, more vexatious. Here, in principle the argument takes the form that whether we deal with products or services, the physician or manufacturer meets his full obligation when all relevant disclosures are made, even if the outcome is adverse. Within the law of medical malpractice, that proposition is captured by the black letter law of informed consent, which emphasizes disclosure of the relevant risks of alternative forms of treatment.[15] Within products liability, that proposition is embodied in the rules on the duty to warn of known defects, which adopt parallel standards of relevance and materiality. There are important differences between the two areas, for the physician (who has greater knowledge of the patient's condition) must tailor the warnings to take into account the personal idiosyncracies of users in order to discharge his duty, while the drug company's warnings are generally directed to generic features of its products. Yet in both cases the central dispute in the common-law cases is over what kinds of disclosures are sufficient to exonerate the defendant from liability.

In contrast with the flaws in medical practice and drug production defects, the problem with warnings is the irreducible question of degree, for there is no single litmus test to determine the adequacy of warnings. The intense disputes tend to belie the original black letter proposition on adequacy, for it is easy to find cases where extensive disclosures have been held (or so a jury could find) to be insufficient. In litigation, it becomes possible under the dominant standards of reasonableness to argue that whatever warnings were given were inadequate as a matter of course.[16]

Once the outcome is known to be bad, some further warnings of adverse side effects must have been needed to discourage the unfortunate course of action. Yet this extreme position only reveals the false confidence of hindsight. When the treatment was undertaken, or the drug administered, there was some probability of a successful outcome and some of an unsuccessful outcome. The ideal warning is that which conveys the proper probabilities and their associated gains and losses. Warnings that are too severe are as bad as those that are too soft, because both tend to distort, if in opposite directions, the relevant patient or consumer choices. The full costs of overwarning would only be known if legal actions were allowed to people deterred from taking needed therapy by excessive warnings. But these losses are now obscured from public view because of their intolerable administrative demands.

In the end, therefore, modern common law creates a serious bias, intensified by the discretion left to juries, toward finding all warnings inadequate when judged by the standards of hindsight. On a selective basis, the theory of improper warnings becomes an elaborate, expensive, and erratic pretext for compensating for bad outcomes alone. As every skillful trial lawyer knows, the question of adequacy of warnings is a form of reverse engineering. First find out what warnings were given, and then tailor the claim on adequacy to render them insufficient.

What, if anything, can be done in order to prevent the risks of overcompensation for bad outcomes when proper information is transmitted? At this juncture an important structural difference between the informed consent cases and the drug cases, alluded to above, influences the correct institutional response. The informed consent cases arise out of one-on-one interactions and are fact-dense. Until the particular situation of each patient is known, it is impossible to have a sense of what disclosures should be made. It seems impossible, therefore, to dictate any single form of words to govern all cases. Thus the best that can be expected of courts, if the doctrine is to be retained at all, is to be aware of the twin perils of overwarning and underwarning. Some comfort may be taken from the causal empiricism of the trade, that it is very hard for a plaintiff to win a malpractice action on a straight informed consent theory. There does not seem to be any institutionalized response that can be used to replace tort law doctrine, even with the notorious difficulties of informed consent cases.[17]

The drug cases, however, do present systematic features that make possible a coordinated institutional response to the problem of imperfect information. Drugs and vaccines are distributed on a mass basis, as was the case with the swine flu and Sabin live polio virus vaccines that were so controversial in the 1970s and the ominous pertussis vaccine problems of the 1980s. It should be possible to *standardize* the warnings in advance in ways that resist legal liability after the fact. What is needed, I believe, is a rule that provides that certain warnings approved by, say, the FDA shall be *conclusively* regarded as adequate in any subsequent lawsuit; the only triable issue on the question will be the simple one of whether the warning as issued complies with the standard form.[18] At this point it becomes necessary to use the administrative process to determine the content of the warning, a task already required under the present rules. To be sure, the public input on the question will have to be stronger, precisely because there is no judicial check on the matter of adequacy. Nonetheless there are huge gains from balanced warnings that do not conceal the net benefits of taking the product. Where there are special cases (as to whether the vaccine should be given to pregnant women or to asthmatics), a sound set of warnings could indicate persons at special risk, for whom consultation with a physician might be appropriate. Any system of warnings could be published in newspapers and distributed through physicians long before the drug or vaccine is used, in order to allow time for study and review. Any warning so prescribed should, of course, be quickly updated as new information is revealed. The system itself should be viable, because its costs can be spread over a large number of production units.

In making this proposal I do not want to suggest that the administrative process is ideal. Indeed, the FDA has been effectively criticized because of its conservative approach to the release of new drugs on the market. Nonetheless, if we are prepared to trust the basic decision of whether the drug will be marketed to the agency, then it seems odd to say that it cannot confront (with an assist from the medical profession) the warning issue as well. Warnings and package inserts are already required by the FDA, so the critical point is only to provide the firms safe harbor when they comply with the demands of the statute. Once lawyers have little to gain from the way the warnings are phrased, one divisive element is removed from the fray. On matters of this sort, it should be possible to find enough persons with independent judgment to minimize the risk that drug companies will softpedal their warnings in order to escape liability. Where companies do withhold or tamper with the evidence, then very severe penalties, both civil and criminal, are warranted, as is indeed the case under current law.

It may be objected that the need for fixed standards is alarmist because the price of drugs is free to move to take into account the added liabilities. Empirically, the swine flu cases and the recent cases of Bendectin and of pertussis vaccine have shown the point to be false. Firms withdraw from the market, even if they are free to set whatever price they choose. The easy way to explain the point is to treat the present rules on product liability as a restraint upon voluntary contractual transactions, at least in one dimension—product warranties. When the price term is free to move while the liability term is not, there need not be a market clearing price which will allow production to continue. The key question is whether the costs generated by the new liability rules exceed the joint gains to consumers and producers under the previous voluntary contract. If in the aggregate the net gains are wiped out by the liability costs, then the product will no longer be made. If some net gains survive, then fewer units will be produced to reflect the changes in rules and some marginal consumers must do without.

The critical question, then, is how to estimate the size of the losses imposed by the present legal regime. Several points suggest that these are substantial. First, there are very heavy administrative costs to make the transfers. No consumer derives any direct benefit from these administrative expenses, even though producers must charge to cover them. Second, there is the possibility (real today) that the damage awards paid will exceed those demanded in private markets.[19] Damage levels for death cases may be too high, and excessive levels of coverage may be provided when collateral benefits (for example, medical insurance) are not subtracted out from recovery. Third, once the defendant is not safe on the warning question, it may be forced to pay for losses that its products did not cause, given the false attribution of disease to the vaccine. This problem arose in vivid fashion in the Sabin vaccine cases.[20] There, the problem arises because the vaccine tends to be called into use when the risk of polio is elevated. It is therefore very easy to charge against the vaccine illness brought on by natural causes. Similarly with the pertussis vaccine: the risk is that severe damage brought on by independent causes is chalked up erroneously as a side effect of the vaccine or that the vaccine only hastens cures that would have occurred anyway. In each case, the erroneous attributions after the fact lead one to overstate the risks of the vaccine and hence to overstate its true cost of production. These errors then work themselves back into the pricing and production decisions. At some point, if the number of false positives attributed to a vaccine rises sufficiently, then the private costs imposed upon the manufacturer diverge from the social costs of the vaccine. Systematic underproduction results. Drug companies are not in the risky end of the life insurance business. If their losses from that line of production exceed the profits that they can make from the sale of vaccines, then they will leave the market. The enormous consumer surplus from the purchase of vaccines can be and has been dissipated by unsound liability rules. The public health benefits are likewise lost. Markets work because the costs to the seller are justified by the benefits to the buyer. They cannot survive when costs are falsely charged onto the buyer for whom there are in fact no parallel benefits.

EXPERIMENTAL SITUATIONS

The proper role of medical malpractice and products liability law in experimental situations is, if anything, more complicated, because the level of information about risks is necessarily lower than in the routine cases just discussed. Nonetheless the same analytical framework applies, because the central function of the legal rules should still be to provide consumers with the (lower) levels of information that are available. Imperfect information is better than no information at all. Within the experimental context, matters are often especially vexing, since controlled studies are designed to isolate the effects of a given drug or treatment. Typically, the size of the sample will be far smaller than with the groups participating in mass vaccination programs. Nonetheless, they will be large enough for the results that flow from them to be of statistical significance. Given these modest economies of scale, standardized warning procedures should be available to reduce the role of tort liability against either physicians or drug manufacturers.

The traditional rules of tort liability function fitfully at best in experimental situations. The standards of customary care, for example, lack specificity when dealing with treatment or techniques for which no customary practices have yet been established. To be sure, it is possible to develop a set of "metacustoms" which are designed to deal with those particular gaps in knowledge, but these rules will have far less bite than specific directives about the use of given products or therapies. In addition, the doctrine of informed consent is under far greater pressure, first because of the persistent conflicts of interest between the physician's experiment and the patient's well-being[21] and second because the greater uncertainty means that there is more to be said about the problems to begin with.

Under these circumstances it is not surprising that the tort approach has not proved adequate for the task. Instead, the dominant institutional response works on two levels. The first is to insist upon individual consent on the part of persons who work in the programs, consent that brings home the fact that they will often be involved in double-blind experiments in which they may not receive the treatment someone thinks (but does not know) is preferred.[22] The second is to insist upon independent review boards, given that many of the risks themselves are hard to convey to individual patients. The function of the boards is to act as independent experts before the fact and to pass upon the desirability of the programs in the abstract. The hard question is always whether this extra layer of protection is worth the costs that it imposes, as measured both by its direct costs and by the soundness and the speed of its internal procedures. That question is extremely difficult for someone outside the medical establishment to evaluate; much may turn upon the particular details of institutional organization, which vary widely from board to board and from case to case. Indeed, even if one could show that the decisions across boards are wildly inconsistent with each other,[23] it does not necessarily follow that the procedures should be condemned. It could well be that the average level of experimentation is higher when there are boards than when investigators are left to their own discretion. Nonetheless, these boards cannot be dismissed simply as an artificial government creation by persons (like myself) who believe in the superiority of voluntary contracts to government regulation. The participants in these experiments might well want some form of external independent review to offset their own ignorance. The risk of government regulation is that it imposes a monopoly of practices that makes it difficult to obtain the information that might lead to informed choices. The relevant variables are many, and certain situations (for example, psychological harm) may not call for as much supervision as others. Yet the insistence on uniform standards prevents the acquisition of additional information by institutional experimentation.[24]

These forms of direct control bear also upon the question of whether there is a place for individual compensation for bad outcomes within the experimental setting. Here my own answer comes in two parts. First, the central purpose of the elaborate mechanisms of disclosure and review up front are a good reason to displace the tort liability system after the fact. I do not have any objection to tort damage actions for injuries sustained because of departures from the experimental design: these cases are too close to the routine cases of inadvertent deviation from custom. Yet by the same token I think that it is mischievous or worse to look behind the experimental design after the fact when the outcomes are bad, as they often will be. As with the warnings in vaccine programs, the gains from experimental work can easily be dissipated by lawsuits that depend upon second-guessing the myriad difficult choices necessary for any experimental design.

Should some other compensation system be set up for participants in the program who have bad outcomes, wholly without regard to improper conduct by the medical personnel? Again, my response is to resist the proposal. One initial point is that it is very difficult to determine the baseline against which compensation is awarded. In many experimental programs, such as those for cancer, the persons who participate are in very dire circumstances to begin with, so bad outcomes will be the norm, even where the proposed innovation enjoys some modest success. Any system of compensation must therefore be able to measure the *marginal* contribution of the experimental input, which may well be small compared to the underlying disease. There are also many forms of implicit compensation that derive from the simple fact of participation in experimental programs, not the least of which is superior conventional medical care of the sort that helped throw off the original investigations into the efficacy of DES (which were corrected by the Dieckmann study).[25] The persons who elect to participate in these programs, moreover, can easily be made to understand that compensation is not forthcoming: consent remains consent, even if the options available to the participant are limited by the disease, for the defendant only expands the patient's set of opportunities which the disease itself limits. There seems, therefore, little reason to bear the very heavy additional costs that a compensation system will impose. The funds saved could be turned to more productive uses.

THE UNKNOWABLE HAZARD

The last case to consider is that of the unknown and unknowable hazard of certain medical or product innovations. As before, the problem is one that can arise either in a medical malpractice or a products liability setting. Arguably the routine use of radiation to treat tonsillitis falls into this category, as does the use of DES, with its untoward side effects. In all these cases the traditional legal view was that liability did not attach where the treatments or drugs met the applicable standards. In the medical malpractice context, the general rule of customary care provided a limitation upon liability: it was no longer necessary to test a procedure forever before adopting it as a matter of general use. Under the law of products liability, the general position was that strict liability principles did not apply to drugs that fell into this category.

The question of liability for unknowable defects has been much mooted in recent cases; while there was some move to hold defendants liable for such risks in at least one state, there has generally been a quick retreat, in the drug cases.[26] There is commendable caution in the limited situation. The critical arguments parallel those in cases of warning for adequate defects. It is simply that the accumulated costs and errors of the system, be they in determining causation or damages, threaten to exceed the enormous gains from marketing new products or using new medical technologies. With drugs, the institutional response is preferable. The obvious idea is to encourage only that level of investment in resources that is cost-justified. The system will keep too many beneficial products and treatments off the market if it insists that they be riskfree. Instead of allowing reasonableness standards after the fact to decide whether liability is appropriate, it becomes critical to answer the liability question in conclusive form *before* products are marketed.[27] I have no great confidence in the ability of the FDA to determine the optimal level of social research in drugs. The point is, given that it undertakes that inquiry as a part of its general licensing procedures, there is little to be gained by running every case through the second filter of common-law reasonableness standards.

Those tests are difficult enough to apply in routine accident cases, and the cost and error in their elaboration only increase when applied to firm and industry behavior that may well have taken place decades ago. Risks are surely higher when dangers are unknown, but it does not follow that the difference in risk levels dictates a greater common-law liability for unknowable hazards. Rather, so long as the information that is acquired has been transferred and all appropriate administrative procedures have been followed, the providers of the product should be spared liability.

The same administrative route is not available in cases of medical practice, given the want of any centralized system of approval. By default, therefore, customary standards are the appropriate ones for litigation. Here, as above, no one should defend the use of custom on the ground that it is perfect. It clearly is not. Most customary practices, for example, are not routinely verified by randomized control trials before they are placed into use.[28] But the best should never be made the enemy of the good. Randomized experiments are costly to operate and difficult to maintain in the face of the ethical objections raised to them (when it is suspected that one course of treatment is superior to another in a given case, for example). The debate over whether they should be routinely adopted is one that can proceed elsewhere, but the important point is that, unless and until that day is reached, customary standards should afford the complete defense, leaving the control of unknown risks to the steady, if erratic, course of medical science.

CONCLUSION

The question of legal liability for medical innovation is part of a larger complex of issues relating to the liability of medical services and products generally. In all of these cases risks are involved, knowable or not, quantifiable or not. There are obviously large social gains that can be obtained from the control or the elimination of these risks. The issue is not whether an investment should be made, but where it should be made. In my view, the place of tort liability within this scheme is limited. Lawsuits are a poor place in which to determine the wisdom of various courses of treatment on which the experts themselves are divided. They are a poor place to review the subjective judgments of individual patients and consumers who now are disappointed with choices that may have been sound at their inception, if unfortunate in their consequences. The best we can expect of the judicial system is to ensure that the standards that are developed elsewhere—be it by statute or administrative order, by institutional review board or ordinary custom—are faithfully applied in the cases that they govern. It is hard enough to perform accurately the translation function, in order to ensure that standards developed elsewhere are sensibly applied within the legal context. It is quite beyond the power of courts to use the amorphous principles of cost-benefit analysis to forge independent standards for judging the provision of medical goods and services. There is great virtue in doing small tasks well.

NOTES

1. For that argument, see Richard A. Epstein, "Medical Malpractice: The Case for Contract," *American Bar Foundation Research Journal* 1(1976):87; "Contracting Out of the Medical Malpractice Crisis," *Perspectives in Biology and Medicine* 20(1977):228.
2. See, for example, Clarence Morris, "Custom and Negligence," *Columbia Law Review* 42(1942):1147, 1164-65; Alan H. McCoid, "The Care Required of Medical Practitioners," *Vanderbilt Law Review* 12(1959):549. Some doubt has been raised on the issue by *Helling* v. *Carey,* 83 Wash. 2d 514, 519 P.2d 981 (1974). While the decline of custom in medical cases has probably enjoyed a subterranean existence, the rule has not spread formally much beyond the glaucoma testing cases that gave it its birth. See, for example, *Gates* v. *Jensen*, 92 Wash. 2d 246, 595 P.2d 919 (1979).
3. The standard formulation of the doctrine reads as follows: (1) the event must be of a kind which ordinarily does not occur in the absence of someone's negligence; (2) it must be caused by an agency or instrumentality within the exclusive control of the defendant; (3) it must not have been due to any voluntary action or contribution on the part of the plaintiff [John Wigmore, *Evidence*, 1st ed. (Boston: Little, Brown, 1905), § 2509]. Note that the standard can be adapted to strict liability cases simply by eliminating the first requirement, so that it calls for a proof of causation by elimination of both third-party conduct (by 2) and plaintiff's conduct (by 3). See generally, Richard A. Epstein, *Modern Products Liability Law* (Westport, CT: Quorum Books, 1980), pp. 162-65.
4. This approach works in other contexts as well. Thus, in order to understand the legal regime for industrial accidents, it is necessary to examine the way in which the principles of products liability interact with the principles of employer's liability both before and after the advent of workers' compensation. For a discussion, see generally, Richard A. Epstein, "The Historical Origins and Economic Structure of the Workers' Compensation Law," *Georgia Law Review* 16(1982):775, which seeks to explain the restricted rights of action against manufacturers as an effort to focus liability for workplace accidents upon the employer in order to reduce litigation costs and general uncertainty.
5. See Randolph Miller and Kenneth Schaffner, "Ethical and Legal Issues Related to the Use of Computer Programs in Clinical Medicine," *Annals of Internal Medicine* 102(1985):529. Miller and Schaffner pose the question of whether computer programs should be strictly responsible for wrongful results when physicians are liable only for negligence. One argument

against that configuration is that it tends to retard the use of computer assists when they are more efficient than their rivals because of the differential burdens their use imposes.

6. This is another example of the Coase theorem, which predicts that, when transaction costs are low, voluntary exchanges that work to the benefit of both parties will take place, no matter how the original liability is set. See R. H. Coase, "The Problem of Social Cost," *Journal of Law and Economics* 3(1960):1.

7. Alan Weisbard (chapter 15) objects to my reliance on the assumption-of-risk defense, which he notes has been widely rejected by both courts and scholars in the industrial accident cases that gave it birth. He is clearly correct about the unkind reception that the defense has received in the twentieth century, but I think he is wrong on the merits. The theory of assumption of risks is that the parties themselves are the best judge of the risks they want to take. So stated, the defense is required by the principle of individual autonomy that Weisbard himself prizes. The weakness of the defense has always been the risk of imperfect information, be it by patient or employee. Yet the system of warnings is designed to obviate just that problem and to allow individual patients to make whatever level of additional search they think appropriate, given their own taste for risk and their desire for information. There is no reason to assume that parties, once informed, would not act in their best interest. In regard to industrial accidents, many large firms developed explicit voluntary compensation programs for their workers before the advent of the compulsory workers' compensation system. The emergence of such programs is wholly inconsistent with the dominant legal view that the employment relationship systematically exploited workers; yet it is wholly consistent with the view that contracts are struck for the mutual benefit of the parties.

8. The "at peril" language occurs even in nineteenth-century cases on the subject. See, for example, *Carpenter* v. *Blake*, 60 Barb. 488, 514 (N.Y. Sup. Ct. 1871), *rev'd. on other grounds*, 50 N.Y. 696 (1872). See generally Dale H. Cowan and Eva Bertsch, "Innovative Therapy: The Responsibility of Hospitals," *Jourrnal of Legal Medicine* 5(1984):219.

9. One possible rule is to make all-or-nothing determinations on a case-by-case basis, and then to award full compensation in some cases and none in others. Another method is to seek to determine the extent of the increased risk and to award compensation on a probabilistic basis. The error rates of both procedures are, of course, very high. See, for example, *Herskovits* v. *Group Health Cooperative of Puget Sound*, 99 Wash. 2d 609, 664 P.2d 474 (1983). Glen O. Robinson, "Probabilistic Causation and Compensation for Tortious Risk of Harm," *Journal of Legal Studies* 14(1985):779-98.

10. There are many cases in which the plaintiff's conduct is critical, as with operators of machine tools and drivers of automobiles. For a discussion of the mistakes that arise when this conduct is downgraded or overlooked, see Richard A. Epstein, "Products Liability as an Insurance Market," *Journal of Legal Studies* 14(1985):645-69.

11. See American Law Institute, *Restatement (Second) Torts* (St. Paul, MN: American Law Institute Publishers, 1965), §402A comment n.
12. There is an extensive literature devoted to the proposition that the optimal negligence standard, defined as taking all cost-justified precautions, will yield the same outcome on care, even if a different result on compensation. The classic formulation is still John P. Brown, "Toward an Economic Theory of Liability," *Journal of Legal Studies* 2(1973):323. But the administrative and error costs of the rule have led (rightly, in my view) to its rejection in these bad-batch cases. On the question of error costs, see, for example, Mark Grady, "A New Positive Economic Theory of Negligence," *Yale Law Journal* 92(1983):799.
13. I have elaborated on the use of custom as an antidote to imperfect information in "A Contractual Approach to Medical Malpractice," *Journal of Law and Contemporary Problems,* forthcoming.
14. See, for example, *Revised Code Washington,* 4.24.290.
15. See *Canterbury* v. *Spence,* 464 F. 2d 772 (D.C. Cir. 1972).
16. For those who doubt the proposition, see, for example, *Givens* v. *Lederle Laboratories,* 556 F. 2d 1341 (5th Cir. 1977), discussed critically in my *Modern Products Liability Law,* pp. 108-11. See also E. W. Kitch, "Vaccines and Product Liability," *Regulation* (May-June 1985):11-18.
17. For an elaboration, see Richard A. Epstein, "Medical Malpractice: The Case for Contract," *American Bar Foundation Research Journal* 1(1976): 87,119-28.
18. Weisbard (chapter 15) takes a different view on vaccines, claiming that it is socially unfair to have one person suffer from vaccine-related illness without compensation so that others may benefit. His view is that, in the absence of some legislative system of no-fault compensation, the tort system should be invoked. He thus defends the current position, as set forth in *Davis* and *Reyes* (see note 20). It is a disastrous social prescription. First, it wrongly assumes that vaccine injury raises a we-they question, where there is some determinate group of persons that benefits and another, separate group that pays. This opposition is a false one, because no one knows *ex ante* who will get what illness, with or without vaccines; but we do know that reducing the overall level of illness leaves everyone better off, even if no explicit compensation is provided *ex post.* Given the choice between a 10 percent chance of the natural disease and a 0.1 percent chance of vaccine injury, who would not assume the latter to be rid of the former?

Second, Weisbard writes as though the imposition of tort liability had no adverse allocative consequences. His position is belied by the massive disruption in vaccine markets: supplies are now being interrupted, and work on new vaccines has been cut back. In consequence, the present tort liability may push us back to a worse social state for all persons: there could be less tort liability because there are fewer vaccines. A vaccine-related compensation system may be desirable, or it may not; but there is no reason whatsoever for courts to impose perverse tort liabilities and punitive damages, against the clear weight of the evidence, because the legislature has not adopted some no-fault compensation program. It is wholly mistaken to act as if vaccines take lives while ignoring the great number of lives they save. There is no one who does not grieve at "the plight of a young girl afflicted with polio," as Weisbard states. It is precisely to minimize the number of such cases that the vaccine makers should not be made to fund a compensation program under the clumsy auspices of the tort system [see generally, P. Huber, "Safety and the Second Best: The Hazards of Public Risk Management in the Courts," *Columbia Law Review* 85(1985):277-337].

19. See the evidence collected in Patricia M. Danzon, "Tort Reform and the Role of Government in Private Insurance Markets," *Journal of Legal Studies* 13(1984):517, 522-30.
20. See, for example, *Davis* v. *Wyeth Laboratories, Inc.* 399 F. 2d 121 (9th Cir. 1968); *Reyes* v. *Wyeth Laboratories, Inc.* 498 F. 2d 1264 (5th Cir. 1974).
21. The point is stressed in Charles Fried, *Medical Experimentation: Personal Integrity and Social Policy* (Amsterdam: North-Holland, 1974), pp. 29-36.
22. Ibid., pp. 32-36.
23. See, for example, Jerry Goldman and Martin D. Katz, "Inconsistency and Institutional Review Boards," *Journal of the American Medical Association* 248(1982): 197-202.
24. Note that it is implicit in this argument that institutional uniformity accounts for far less here than it does in any mass distribution of drugs or vaccines, which I believe is the case. The variation between programs is greater, and there is no concern with inconsistent results, because the separate programs need not be subject to litigation under a common rule.
25. W. J. Dieckmann, M. E. Davis, L. M. Rynkiewicz, and R. E. Pottinger, "Does the Administration of Diethylstilbestrol During Pregnancy Have Therapeutic Value?" *American Journal of Obstetrics and Gynecology* 66(1953): 1062-81.
26. See *Beschada* v. *Johns-Manville Products Corp.*, 90 N.J. 191, 447 A. 2d 539 (1982), which laid the risk of unknowable hazards on manufacturers in asbestos cases, followed by the quick (and impenetrable) retreat in *Feldman* v. *Lederle Laboratories,* 97 N.J. 429, 479 A. 2d 374 (1984).
27. The received wisdom is otherwise. See, for example, *Stevens* v. *Parke-Davis & Co.*, 9 Cal. 3d 51, 507 P.2d 653, 107 Cal. Rptr. 45 (1973). My quarrel with that decision is not with the proposition that all adminstrative procedures are ideal, but that the costs of finding out which determinations are right and which are wrong is so fraught with error that we are better off not incurring the costs that the inquiry entails. For a defense of the cost-benefit analysis of warnings, see Alan Schwartz, "Products Liability, Corporate Structure, and Bankruptcy: Toxic Substances and the Remote Risk Relationship," *Journal of Legal Studies* 14(1985):689-736.
28. See, for example, John B. McKinlay, "From 'Promising Report' to 'Standard Procedure': Seven Stages in the Career of a Medical Innovation," *Health and Society: Milbank Memorial Fund Quarterly* 59(1981):374-411. Notwithstanding the strong criticisms of the current procedures used to

assess new drugs and therapies, McKinlay does not raise the possibility that tort liability should be imposed upon physicians who follow customary practices. For a more guarded reception of randomized controlled trials, see Fried, "Medical Experimentation," pp. 50-67.

12

The Role of Causation in Several Legal Systems

Charles M. Gray

This chapter is essentially a meditation on the usefulness of nonproximate history for practical philosophy. Practical philosophy is systematic reflection about what ought to be done in a particular situation; it raises the question free of the constraints that define rhetoric, politics, and law. Situations usually come about by stages, and that may also be true of the ways in which they are talked about—often within the constraints of rhetoric, politics, and law. That is, currently troubling situations and terms of discourse about them have proximate histories. I do not think it is obvious that working out those histories carefully and disseminating awareness of them greatly assist practical philosophy, but I think there is considerable faith in our culture that they do. What is strongly believed can turn into what is "only common sense": surely knowing how we got into this mess is the first step toward figuring out how to escape it.

I will agree that a feeling of command over the proximate history—the sense that something one is worried about is intelligible in the peculiar and elusive way things seem intelligible when their antecedents have been painfully dug up from oblivion and ordered by historians—is psychologically heartening. Perhaps that is because of the odd (paradoxical and inextricable) mix of contingency and necessity in historical explanation. Contingency and necessity are rival comforters so old they have lost the rivalry they must profess, like suitors who cannot publicly admit the arrangement they have fallen into for sharing the lady may have advantages over total conquest. "Where we are we could not help but be" and "We are where we are because of a series of accidents" are both thoughts conducive to the calm and sobriety requisite for practical philosophy. Not to blame the past, to feel with a kind of resignation that all one can do is take it from here, given the inevitable givens; not to feel trapped by ineluctable forces, so that reasoning about "oughts" appears a comedy staged for gods who have already made up their minds: both attitudes have pragmatic value.

The tendency of good historical explanation is to foster both—contradictorily enough—but the sense in which history is most an art is that, at its best, it contrives to hide the contradiction. In this respect, it is an art like poetry. Its goals are to show strong forces at work and human actors who quite evidently could have done differently than they decided to do, and to weave these two into a texture such that the warp and the woof do not seem to be at cross-purposes.

Criticism can unmask the fraud, and that too is an honorable office, but exposability does not detract from an art that consists of fending off immediate exposure. Like good poems, good histories induce a feeling of satisfying complexity, and that is what renders them intelligible; explanation by simplification has its very large place, but it is not historical explanation. Picked apart, historians' complex textures can always be shown to be less than satisfactory. There are too many pieces to be placed and related for anyone's arrangement of them to be a sure picture of things as they were, and no one's delimitation of the spheres of necessity and contingency is definitive. History in the sense of what has happened over some span of (undefinitively demarcated) time in some (inconclusively isolable) area of human life is too complex to be known—but not to be explained through the apt representation of its complexity. How we got where we are cannot be demystified, but there is such a thing as an intelligible mystery.

Philosophers are *ex professione* too wise to be cheated by bad history that tries to demystify, but perhaps they are capable of partaking of the supposed benefits of that sense of intelligible mystery that history can convey. And perhaps there is a stronger point to be made: Who *if not* the philosopher, especially in his practical role, stands particularly to gain from apprehending the moment in which he stands, with its hard problems of correct judgment and justifiable prescription, as the product of a complex past—a past too complex to be subdued, but not too complex to make a kind of sense, to have a kind of intelligibility as what had to be and need not have been, as something whose complexity is not acknowledged in the abstract but seen concretely in a representation adequate to the mysterious reality, though never the thing itself stripped of mystery. Culturally popular and institutionalized activities, of which history is one, can seem their own excuse for being, but I doubt that they usually are. If some warrant for the immense trouble of historical investigation and writing is to be found, I suspect it is mainly in the possible dependence of practical philosophy on the sense that the situations that engender it are historically intelligible. I have already said that the dependence is not obvious.

I am sure there are many historians who could make intelligent contributions to the immediate history of the situation we confront, but I am also sure that its history has not been written. Writing it would be a tall order. It would involve combining the history of modern medical science and technology with the history of modern tort law and setting both of them in the history of modern Western economic development. One would certainly have to add the history of the medical profession and medical institutions; perhaps the most interesting chapter would be that which attempted to pin down changing conceptions of health and attitudes toward medicine in various modern societies. The history of ethical discussion about medicine and the recent history of discourse about policy in the light of ethics could hardly be omitted; and so forth, no doubt.

Tall orders in history are not unusual, however. History would never be written if historians had to know enough about all they try to encompass. Much of the trick for generating significant history is getting an idea, and ideas are none the worse for seeming formidable at first sight. Given an idea, historians have their ways of making do with their own ignorance, partly by discovering the relevance and usability of related historical work that has already been done and, most essential, by applying their fundamental skill: that of making out what documents have to say. If historians, who are necessarily amateurs in everything they touch, can claim anything, it is that they can see possibilities in documentary evidence that might elude professionals. A related skill is their ability to select documents, their feeling for what can be managed and when to stop without stopping short of significant ranges of evidence.

Not infrequently the aspiration to bring everything together falters in the face of limited time and infinite complexity, and history ends where it in principle begins—in analyzing some documents and forming hypotheses on the basis of them. Curiously, this fragmentariness—the tendency of "perfect history" to turn into "commentary"—does not destroy the psychological benefits of history. It is as if no one really expected stories to be complete, so long as they are not simple, which they will not be, since they are grounded in documents. History written under the wing of a priori theories about how things happen in the world may furnish other gratifications, but it does not furnish the sense of cleared mystery or deepened mystery as to how we got where we are (on which something of our capacity to deal with where we are seems to depend).

I have insinuated a few thoughts on causality in history because history is one of the arenas, like science and law, in which causality is a common topic and because the meaning of causality is different in each.

NONPROXIMATE HISTORY

Nonproximate history is a species of ethnography. It is interested in capturing whatever difference defines one set of cultural ways as opposed to another. Nonproximate history is often attracted to the temporally remote and the visibly "other," to times and places unlikely to figure in sensibly limited accounts of how we got to where we are. That is not necessarily so, of course, just as proximate history does not have to take as its endpoint some present situation. The two kinds of history are certainly interdependent, for what I call (vaguely enough) "cultural ways" are among the most important and most easily overlooked stations on roads from A to B, and, per contra, configurations of such ways will not always stand still long enough to be caught: one's picture of them must be a compound of moments glimpsed along some such road.

Nonproximate history is of greater intrinsic philosophic interest than proximate history. I have already said by implication that I do not think somber brooding on causal explanation in history will help very much with the delicate problem of linking causality as it is understood in modern science to appropriate ethical responses. Proximate histories tell causal stories; that is, they try to make it convincing that one thing happened because of another thing. Their convincingness depends on the kind of everyday intuition whose natural genius is not to be unduly critical of itself. Nonproximate history raises problems of translation: What is it to say in this culture's language what that culture is "saying" as it goes about life and talks about it?

That sort of problem is not strictly in the province of practical philosophy. It impinges, however, because practical philosophy has an appropriate interest in whether people at some presumptive distance from our circumstances, our dilemmas, and our vocabulary might have something useful to say to us. I think the ethically perplexed in our culture are drawn to the remote in two ways—one suspect, the other quite respectable. The disreputable craving is for the refreshment of ethical relativism, the relief of seeing that the values and imperatives oppressing one with contradictory claims demanding to be reconciled do not have to be: life has proceeded under other regimes, even better ones, perhaps. I do not mean the desire is criminal, just delusory and a shallow comfort, like other fantasies—useful for getting through the day, but only temporary relief. For our freedom to dispose our values and consciences is distinctly limited: they can at best be kept in perspective and prevented, by normality and in extreme cases by therapy, from driving us mad. The second and more promising impulse is to see alternatives to how we think, to appreciate the contingency of the ways we do and possibly to become a little freer to think otherwise. Or, and the contrary is a real possibility, one might discover that the way we think is pretty much the way to think, that when differences of consciousness, of value, and of vocabulary are pared away, apparently remote cultures are playing essentially the game we play. In that event, the disappointment of discovering that there is no liberating other way to take hold of our problems would be offset by the assurance that we are on the right track and that its asperities must simply be faced.

I am aware of the paradoxicality of saying that people, even practical philosophers, are more prisoners of their culture's ethics than of its ways of thought, and I am aware of the tenuousness of the intuition that leads me to assert it. The paradox, if it is that rather than mere error, runs deep, for ethics more obviously change, belong more evidently to the realm of flux. My suggestion is that what belongs to flux must largely wait on flux, on insensible alterations in what people care about, feel guilty about, and admire—slower change than journalists and prophets with a stake in heralding the new (usually shocking) sensibility care to admit. The shock value of the new sensibility, after all, depends on the continuing vitality of the old; life in the midst of ethical flux, afflicted by competing ethical responses, is what we cannot escape by taking thought. Ways of thinking, on the other hand, while more durable and possibly in some aspects indefeasible, would seem to have a sort of prima facie susceptibility to the effects of thought. Even how you must think can hardly be the same when you see you must.

I have had a growing—I am sure a still inchoate and confused— interest in how some remote cultures within the historian's range (as opposed to the anthropologist's wider one) thought about the relatively simple and homespun matters that law deals with. This interest represents, in my case, a legal historian's effort to stand back a bit from the legal tradition that is ours—the history of the common law—ultimately in order to see whether elements in that tradition (at some distance from the modern world in time) will look different or clearer in the light of some experience beyond it. As it were, could one think about the common law better by learning to think a bit less like a common lawyer, or at any rate by having to think about legal documents, concepts, and situations that may put some strain on a common-law mentality? I can report no results from that experiment, only perform a lesser demonstration-experiment illustrative of the sort of thing I am trying to do.

I have been attempting to keep two legal worlds with the quality of "otherness" in view at once: that of ancient Greece (Athens, in effect, by reason of surviving evidence) and that of the Germanic barbarians. An attractive feature of this combination is that, on top of the many other differences between the Greeks and the barbarians, their legal orders are very differently documented (and neither system having had lawyers, neither is documented by the treatises and cases on legal issues—the lawyer's law—of the common-law tradition, nor by the treatises and commentaries of Roman lawyer's law). For Athenian law, we have abundant direct evidence of litigation in the form of speeches before the courts, preserved because they were among the works of famous rhetoricians. On the other hand, there is very scanty evidence of what the written law (conceived by the Athenians, at least on the conscious side of their minds, as "the law") said, and much of that is what the speechmakers say the law said. We have, in short, case law—but that of a lawyerless, informal system without any clear notion that decided cases make law and without any technique for defining the question before the court or separating legal and factual issues. Basically, the parties told a huge jury of hundreds of citizens (selected at random from among those who volunteered) whatever they thought would do them good: their versions of the law and the facts, piteous pleas, and dust in the jury's eyes. The party who got a majority of the jurors' votes won. Through this welter of rhetoric one has to pick one's way to a sense of how those issues that do not reduce merely to what happened were perceived.

Early Germanic law, by contrast, is largely documented by law collections. (They are sometimes called codes, but modern suggestions of the word, of comprehensiveness and of a claim to be the source from which all determinations in particular cases can and should be drawn, are extremely misleading. The neutral "collections" is as good a term as any: we have lists of laws, in the prescriptive form associated with legislation in our world.) These were typically issued and proclaimed to be the law by some tribal king. Why a particular rule occurs on these lists is never wholly apparent, since they usually do not touch everything the society is likely to have had rules about. The lists include some unmistakable acts of legislation, changes in the law made on the king's authority, usually with at least the recited pretense of consultation and general consent. It is unlikely, however, that legislation predominates over mere restatement of what was understood already to be the customary law: what is change and what is only the writing down of long-standing, agreed-on rules is always problematic, and there is little beyond internal evidence to judge by. The collections may come closer to case law than they appear to, if the occurrence of doubtful cases encouraged the propounding of rules and thus tends to explain the makeup of the lists. But these sources fail to supply just what the Greek speeches do supply—action shots of litigation, a view of what it was like to be in actual legal combat. In the one instance, we have an abundance of rules and a hard job of constructing the character of litigation from the rules (without knowing for sure even that much attention was paid to the king's pronouncements). In the other instance, we have plenty of courtroom action and a hard job of making out the rules (overlaid with uncertainty as to how firmly committed to the rules, as opposed to rough justice and free interpretation, the Athenian citizens who decided the cases were).

We owe the Athenian speeches to the fashionableness of rhetoric in antiquity, not to any felt need to preserve the record of litigation for its own sake. We owe the barbarian collections to the urge for writing down the law that took hold of German chieftains after they had moved onto the territory of the Roman Empire (it was fashionable to do as the civilized Romans were supposed to have done). In the Greek case, inferences about ordinary law have to be made from the exceptional speeches preserved for their reputed power to teach the linguistic arts; in the barbarian case, inferences about the earlier law of the unlettered tribes must be drawn from products of their later, Romanized phase. Barbarian law is top-heavy with torts— with rules for dealing with various forms of injury to the person and, in lesser degree, to property. It therefore provides plenty of material bearing on our concern with accidents and liability. Athenian law is thin on torts compared to such subjects as inheritance and commercial transactions. There are nevertheless some tort cases, and it is with one of these that I shall begin. I shall from this point perform my demonstration-experiment in two parts: first by analyzing a single Athenian case that deals with fixing liability and assigning cause for an unintended bad outcome, and then by inspecting a selected miscellany of barbarian laws touching the same matters.

THE GREEK CASE

My Greek case comes from the so-called *Tetralogy* of the rhetor Antiphon.[1] There is great doubt as to whether it is a real case, or one made up for the purpose of teaching forensic rhetoric. A suspicious, though valuable, feature is that we have speeches for both sides, whereas usually—and usually there is no reason to doubt the reality of the cases—we must make do with what one side said and construct the other side from that. (Virtually never do we have information on which side won.) But whether the case is real does not make much difference: if it is fictitious, it is a practical fiction and therefore informative as to what an experienced practitioner thought could be said to an Athenian court with some hope of success. The case is accidental homicide: in brief, a boy threw a javelin in the course of gymnastic exercises, hitting and killing another boy. Before describing the case more particularly, I must set down a few preliminaries.

In general, liability was attached to unintentional killing in Athens.[2] This is well-attested and was assumed by both sides. Just what that liability meant is the essence of this case, to which I shall return. For the moment, I will simply say that liability was not straightforwardly confined to negligent unintentional killing (and its more culpable relatives, such as reckless killing and causing death as a result of acts intended to injure but not kill—to which killing in a state of passion can possibly be added, since there is some question as to whether Athenians classified this as intentional or unintentional. I should also say that I am using the familiar words "intentional" and "unintentional" as equivalents for words that mean more exactly "willed," "willing," "willful," "voluntary," and their opposites.) Incidentally, under the law in Athens, physicians were exempt from liability for causing the death of a patient unintentionally in the course of treatment. Whether this exemption rested on an assumption of risk theory or some other ground, it removes anything that can be learned about Athenian thinking on accidents generally from applicability to "malpractice" in Athens itself.

What sanctions would the defendant in unintentional homicide be subject to if he were held liable? Outside sources suggest that he was to be exiled from Athens for an indefinite period and that he could be readmitted when the relatives of the victim agreed. If that was the system, it looks like a peculiar form of assessing damages—as if, having been convicted, I were obliged to withdraw to Indiana until I could agree with the victim's kin on the price for which they will assent to my return to Illinois. The relatives in Athens were probably under moral pressure to be reasonable rather than vengeful, more so when the killer was less at fault (taking it that liability was at least close to absolute, so that the convicted would range from the negligent or worse to the totally or nearly faultless). Even if the relatives were insensitive to moral pressure, they would have considerable financial motive to settle: you can send me to Indiana or take the $1,000 I offer you now. You may calculate that in six months I will be desperate to come home and will offer you more, but that is not the only possible effect of the running of time, and meanwhile you must do without $1,000. (Perhaps decency requires me to signify my regret and respect for your feelings by withdrawing briefly and perhaps you owe it to the dead to make sure I do so; that need not delay settlement long or prevent present settlement in the form of a contract that I will leave Illinois for a month, after which I am free to return, in consideration of my present payment of $1,000.) Plausible alternative constructions of the Athenian system would posit a short period of mandatory exile, or a period within which either the relatives must release the killer or he is free to return without their assent, or both.

In any event, there is every reason to think that Athenian sanctions for unintentional homicide were far removed from the mandatory death penalty imposed upon conviction of intentional homicide, to which the only alternative was voluntary perpetual exile prior to conviction with loss of property. An added feature of our case is that some language suggests that the defendant (the father of the juvenile javelin thrower) is pleading for his son's life, but I do not think it has to be so taken. The hint to that effect can probably be construed as hyperbole, which could be a significant indication that not being convicted for homicide was important in Athens, even if the risk of liability's being costly was slight—conviction being a disgrace and carrying the implication that the taker of a life owes a life, even though in current law the price was not exacted.

A second question: How unique is homicide? It was certainly unique in several ways in Athenian law. Fear of pollution demanded a societal response when someone was killed, and the ghost of the victim demanded action from his kin. On the assumption that pollution is quasi-mechanistic and that ghosts are angry at being dead by human hand without a nice concern for the doer's fault, one is inclined to infer strict liability in homicide (although through the case I shall be suggesting grounds for caution on that). There is no necessary reason to extend it to other harms. The pollution and ghost-involvement that tend to set homicide apart attract observers' attention, and so they should, but it is also true that what they express can be rather easily secularized. Even in modern societies, death is sobering when it is not natural, neither "in due course" nor by natural disaster, but when human doings that could have been different are in the picture. Emotions felt and decencies demanded are not the same as when other injuries occur. Yet deaths involving human agency seem in the end to get sorted out along the lines of tort law in general. I do not think there is any reason to suppose that was not true in Athens. There were sanctions and procedures peculiar to homicide, but the basic distinctions were probably applied across the board—intentional versus unintentional (roughly); acting directly with intent to harm versus pursuing such intent by conspiracy or accompliceship; being connected versus not being connected with an accident in a way that can be thought of as "doing" the harm. Within the area of the unintentional, there are reasons to expect disregard for the doer's fault in homicide (whether or not it was in fact disregarded). I do not think there are evident grounds for doubting that the same problem—Do we take account of fault *quoad* liability, not only *quoad* damages?—would arise in case of other injuries, nor for supposing that a different answer would have been reached systematically. In short, I do not think that the javelin case is necessarily vitiated as evidence for more general ways of thinking about liability by being a homicide case. We have no good cases on other sorts of accidents.

The facts of the javelin case do not appear to be at all in dispute: the defendant's son took his regular turn in javelin practice and made a completely competent throw. Whether or not it was an absolutely perfect throw, the javelin was headed at the target; the throw could not be criticized as even slightly wild. The victim was standing on the sidelines at the target end of the range, together with other onlookers, including the coach (*paidotribes*). Probably these onlookers included, if they did not consist entirely of, javelin practicers in another squad who had already taken their turns at the throwing end or were waiting to do so. Nothing, however, is made of whether the victim had in some way assumed a risk, was in a special position to know the danger of the sport in which he was participating, or could otherwise be differentiated from a spectator. Though we are given no physical details, there is no dispute that the onlookers standing on the sidelines were outside any significant danger of being hit by a javelin thrown with anything like normal competence. The coach told the victim to go pick up javelins lying around the target. In performing this errand, he ran across the path along which the throwers were making their throws and was fatally hit by the javelin thrown by the defendant's son. There is no suggestion that the defendant saw the victim start, or poised to start, on a potentially lethal dash, nor that the victim noticed the thrower on the verge or in the motion of throwing. Either could presumably have avoided the accident by paying a moment's more attention to what was going on at the other end of the range, but "he just forgot to look" seems more applicable to the victim than to the boy concentrating on his throw, who had every reason, in the setting of the activity in progress, to expect others to be careful.[3]

The issue in the case is the meaning of the principle of Athenian law that liability for homicide is not confined to intentional killing. There is nothing to suggest that the principle was anywhere in the texts of the law stated so as to make any distinctions within the class of unintentional homicide. The present case represents the law as saying "Killing is forbidden whether it is just or unjust." Whether "unjust" is equivalent to "intentional" seems open to question, though most cases of killing on purpose would be unjust. Perhaps killing negligently—by departure from the standard of care that is regarded in the community as customary, reasonable, or in the general interest—would be considered unjust (as well as such cases as reckless killing or, more questionably, killing when possessed by strong passion). Proclaiming it a matter of indifference whether a killing is just or not perhaps points more clearly to a strict liability system than proclaiming the indifference of whether a killing is intentional, since the latter leaves it open whether liability attaches to *all* unintentional killing.

The parties in our case *essentially* assume strict liability. If A killed B, there is liability, and some detriment should fall on A, assuming that A alone was the killer and B was simply killed (that is, that he was in no way an active contributor to his own death). There is no overt argument that A's non-negligence should absolve him. I shall show that one line of argument in the case seeks in a subtle way to qualify strict liability, without contesting it *per verba*. This may come closer to insinuating a negligence standard than appears on the surface, but for the moment let us take the system as what it at least nominally was—strict liability. There is nothing shocking or primitive about that, and it is not shocking in homicide if the sanctions are essentially compensatory. For the case farthest removed from death, pollution, and ghosts: there is no obvious reason why the unlucky, wholly blameless breaker of a window should go unscathed while the unlucky wholly blameless householder is out $10, just as there is no reason the other way, unless at some level of policy or subtlety beyond the obvious. The only thing that is *plain* reason is that the loss should be shared somehow, if not more widely, at least between doer and victim.

Whether this is a drawback or a strength, strict liability focuses causality problems as it eliminates standard of care problems. The victim's contribution is one form of causality problem, the one that is relevant in our case. Was the javelin thrower's act the cause of the victim's death in as real or significant a sense as the victim's own act? Should we say that the thrower killed the victim and therefore is liable even though he did not mean to, or that the victim killed himself, equally unintentionally, wherefore there is no killing for which anyone can be meaningfully held liable? This is essentially what the parties are arguing about. The question is, On what basis can one say which party really or significantly caused the death? Can this be done without referring to blameworthiness, that is, without allowing the moral or judgmental vocabulary that strict liability appears to eliminate to reenter the discussion? If A and B jointly caused B's death, and A was not negligent while B was negligent, can we resist the conclusion that B was more significantly the cause of his death? If we cannot, if we have to let negligence in by the back door, is it coherent to bar the front door to it? Do we really mean that liability does not derive from negligence? If the non-negligent participant is released from liability because the other party was negligent, should he not be released from liability *simply* because there was no negligence on his side (though it may be advantageous to presume negligence—that is, throw the burden of making out that there was none on the defendant)? In their Greek vocabulary and with their Greek sensitivities, the parties in the case are struggling with these questions. The most important fact about their vocabulary is that negligence is not the critical word for something like *culpa,* some sort of deviation from acting just as you ought in some sense of ought.

The defendant's essential contention is what we would expect: my son would be liable if he had killed the victim, but he did not kill him; his death was the result of his own actions. Those actions were the real, or significant, cause of his death, so much the more decisive contribution to the result that we cannot for legal purposes be said to have killed him or caused his death. But this is not quite the defendant's way of putting it. Rather, he says that his son did not kill the victim because the victim committed *hamartia* "with regard to himself." Herewith, at the start of the defense, the most important word for the discussion is introduced.

We would expect the defendant, were he to depart from the spare language of causality, to say the victim perished because he was negligent. *Hamartia* cannot, however, be translated as simply "negligence." It is a complex word in Greek, with usages ranging from the paradigmatic "missing a target" to grave moral offense. (When it occurs in the New Testament, it is translated "sin.") We shall see several meanings in the javelin case. It seems to me, however, that the word does not require radical "family relation" analysis; usages have the common ground, "deviation from—or lack of complete success in fulfilling—a course of action one has in mind or intends, actual or putative."

Defendant's first use of *hamartia*, then, is to say that the victim committed it and died as a result. Clearly the victim meant to do his errand of picking up the javelins without getting hurt, and in this project he failed. Perhaps that is enough to lay *hamartia* on him, but it is obvious in addition that his misjudgment or inattention partly explains the failure (the thrower's throwing just when and how he did being the rest of the explanation). If we impute to everyone the intention of carrying on one's activity within the community's standard of care, the victim failed to (on any sane construction of the standard); his *hamartia* would amount to negligence. Negligence systems could be said to pick out deviation from this putative intention as the significant form of *hamartia*.

The defendant next concedes that he would be liable if his javelin had gone off course. There is no suggestion that this is a possibility rather than a certainty, that is, no qualification of the form "if victim had not also made mistakes (or been negligent)" or "if victim's acts had not in some more vivid sense than the thrower's caused the accident." The suggestion is rather that once *hamartia*—in some sense that is significant, and the most primitive sense, "misthrow," is one—can be pinned on a contributor, no further questions need be asked: liability is established. The defendant proceeds to generalize: the *doers* of unintentional ("not willed") things are those who commit *hamartia* as they *epinoesosi* (intend, have it in mind) to do something. I believe there is a conceptual point: you can't say A did something to B unless you mean either (1) A had it in mind to do that to him and succeeded or (2) A made an error—committed *hamartia*—in doing something else he had in mind to do (or in failing to do what he had in mind as he meant to do it), as a result of which B suffered. That A made a causal contribution to B's injuries, which injury he in no sense intended, is not represented as the *first* reality, after which it is necessary to ask whether A did anything wrong, wrong in what sense and degree, whether B's acts partly explain the injury, whether they were in any way wrong, and so on. Rather, there is nothing to start with, no possibility of saying that A did anything to (or acted on, or caused a state of affairs in) B unless something that would count as *hamartia* can be attributed to A. Without that, all you can say is that something happened to B. I cannot arbitrate whether this apparent conceptual point is about ordinary language or legal ideas. ("It's funny Greek to say A killed B unintentionally unless you mean there was some *hamartia* on A's side" versus "In contemplation of law, an unintentional homicide is a death resulting from an action tainted with *hamartia*.")

The defendant then makes his minor premise explicit: the thrower did everything *orthos* (correctly) as he intended; therefore he "did nothing unintentional." He failed of his goal (hitting the target) only because something (the victim's act) prevented him; not hitting the target was something that happened to the thrower, not something he did. In addition, however, the bare sense of "no *hamartia*"—no misthrow—is supplemented by language sounding in moral rectitude of a sort; the thrower was also in no way doing what he should not have been where and when he was doing it, in no way departed from the general path of usual, approved, expected, comme il faut behavior. The suggestion is that some irregularity, such as going out of turn, though free of either technical error or negligence, could still count as *hamartia*—but there was nothing of the sort. Then the defendant reiterates that the victim did commit *hamartia*, describing this in the minimal terms that require no reference to a putative intention to take "reasonable" care (he mistook the moment at which he could have run across the range without getting hit).

Note the static between this return to a focus on the victim and the conceptual point: one suggestion is that, without *hamartia* in the thrower, the question of his liability does not arise. Refocusing on the victim suggests that, even if the thrower were without *hamartia*, the question of his liability would arise, were it impossible to pin *hamartia* on the victim. The thought behind the second possibility is intimated. I believe it can be spelled out as follows:

The victim's acts were tainted with *hamartia*, therefore he "killed himself" or caused his own death. Unless we can say somebody killed somebody, all we can say is that somebody's death "just happened." One might then be tempted to say so be it: a death with the appearance of having occurred through human acts that could have been different may turn out, because none of the human acts were tainted with *hamartia*, to be a mere unfortunate happening. The law has no interest in those. The trouble with this is that it leaves a death unresponded to or unpaid for (although that may be necessary when the death is the gods' doing, the doing of those from whom the dead and their connections have no power to demand requital). Such unresponsiveness was not quite acceptable to Greek sensibility. For example, Athenian law, like many other systems, provided a ritual analogous to condemning and punishing the doer when death was attributable to an animal or inanimate object. "If you can find someone or something to take payment from, take it" seems to be the operative maxim. Therefore, in a case involving human activity, where, for want of *hamartia*, there is nobody who did it, it may still be preferable to respond, to take payment where it can be taken, out of the involved human beings who are still alive. The primal justice of seeing that death is requited, if it can be done without making futile, improper, or dangerous demands on the gods, outweighs justice as fairness by graspable human standards.

The answer to this line of argument is to say that, where the victim alone has committed *hamartia,* primal justice is satisfied by his suffering—and this, in effect, the defendant says. If there were *hamartia* on the thrower's side, he would pay, probably without reference to *hamartia* on the victim's side. If there were no *hamartia* on either side, the thrower might still have to pay (on the basis of the argument above). If there is *hamartia* on the victim's side only, then requital has been made in the same sense in which requital would have been made if there had been *hamartia* on the thrower's: someone errs, someone "does something" to someone, and the erring and "doing" person pays. Here the victim erred, therefore has done something to himself, and by dying he has paid for "error causing unintended harm." It would be superfluous to exact more.

If this sounds tortuous, the plaintiff thought so too. He accuses the defendant of sophistry, and the defendant later admits that he has spoken with exceptional subtlety and precision—in the interest of justice and correct application of the law, of course. It is noteworthy that the defendant is arguing for an interpretation of Athenian law that we might think the more civilized: (1) liability absolutely without fault is dubious (though "fault" need not be given the sense of "negligence"); (2) if in some circumstances liability without fault is a lesser evil than letting the losses fall where they may, fault in the victim should at any rate exonerate faultless persons involved in the accident. But saying these things in Greek was not easy; it sounded sophistical.

Perhaps the trickiest point in the defendant's position is his argument that what resulted from the victim's *hamartia*, his death, also counts as payment for his *hamartia*. (Consider the solo actor who errs and perishes. One may feel no urge to say "justice was done" or "he paid for this mistake," but if one does it is necessary to count the same state of affairs as both the result of the error and the requital. In his speech in reply, the plaintiff does not in any event pounce on this difficulty. He mainly contends that it is common sense to say the thrower killed the victim, and not common sense to say the victim killed himself; to contrive an objection to the ordinary way of speaking is sophistry. The plain meaning of the law, per plaintiff, is that killers in this ordinary sense pay. Why else would the law insist that the "justice" of a killing is irrelevant for liability? I presume the plaintiff would say, though he does not enter deeply into the metaphysics, that the law's rationale is that killings should be paid for when there is some person or thing that can be reached and made to pay (even if only symbolically, in the case of nonhuman things). Human causers, in however rough and everyday a sense, are the obvious payers. To get fancy in order to avoid a payment or response is to cross the law's purpose. No amount of talk about whose *hamartia* was the cause can break the pattern common sense perceives and the law assumes or endorses: the thrower did something, the victim had something done to him, and primal justice asks that something be done back to the doer.

Apart from this principal contention, the question arises as to whether the plaintiff also concedes something to the defendant's argument and tries to show that it is nevertheless rebuttable. I think he does, though the logic does not stand out sharply from the text. The plaintiff makes an effort to pin something that would count as *hamartia* on the thrower, as if to concede that there might be an oddity in saying "A killed B without wanting to" unless one meant to assign *hamartia* to A. The plaintiff urges that the thrower did, after all, mistake the moment at which someone was going to pick up the spent javelins. This amounts to using the vocabulary of *hamartia* to state the principle of absolute liability: until the contrary (a lethal intention) is alleged and proved, everybody has a putative intention to act in such a way that no one else gets hurt, including those who recklessly expose themselves to danger; miscarriage of this intention counts as *hamartia*. In addition, the plaintiff uses, without elaboration, one more judgmental word to characterize the thrower—*akolasia*, or unrestraint, indiscipline, abandon. The suggestion in the word is not developed into a claim that the thrower was abnormally disregardful of the risk that someone might get in the way; perhaps it need not mean so much that the thrower was culpably inattentive, as that he was just going about his business without checking himself and therefore *in fact* not noticing what was going on at the other end of the range—*hamartia* enough, according to the plaintiff. The word is in any event presumably meant to help the jury think that it goes too far simply to clear the thrower of *hamartia* and thereby to bring in question the intelligibility of calling him an unintentional killer.

If this point is won, the plaintiff is in a position to make a stronger concessionary argument: very well, there was *hamartia* on both sides. So what? There is a concession to what the plaintiff does not believe, that the victim can be said to have commited *hamartia*. His real belief is that the victim's obvious mistake was not legally significant *hamartia*, because a miscarriage of the putative intention to do what one does without injury to oneself does not count. This only reformulates the position that being "done to," at any rate done to death, demands a responsive "doing" to the doer, whatever the explanation of the accident may be. The victim's freedom from *hamartia* in this sense is reinforced by the plaintiff's observation that he acted on the coach's order. The plaintiff may fear that the jury will not buy the relatively abstract argument that error with respect to one's own safety is never legal *hamartia*; it may be taken as such if the erring victim is seen as departing from the standard course of good behavior (the putative intention to behave as mores require a person in a given role or situation to behave); it therefore helps to show that the victim was being a good boy, obeying the teacher, however ineptly. (This part of the argument corresponds to the defendant's felt need to clear the thrower of any misbehavior, over and above clearing him of mistake in the immediate act of throwing.)

Granting that there was *hamartia* on both sides, what then? According to the plaintiff, both parties erred and by erring jointly caused the accident. Both should pay. The victim already has, as the defendant maintains, and now it is the thrower's turn. The plaintiff has in effect embraced, as his fallback position, the theory that costs should be shared between co-causers, without tortuous attempts to make out that there was more causal weight on one side than the other. (A simplification is to share costs between victim and doer, thereby avoiding attempts to distinguish between actively contributing and merely passive victims.) The plaintiff's preferred position, however, is that the victim was not a co-causer, for want of *hamartia* with regard to anything but his own safety. (This position generalizes to "whenever someone suffers injury as at least the partial direct result of other people's doings, he should be compensated, no matter what; whatever can be said for collective compensation, it is at any rate better that the other people involved bear the full cost than that the injured bear any beyond the incompensable pain of having been hurt, of simply having been on the losing end of human interaction.")

The final speech, the defendant's replication, contains three new elements with a concession-and-rebuttal structure. Its main purpose, however, is to restate the defendant's original position in a way that displays sensitivity to its vulnerable points. The defendant recognizes the oddity of saying the victim killed himself. He is now careful to refine that almost to a manner of speaking: all we mean is that the victim *acted*—with *hamartia*—and as a result perished. The implication is that there is a category of passive victim whose causal contribution to the accident by merely being where he was does not count in the legal calculus. Such a passive victim would either be killed by the active party or by nobody (if the actively involved party must be touched with *hamartia* in order to say "he killed unintentionally"). Perhaps a *hamartia*-free active party would have to pay, on the ground that somebody's paying is a lesser evil than nobody's (possibly even if the passive victim's being where he was could be tainted with *hamartia*: Possibly you should, and do, pay for killing yourself, but perishing by your own fault would be different). But in this case the victim was not passive.

For the concessionary points: first, the defendant is willing to entertain the possibility that the coach was the killer rather than the victim himself. The plaintiff says the victim was free of *hamartia* because he was obeying the coach. Very well, why isn't he suing the coach, who is presumably subject, as the thrower is not, to the claim that he misperformed in his role and failed in his putative intent to see that the practice session proceeded safely? (Note the apparent absence of concern about intervening human action. The coach is not ineligible as the killer because, however inadvisedly he acted in giving his order or giving it without sufficient warning to take care, avoidable mistakes on the victim's part were closer to the accident than the coach's error. Juvenility in the intervening actor may be held to defeat the effect an intervening mistake would normally have. It is hard to say whether the age of the principals complicates the debate. Nothing is expressly made of it in such form as saying that what would be *hamartia* in an adult need not be in an adolescent.)

Second, the defendant makes an argument that adheres to his position that no *hamartia* can be placed on the thrower as an individual, but he concedes that the victim's *hamartia* might be irrelevant—in other words, he concedes that a payment is due, whatever can be said about the victim's contribution. But from whom is payment due? The defendant's answer: all the participants in the practice session. Since the thrower whose particular throw resulted in the death cannot be singled out for having made a mistake or having violated the good order of the enterprise in process, the only place to put the blame or liability is on the enterprise as a whole, assuming the victim cannot be exclusively blamed or be said to have paid for his error. All participants partook of the unfortunate outcome; none is more chargeable with *hamartia* than another. If there was *hamartia* in a minimal sense, that something turned out otherwise than it was meant to, then it was simply the enterprise, the whole way it was conducted, that went wrong; everybody who was part of it should be in the defendant's seat. There is no elaboration of how the enterprise could have been "more correctly" conducted, that is, conducted so as to reduce the risk that the putative intention of having safe javelin practice would fail, but of course ways can be imagined if there is any need to think beyond the fact that the enterprise went wrong. The defendant's concern is only to show that it makes no sense to single out a cog in the machine, a cog that worked exactly as it was supposed to. He does not go into the practical and procedural feasibility of prosecuting all the participants jointly or severally, for his concern is only to show that it makes no sense to be prosecuting him singly.

Third, the defendant at last comes around to language that sounds in negligence. He does not say that the victim's *hamartia* consisted in negligence, but that there was not only the *hamartia* of the boy, but also the *aphylaxia*. *Aphylaxia* means not being on guard, not watching out—very close to not being as careful as one can reasonably be expected to be. The defendant goes on to use the language of negligence and last clear chance, with which we are familiar. The thrower saw no one running across his path, so how could he have watched out so as to avoid hitting anyone? The victim did see people throwing at the other end and could easily have watched out so as not to run across.

What does this argument mean in context? It will not defeat the plaintiff's ultimate position that "someone is dead with human agents involved, and someone other than or in addition to the dead man must pay." But the argument alters the way in which the question—Do you really, gentlemen of the jury, think the law has *that* dire a meaning?—is posed. It changes the balance between the parties in a concessionary manner: the plaintiff wants to pin *hamartia* on the thrower. Very well, let him; but there is something else—*aphylaxia*—of which he is free. The plaintiff wants to render the victim's *hamartia* irrelevant, but need the more specific fault—not being as careful as he should have been—also be irrelevant? Say there was no *hamartia* on either side or there was *hamartia* on both sides and perhaps the contributing party who has not suffered must pay. But need we come to the same conclusion when the parties can be unbalanced in terms of *aphylaxia*?

While I can only guess at this final point, I suspect that in reaching *aphylaxia*, in making explicit what no one sitting there listening to the speeches could fail to be thinking, the defendant would have done himself good. Who would not, sitting there, feel it rather a pity to convict a well-behaved and faultless young man for a damn fool's death (or perhaps a rash kid's, for which perhaps a careless coach should share the blame)? Am I slipping into anachronism or out of Greek when I ask that? I am not sure. Athenian tort law was not a negligence system. One could not stand up and say in the first instance, No *aphylaxia*, no liability; or the victim had the last clear chance to avoid catastrophe and failed to watch out—the defendant is clear whatever else. But then Athenian law was not very rigid and was not lawyerized. If you were not negligent, or if your victim was, were you *in fact* very likely to be convicted? We have no way of knowing. Clearly the law and the language required you to *talk* a different and more complicated game.

THE BARBARIAN CASES

Whereas personal injury and accident are rarely the subjects of the Athenian cases we know about, torts, though not accidents as such, dominate in the collections of Germanic law. (The survival of evidence for Athens says nothing about the actual incidence of kinds of litigation, for the fame of the speechwriter is the reason the speech was preserved. On the whole, it made more sense for a person who stood to lose a large inheritance to employ Demosthenes than for a person who had suffered a broken arm.) For my brief contrasting sketch of barbarian law, I concentrate on situations in which establishing liability or identifying the causer of damage is problematic. They shed such light only marginally. A few fundamentals of early Germanic law need to be described in order to set the context.[4]

The single largest element in the law collections is the prescription of specific monetary compensation for specific injuries. The injuries are mainly bodily, but insults and offenses to dignity of various specific sorts (for example, hair pulling and provoking or committing a fracas in someone's house, whether or not any damage is done to him or his furniture) are included, as are some particular offenses against property. These laws are of the "If a man breaks a man's nose, let him pay $20" sort. The tariffs of compensation are often worked out minutely: so much for a front tooth and so much less for a molar, a separate price for each finger, and the like. (Barbarian law is only one historical precedent or comfort for modern insurers and governments that feel compelled, for their purposes, to specify what they will pay in compensation for, or toward the treatment of, particular medical "bad states.") The promi-nence of such price specifications in barbarian law does not mean that mone-tary compensation by assessed damages was unknown: it was used in most cases of damage to property, where how much the owner is injured depends on what the stolen or destroyed property is worth or how much repairs will cost. Neither the tort-centeredness of the law nor the heavy use of fixed compensations implies an exclusively civil or compensatory system. The barbarian societies had criminal law in the form of payments to the king and other penalties over and above payment, fixed or assessed, to the injured party. In addition, express penal damages payable to the party (a multiple of assessed damages) were due for some torts, and there was almost certainly an element of penalty in the quantification of fixed compensations. By and large, prosecution rested with the injured, even when an offense was penal as well as compensable. (Athens also lacked public prosecution, though it permitted persons not injured to prosecute for some offenses, keeping all—or, as the case might be, part—of the discretionary or preset penalty.)

The background of precise compensation setting in written barbarian law was probably a self-help, or "feuding," system. When someone suffered what was perceived as damage, he was entitled to take satisfaction without the endorsement of anything so formal as a court or similar institution. It is a fair guess that in early Germanic society "entitled" was close to "obliged": societies vary in their estimate of the duty one has to respond when harm has come upon one from someone else. Although we know little of Germanic law behind the written collections, it is a virtual certainty that a system permitting self-help will be hedged about by at least general moral beliefs as to how a person entitled to take satisfaction or revenge from an injurer should conduct himself. He will probably be expected to demand satisfaction from the injurer before taking it (to give the injurer a chance to pay up and make peace voluntarily or to propose another amount or mode of satisfaction than that originally demanded). He will probably be expected to haggle for a reasonable time if settlement is not immediate. Both sides will be regarded as normal and decent only if they bring their friends and relatives into the negotiations, an expansion of the argument that will permit a testing of public support for the adversaries and give the natural backers of each a chance to urge restraint on their overeager connections. Willingness to consider arbitration if settlement is sticky will be regarded as at least commendable. There will be at least rough notions of what compensation is reasonable for a particular kind of damage. (For the early Germans, there is every reason to suppose that seeking a penal or vengeance satisfaction over and above reparation of economic loss would have been approved when the damage was done on purpose and that satisfaction for insults was at least as properly demanded as material reparation.) The parties' conformity to such general standards is likely to have a great deal to do with the de facto outcome of a tort case. Even when social tolerance of or taste for feuding is relatively high, people will not generally be willing to defy the opinion of the community by taking unreasonable satisfaction, refusing reasonable satisfaction, or helping themselves without the due process that even courtless communities have a form of. If they are disregardful of their reputations, they must think twice lest third parties come forcibly to the aid of the other side and lest even their friends and kin desert them. (This may take a while where loyalties to relatives, protégés, and protectors are strong, but loyalty to chronic troublemakers can wear out.)

It is uncertain how far the Germanic tribes had advanced beyond a pure self-help system before their occupation of Roman territory. It is likely enough that they had arrived at some institutionalization of the simple truth that formalizing legal process helps; that is, that there will be fewer unwarranted attacks by persons seeking satisfaction and fewer counterresponses escalating to feuds if the offended are required to make their demands for satisfaction publicly—to or in something like a court—and if there is a more regular procedure than negotiation for clearing up at least some of the disputes that can arise (as when an accused person disclaims responsibility for what has happened to the accuser). How effective attempts to insist on public process—as opposed to mere reasonableness in private dealings—will be depends on the strength with which communal opinion condemns those who pay no attention to the process (who may otherwise be perceived as justified and well-behaved) and on the muscle of kings and chiefs who set themselves up as the sponsors of public process.

A further step in the right direction is for a court at its discretion (or the law, by anticipation of cases and specification) to say just what an accuser who can establish his entitlement to satisfaction is entitled to. This is a trickier step than it appears to be and one which was not unambiguously taken by Germanic law even in the historical period, when the written laws were promulgated. (The still further step—collection or infliction of the court-awarded satisfaction by a public official, as opposed to the entitled party's using such means as he can and such force as he needs—shows little sign of having been contemplated in the period of the written laws, as it was generally not in Greek and Roman law.) We cannot know how specific people's ideas of reasonable satisfaction were before we find compensations specified in the written laws. But the best hypothesis is that extreme specification is precisely the function and the advantage of law laid down by a king and written down at his behest. In other words, people are unlikely to carry around in their heads figures expressing the exact proportion between the price of a cut-off middle toe and that of a fractured tibia, though they may well have general notions of what would be a reasonable or an outrageous demand.

Quantification need not have waited on writing and the supposed imitation of Roman ways, and it almost certainly did not altogether. All that is necessary for precise figures to enter the customary bloodstream, as it were, is frequent resort to arbitration: an arbitrator says, You must let the man who broke your nose off if he pays you $20; the figure sticks in people's minds and becomes the reasonable sum when similar cases occur. If kings and chiefs often find themselves in the arbitrator's role, or use their prestige and muscle to see that they do, the function of deeming how much a reasonable man will ask and give may be highly associated with those personages, and they may begin to accumulate a body of judicial precedents. It seems nevertheless likely that both writing and kings (in the self-conscious posture of setters-down of law) were great encouragements to the settlement on and proliferation of precise figures. There is nothing like writing to keep memory from going vague and nothing like sitting down to say, These are my laws to encourage a king to extend a useful institution. That is, the king is encouraged to pronounce that I, the king, *will* expect men who have lost an ear to be satisfied with $50, even as I record that the victims of broken noses *have* been told—perhaps so often that it is engraved in communal notions of reasonableness—that $20 is enough. I am, of course, saying that the written law collections in their most typical aspect are likely to have a distinct, though not exclusive, legislative side.

The best argument for what I have just said is an article from the earliest written Lombard laws which straightforwardly says the king is raising the prices of various torts because the old prices were too low to prevent feuding. [5] This is manifestly legislation—departure from prior custom for a reason—not the recording of custom. The article also goes to show that quantification antedates written law. Whether *as much* quantification as is pretended raises a question: Were there really already certain prices for a large number of injuries to be revised upward, or a mixture of some outdated settled prices and areas of vagueness now for the first time settled at currently realistic sums? Finally, the article demonstrates the end and the peril of the game: the goal is to lay down what the offended party must take if offered, and to hit a figure that the claimant and the public will consider sufficient; otherwise the offended will help themselves anyway, and communal sentiment and force will be on their side. The king is under no illusion that he commands the force to compel men to accept significantly less than they think their just due.

By and large, barbarian compensation law states what you must be content with if the injurer will offer you that. If he will not or cannot come up with the money or negotiate an alternative, you may help yourself. While moral restraints would probably hedge what you may do, you would not, on the whole, be in the position of someone who is simply owed $20 and is entitled to take whatever steps the law authorizes to collect simple debts. There are signs that barbarian law distinguished, morally and procedurally, between debt collection and vengeance, or rightful self-help to obtain satisfaction for a per-ceived injury. Although the debt-collection law is hard to reconstruct, it was probably in the nature of distraint: the right to seize property and hold it hostage until the debt is paid (not to liquidate it). An injured person left unsatisfied by the legally endorsed payment was not so confined; within reason, anyway, he could inflict retaliatory injury or seize and liquidate property without a nice concern for its equivalence to the compensation he would have had to put up with if it had been forthcoming.[6]

One basis for positing a distinction between debt collection and vengeance legitimated by refusal to pay the legal compensation is that it was sometimes used to implement a distinction between intentional and accidental injuries That is, there are some laws that permit the offended to feud if they are not properly compensated for intentional injuries, while the victims of humanly caused accidents are confined to collecting the compensation as if it were a debt. Such laws are evidence of what there is no reason to doubt: compensatory response was expected whether or not the injury was inflicted on purpose. The laws fixing compensations do not on the face of it interfere with the assumption that the nose breaker must come up with the same $20 whether he meant to do it or not. Within the class of unintentional harms, there is nothing to suggest that a line was drawn between a pure accident in which a human hand is visible and injuries resulting from negligence or from some more inclusive or slightly different "deviation from the intended, the expected, or the proper," which the Greek word *hamartia* captures. In short, we have again to do with what can be called *essentially* a strict liability system. And again we shall be faced with the problems raised by such a system, including the question of whether it was true to its essential principle in practice. That question cannot be approached without referring to procedure.

Judicialized barbarian law relied primarily on oath helping. When someone was charged with a wrong (subject to whatever procedure there was for scrutinizing complaints and screening out frivolous ones, an obscure point for most barbarian systems), he had to find swearers to back up his own oaths disclaiming liability. The amount of swearing power needed to clear a particular class of person from a particular charge was minutely regulated in some barbarian systems. The oath helpers were not witnesses to facts but affirmers of their belief in the defendant's truthfulness and in the justice of his case. How oath helping worked in practice is not directly accessible. The critical feature is that the defendant had to go out and raise his own support. The interesting questions are how difficult that was and how people's consciences—reinforced by fear of divine vengeance for false swearing and loss of reputation and legal capacity if it ever came out—directed their willingness to serve as oath helpers. This bears on the realistic meaning of strict liability. Would people in fact help clear defendants because they thought them faultless? Did helpers, and defendants themselves, clearly conceive it as their duty to swear away the charge *only* if they believed the defendant did not cause the harm? Would they swear on the basis of a vaguer, more impressionistic belief in the defendant's "in-the-rightness," which might include the belief that he was so clear of blame (including negligence) that the spirit of the law demanded no compensation? If that goes too far, would they have felt comfortable about narrowing the range of causation, thinking, Oh well, I can swear in this case—it doesn't seem to me that the things this defendant did have to be considered *why* the plaintiff suffered the harm? We have little basis for resolving these questions, though the formal law does provide evidence, of which I shall give some examples, that some human acts that would be thought of now as legal causes were not so conceived. Ideas of causality do not, presumably, come first historically, and they are not born as full-blown abstractions. Causing emerges out of blaming; and perhaps the question, Was he really to blame? is easier on consciences than questions framed in causal language (granted he was involved, he is my cousin and a good deal of pressure and preference may be on the side of my finding excuses to go ahead and swear).

Some written laws reflect dissatisfaction with oath helping, to which the response was to introduce ordeals for certain sorts of accused wrongdoers or to limit the defendant's choice of helpers. Too easy clearance, too much perjury, must have been the problem. I suspect that notorious intentional offenders were at the heart of that: bad eggs who had escaped suspiciously often by finding other bad eggs to swear for them. But it is not out of the question that lax application of strict liability principles provoked some of the dissatisfaction with oath helping and its milder reforms: too few victims of accidents got compensation; ordinary respectable people found it too easy to swear for their friends and relatives when there was no sharp culpability. The harm in that may be that the uncompensated would take compensation into their own hands.

I have said enough to make the point that, although explicit barbarian law often does not make any distinction between intended and unintended harm, it does, in quite a few places, recognize the accident. There are some harms, mostly to property, where the injured's compensation is penal only if (or more penal when) the harm is intentional. Particularly in Lombard law, the system's procedural reliance on swearing was sometimes enlisted to permit the defendant to disclaim intention by an unsupported oath (that is, without helpers), and thence to enjoy the benefits of being the merely accidental causer of the harm.[7] Perhaps one can say there is just enough express differentiation of accident in the laws to make it somewhat puzzling how the societies managed without differentiating it more systematically. Hypothesizing that distinctions tended to be made behind the veil of the oath-helping system is the likeliest solution. If the injured holds out for the full fixed compensation in an accidental case, especially one where culpability is low, he may get nothing at all: people will swear for a defendant who has behaved well and offered part payment proportionate to the circumstances. My guess is that, if you wanted help, you had better not try to get away with paying nothing on the ground that you were not even negligent. By and large, negligence was not a category of the barbarian systems, perhaps because compensation was as realistically flexible as it was nominally rigid. If it is possible to award a good deal less than even economic damages—perhaps amounts tending to settle around equal cost sharing between doer and victim—there may be no point in talking about negligence in any formal way. If a doer pretty obviously was not watching what he was doing, he will pay more—the full tariff if he is not alacritous with apologies and a generous offer—and the negligent plaintiff may get nothing. Even so, something like negligence appears here and there in the laws.

Burgundian law has a neatly drafted article on how a wolf trap must be constructed if the trapper is to avoid liability when someone accidentally gets caught.[8] In addition to observing the construction standards, the trapper must give notice of his setting the trap. Even so, if a free man is killed, the trapper must pay some fraction of the set compensation for death; there is no liability for a killed slave, and apparently none for lesser injuries. There are a few laws of the same type in other collections (if a fence is constructed or a wall protected in the prescribed way, the owner is not liable for accidents).[9]

Such laws testify to the accessibility of the idea of a standard of due or reasonable care and to the instinct that necessary or useful activities carried on within that standard should be free of the threat of liability, although we do not find those thoughts articulated in the abstract. Rules laying down precautionary standards for concrete situations have the look of legislation (perhaps prompted by problem cases). The most important question about them is where they come from, what mischief they correct. Are they curtailments of strict liability or extensions of the range of causality beyond its normal territory, as that was perceived by the intuitions current in these societies?

One possible scenario: people feel that, if someone gets caught in a wolf trap, the trapper is liable and must compensate to some degree, subject to whatever mitigation may be mediated through the procedural system (insofar as the trapper has used a relatively safe kind of trap and put it in a relatively safe place, or the victim is fairly chargeable with not looking where he was going). The king perceives that this accepted law is too discouraging to the useful end of wolf control and changes it: henceforth, if trappers take the specified precautionary steps, they need not compensate victims. (One can then speculate on the effects of ad hoc introduction of a negligence standard. Will prospective oath helpers in other situations be a little more willing to clear a defendant when they think that he was approximately as careful in his activity as the trapper is required to be in his, and will victims in other situations be quicker to settle for less compensation lest the analogy be invoked? The answer may, of course, be no: ad hoc measures for situations where there is a strong societal interest will be perceived as ad hoc.)

An alternative scenario: getting caught in someone's trap is generally thought of as bad luck. Merely putting out a trap into which a person stumbles is not "doing something to him," as long as the place and mode of the trap setting are not flagrantly dangerous. The king is confronted with wolf-trap accidents that seem obviously avoidable and responds by setting standards for trappers sanctioned by the threat of liability.

The second scenario is encouraged by a few barbarian laws that seem causally odd; that is, they seem to find reasons, or express an instinct, for holding that an apparent causer is not really the causer.[10] If strict liability systems provoke whittling on the causal front—attempts to show or a tendency to think that everyday causers are not what the law means by "doers of unintentional harm"—there are some barbarian illustrations of the principle to put alongside the Greek. Some barbarian laws distinguish between a victim impaled on a spear stuck in the ground and one held in a person's hand: only the man holding the spear is liable.[11] With, no doubt, a good deal of license as to probable circumstances, one can make the principle sound shocking: someone sticks a spear in the ground where there is a crowd of people rushing about and goes scot-free; another is standing in a deserted place holding his spear when a damn fool on the run blunders into it and he pays. (It is hard to find contributory negligence on the surface of barbarian law.) It seems that a certain noninvolvement of the actor's *person* with the accident makes it difficult to see him as the doer, or easy to find an excuse for not so seeing him.

A Lombard law provides that if a hunter wounds a wild animal and does not pursue it he is not liable for injury done by the enraged animal; contra if he persists in the hunt.[12] Again, it is easy to invent a horror story: an indifferent marksman takes a shot at a bear and observes that he has wounded but not killed it. Perhaps he would normally have followed up, but as it is he knows that his neighbor's little girls are blackberrying in the woods below. He calls off his dogs and goes home. He is not liable for the innocent devoured. Perhaps there are arguments for and against the rule on various premises. It seems to be best taken as evidence that it was hard to find someone liable who was not there, hard to escape the paradigm of the intentional harmdoer, who in normal circumstances *is* there and does the evil he means to. That is, the accidental harmdoer tended to be seen as the case shading off the paradigm—the person who, like the intentional tortfeasor, is, as it were, present with his weapon in his hand, but who, instead of fulfilling his malign intention, slips up, with harmful results.

If however, some laws seem to excuse persons who were not there a little dubiously, so as not to encourage careful or responsible behavior, quite a few excuse them when we would expect it: either when there is someone else to blame or there is an unpredictable intervening factor. The need to lay down such laws suggests the opposite of a tendency not to see causal involvement when it is not immediate—rather, it suggests a willingness to extend causal range, to believe that it is better that someone pay even when he is not very close to the accident, not to mention blameworthy, than that injury should go uncompensated. Thus, in Lombard law for example, you are not liable if you lend your weapon or your horse to someone and he does damage with it; only the borrower is liable.[13] A householder is not liable if an object being used in a hired-out construction job falls off the building and hurts someone; the master builder and his workmen are liable (in this case for the interesting recited reason that the contractor is paid for the job. There is a hint of need to *find* a reason, as if normal feeling would be that I am so associated with my house that I should pay for damage that comes from it, or from things being done to it by my contrivance).[14] The person who incites my dogs so that they hurt someone is liable; I am not.[15] If I hire laborers and one of them dies on the job by an act of God, I am not liable; if he is killed by my servant, the servant pays, not I.[16] (For the case to arise, someone must have thought that responsibility falls on me merely because I created the situation in which a death occurred.) If my domestic animal suddenly goes mad, I am not liable for the damage it does. (On the other hand, Lombard law does not, like some archaic systems, see domestic animals as so endowed with something like personality that the owner cannot generally be thought of as the doer of the damage they do. Owners in possession of normal animals are liable, without regard to foreknowledge of dangerous propensities or precautions taken.[17] Trappers, incidentally, are liable for damage done by the trapped animal, whatever the Lombards would have said about damage done by the trap.[18]) One of the few laws to speak of negligence, as opposed to the several that speak of accident, provides that a person whose negligence causes a fire is liable—*unless* the fire does something unpredictable—spreads across a road or river.[19] Such laws argue for a historical process of narrowing the range of liability relative to a more primitive belief that anyone plausibly associated with the accident is fair game. One can perhaps see in barbarian law what we have seen in Greek: crosscurrents, confusion in both moral beliefs and causal perceptions, cases that can be argued both ways with the resources of the societies in question and that need not be decided consistently.

I should like finally to mention one piece of Lombard evidence illustrative of something we encountered incidentally in the Greek case: a willingness to see the cause, or perhaps simply the most nearly just resolution of the cost-bearing question, in the enterprise itself rather than in the individual whose acts literally led to the damage.[20] If several men are cutting trees and a passerby is accidentally injured, the compensation is shared equally among the workers. If one of the co-workers is injured, the compensation is equally apportioned among all the participants, including the injured. In neither case are the questions asked, Which worker actually cut down the tree that fell on the victim? Were some of the workers having coffee on the sidelines? Was there fault anywhere? While there is little sign of generalization of this approach in the law that was successful, the law that reached the books, a version of looking to the enterprise rather than the individual is perhaps visible in options entertained and rejected. (Am I not part of the enterprise of having my house repaired, so that I should at least share with the contractor and his workers? We noted the resort to contract law to escape from that one, as if the answer might be, "Yes, except the contractor has implicitly undertaken to save the householder harmless, for which he is remunerated." When I hire a gang of laborers to do my work, can we not say my enterprise has gone awry when someone dies, even if it is only bad luck, or even someone else's fault? Even if I should not bear the whole cost, should I not at least bear some?)

CONCLUSION

From this limited look into the nonproximate past, I do not propose to extract useful lessons. The moral in a much looser sense is perhaps banal: how to deal with unintended bad outcomes is problematic in societies vastly simpler than our own and equipped with different moral ideas and perceptual habits. Despite those differences, the concepts we struggle with tend to turn up in one guise or another. One does not find simple societies with notions about responsibility which, if repulsive to us, at least have the virtue of simplicity. One finds uncertainty and arguments, competing ideas about how situations should be sized up and justice done. One finds nominal law, principles more or less recognized as the key to the system; but one is also constantly reminded that nominal law is deceptive, that an eye must always be kept on likely results in the real world. (In a system of strict liability, is a non-negligent defendant really likely to lose or a negligent plaintiff to win? How are non-negligent doctors or corporations likely to fare in a negligence system? How well does the nominal law survive the procedural system: Athens' large assemblies without direction except from orators; oath helping; the American blend of trial by jury and lawyers' law? Besides, people are good at subscribing to the nominal law and then discovering that its real meaning is not what one might think, and, of course, that could be so. The discovery does not depend on lawyers.)

If there is anything more specific in what I have said whose appropriation might be worth considering, I think it would be the following. First, *harmartia*, although unsettled and malleable in Greek hands, has a certain attraction compared to "negligence." If we do not really have a negligence system, the pretense of having one leads nonetheless to such painful and invidious results as good doctors being found wanting in due care. If the alternative of compensating victims, no matter what, seems unacceptable, perhaps it would be useful to learn a language with slightly different tonalities and practical implications. Think of the failed project, for which it may be needful that the person whose project has failed should pay, but do not strain to make out that the failure is one of not watching out or departure from appropriate cautionary standards. *Then* think about what failure *is* with respect to different kinds of projects—it may not be simply throwing a javelin so that someone you wish no harm gets hit, but throwing one poorly, or heedlessly, or out of turn. Nor need every medical project fail when the patient does not recover or suffers side effects; it depends on how the project is conceived. I am not sure that this helps, but it may.

Second, we have seen that it does not take highly complex enterprises to suggest the notion that liability might more intelligibly or more justly fall on the enterprise as a whole than on individual cogs. Javelin practice and a few woodcutters were enough to inspire the thought that costs should be shared among participants, including the victim. Apart from other implications, the sense in which the patient is a participant in an enterprise that is subject to mishap is perhaps worth taking more seriously. If individual blame were dropped, save perhaps for cases of sharp culpa bility, and the basic principle of compensation without regard to fault were adopted, there might be a moment's worth of profit in reflecting on What is the enterprise? Is the simple socialization of costs—with, I should think, the consequence of fixed payments for given types of "bad outcomes," as in barbarian law—preferable to a system with payment of actual damages shared among the participants in a more delimited enterprise than society at large? The answer may be that it is: singling out an individual to litigate against and social assumption of the whole compensatory function are the only practical alternatives. (The Athenian jurors might have thought it pretty impractical to imagine proceedings against all the javelin throwers; the Lombards seem to have had no trouble with suits against a handful of woodcutters.) There would, however, be nothing mechanically impractical about taxing doctors, hospitals, drug companies, and consumers of medical services to raise a fund for compensating medical victims (up to, say, a certain percentage of actual damage, the victim as participant bearing the rest).

Finally, a Burgundian king, within a system in which negligence was not, at any rate, a generalized or explicit operative concept, was able to lay down standards for relatively safe procedure and design in the specific activity of trapping wolves. There is an encouraging cue here for the administrative approach to torts, for looking away from principles of law applicable (but perhaps only mythically) to *anything* that goes wrong and concentrating rather on particular activities about which it is feasible to say fairly exactly how they should be carried out. Liability can be used as an incentive to see that such activity-specific standards are met and kept from being a disincentive to engaging in certain socially beneficial activities (or from engaging in them only in super-cautious, uneconomic ways under an indefinite threat of liability). Whether victims have a claim on some sort of social compensation when such standards are observed is a further question; perhaps it should be called a political one. Private justice in archaic Burgundy seems to have been satisfied by telling the public, "There is some risk of your walking into a wolf trap and receiving no compensation—we have done all we can for you by insisting that trappers serve notice of their intention to set a trap and construct it in a way that minimizes danger without impairing the trap's efficiency for catching wolves."

NOTES

1. I shall not document the case in detail. The speeches can be read in a few minutes, and reading them whole is the best way to judge whether what I do with them is reasonable, at least prima facie. As with any Greek text, the fine points can be picked over with the end of understanding the meaning more precisely, and perhaps with the result of understanding it less confidently, than when one started out. I have tried to do my share of picking over; it would be tedious to encumber this chapter with that process. I do not think anything major eludes the reader of a good English translation, such as K. H. Maidment, *Minor Attic Orators,* vol. I, Loeb Classical Library no. 308 (Cambridge, MA: Harvard University Press, 1941).
2. For all general points on homicide law in Athens, See Douglas M. MacDowell, *Athenian Homicide Law in the Age of the Orators* (Manchester: Manchester University Press, 1963), where the original documentation is thoroughly surveyed and generously reproduced. The same author's *The Law in Classical Athens* (Ithaca, NY: Cornell Unversity Press, 1978) is the best introduction to the system as a whole. I would emphasize a bit more strongly than MacDowell the value of Plato's *Laws* among the original sources (book IX, 864c and following for homicide specifically). The best evidence, for example, that classifying "crimes of passion" was problematic for the Greeks comes from Plato's discussion of the subject.

    I should emphasize that the interpretation below of the sanctions for unintentional homicide as a monetary compensation system in effect is mine, not MacDowell's. I do not want to suggest that there is a scrap of direct evidence for the interpretation. The argument is simply that it is probable—since what most legal systems want out of accidental killers (if not intentional ones as well, and there the Athenian system does seem to have been more severe) is compensation (plus, as I say, "decency")—that the system of "releasable exile" lead to bargaining between the parties.
3. I have not discovered, though perhaps it is discoverable, just exactly what

javelin practice consisted of. It is clear from the documents that there was a target, suggesting that the point of the exercise was like our archery, rather than like our field event. The archery model implies a relatively short range within which it is possible to throw a (relatively short) javelin with some hope of hitting a target. It is not impossible, however, to imagine a sort of combined accuracy and distance event, where the target is set at a distance that only a very good thrower could reach and the object is to get as close as you can, perhaps with points subtracted for deviations from the straight line between the throwing box and the target. In that case, there could be a fair space between the people in the vicinity of the target and the throwers.

4. Some barbarian law can be conveniently studied through original texts, thanks to modern translations. Secondary works, on the other hand, are mostly rather old-fashioned, though they include major achievements of the largely German scholarship of their generation. I shall take my illustrations from the two most accessible books: Katherine Fisher Drew, *The Burgundian Code* (Philadelphia: University of Pennsylvania Press, 1972) and the same author's *The Lombard Laws* (Philadelphia: University of Pennsylvania Press, 1973). Aside from the texts thmselves, Drew's introductions and bibliographies are the best first step into the subject. The extensive Anglo-Saxon laws are also available in modern English—most conveniently in Dorothy Whitelock's *English Historical Documents,* vol. 1 (New York: Oxford University Press, 1955) (these are selections—older complete versions need reprinting). T. Rivers, *Laws of the Alamans and Bavarians* (Philadelphia: University of Pennsylvania Press, 1977) is the latest addition to the store of modern translated editions. Numerous other bodies of barbarian law are well edited in the original languages, mainly Latin.

5. Drew, *Lombard Laws* (Rothair's Edict No. 74), p. 64.

6. I concede that establishing a general distinction between mere "compensation money owed" and an indefinite right to take vengeance when compensation is not received presents problems I have not solved. I think the hypothesis of such a distinction is much encouraged by laws that *explicitly* ban feuding on the *stated* ground that the damage was accidental or nonmalicious. *All* laws appointing a fixed compensation are attempts to stop private vengeance by saying, If you get your money, it is wrong to take vengeance. Laws which say, You must not take vengeance in this case because you are merely the victim of an accident, make sense only if they are assumed to refer to the eventuality of the money's not being received—to be a matter of saying, in *this* case there is no excuse for vengeance *even* when the money isn't received—you have no rights beyond those of someone who is simply owed that sum of money (bear the risks of insolvency, whatever those may be in a given society/may not act against the debtor's relatives, to the degree that vengeance may be taken against others than the tortfeasor himself). For examples of such laws, see Drew, *Lombard Laws* (Rothair's Edict No. 326), p. 115; (No. 344), p. 119; (No. 387), p. 129; (No. 75), p. 65. For debt collection, see, for example, Drew, *Lombard Laws* (Rothair's Edict No. 245), p. 101. Also of interest in this connection is Rothair's Edict No. 143 (Ibid., p. 74), appointing severe sanctions for feuding after

receiving compensation *and* having taken oaths to call off the feud. There are two implications: (1) if, after conviction or confession, the wrongdoer doesn't pay up, there is nothing wrong with feuding (in the ordinary case of deliberate wrongs, which most of the laws contemplate); (2) although (if the laws are to make sense at all) you have no choice but to take the compensation if it is forthcoming, calling off the feud is conceived in theory as a voluntary act of peacemaking which the parties must confirm by oath—as it were, the injured's right to vengeance arises from his being injured and can in strictness only be taken away by his own act. You are no doubt an enemy of society if you refuse to settle for the legal compensation, but specific sanctions come upon you only if you do settle and then renege.

7. Rothair's Edict No. 344 (Drew, *Lombard Laws*, p. 119), is explicit: set compensation per head plus actual damages for turning one's animals into another's field on purpose; actual damages only if the animals got in without their owner's intending them to (nothing to distinguish negligence); determination by unsupported oath as to whether there was evil intent.

   Numerous laws require compensation for actual damages in addition to the set compensation without saying anything explicit to distinguish intentional from accidental cases, but it is quite possible that it should be understood that the set compensation is due only in the intentional case. For example, Rothair's Edict No. 345 (Drew, *Lombard Laws*, p. 119) is about pigs, whereas No. 344 is about horses and oxen, but otherwise they concern the same problem. By the letter, No. 345 does not say the animal owner is liable for actual damages even if he can swear off bad intentions, but this article must surely carry over what is spelled out in No. 344. Separate laws for different animals of similar propensities probably point to the way the barbarian codes were made rather than to any real distinction. (A pig case arose after a rule was propounded in terms covering horses and oxen and required a separate ruling, which somehow got incorporated into the collection as a separate article.) Be it said by way of reminder that the making of the codes—why what appears on the pages of the manuscript appears in the form it does—presents grave problems.

8. Drew, *Burgundian Code* (No. XLVI), p. 53.

9. For example, Rothair's Edict No. 303 (Drew, *Lombard Laws*, p. 112), concerning fences; No. 305 (p. 112), concerning ditches; No. 306 (p. 112), concerning wells, where the well owner is free from liability altogether on the ground that "the waters of a well should be for the common usefulness of all." That is, the social benefits of having wells outweigh the risk of accidents, and it is apparently felt that the burden of relatively safe construction is too much to put on the social benefactor.

10. It is also encouraged by a more general article on traps in the *Burgundian Code*, No. LXXII (Drew, p. 69): if the trap is placed in a deserted spot outside cultivated land, there is no liability. See note 18 below for a different Lombard law on a closely related point.

11. For example, Burgundian code No. XVIII, section 2 (Drew, *Burgundian Code*, p. 35), with, however, the proviso that the person who stuck the

spear in the ground did not intend to do harm. Intent does not matter if the weapon is held in one's hand, but there is a proviso that, for the party to be liable, the spear must be held "in such a manner that it could cause harm to a man." Some barbarian laws on this subject are less qualified.

12. Rothair's Edict No. 309 (Drew, *Lombard Laws*, p. 113).
13. Rothair's Edict No. 307 (ibid., p. 112). Compare Edict No. 308 (ibid., p. 113); same law where the weapon is taken without the owner's consent—it is still necessary to lay it down that the owner is not responsible.
14. Rothair's Edict No. 144 (ibid., p. 75).
15. Rothair's Edict No. 322 (ibid., p. 115).
16. Rothair's Edict No. 152 (ibid., p. 77).
17. Rothair's Edict No. 324 (ibid., p. 115), concerning mad animals. See Edicts No. 325 and No. 326 (p. 115) for the general rule of owner's liability for damage done by normal animals. Burgundian code No. XVIIII, Section 1 (Drew, *Burgundian Code*, p. 35) adopts the rule that the owner must hand over the animal that did the damage to the victim. That is, if the damage is greater than the value of the animal, liability is limited; if it is less, the victim still apparently has a claim on the animal—the "separate personality" that did the damage—unless he can be talked into accepting monetary compensation for actual damage. This article appears to be a reform of the law away from the older rule holding the owner liable for at least full damages.
18. Rothair's Edict No. 310 (Drew, *Lombard Laws*, p. 113). Compare Edict No. 311 (p. 113): the trapper is not liable if the injured goes out of his way in a wrongful attempt to take the trapped animal for himself.
19. Rothair's Edict No. 148 (ibid., p. 76): the word in the original is *neclegenter*. Compare Edict No. 147 (p. 76), which, without speaking of negligence, in effect sets something like an activity-specific standard of care: if one carries a firebrand more than nine feet from his hearth and causes damage by fire to someone else, he is liable; otherwise he is not. This article insists in terms that a liable party should *only* have to pay for actual damage, "since he did it unintentionally."
20. Rothair's Edict No. 138 (ibid., p. 73).

Section 4

Developing a Public Policy for Compensation

13

Liability and Insurance for Medical Maloccurrences: Are Innovations Different?

Patricia M. Danzon

This chapter addresses two questions: Who should pay for the adverse effects of medical innovations? and How is the answer to the first question affected by "imperfections" in insurance markets? In discussing alternative liability rules, I shall be concerned with their prospective impact on incentives for injury prevention, on allocation of risk, and on the rate of innovation and adoption of new technologies. I leave to others the even more difficult issues of equity and fairness.

To distinguish the effects of innovation from other sources of risk, I first analyze the optimal liability rule for innovative therapies compared to established therapies, under the assumption that insurance is available to all parties at actuarial rates. I then examine how imperfections in markets for first-party and liability insurance affect the conclusions. In the final section, I examine the problems that have occurred in liability insurance markets for medical maloccurrences and evaluate the case for special compensation funds for victims of vaccines and innovative medical therapies.

The principal results of the analysis are as follows. The distinction between incentives for care and incentives for innovation is crucial. Liability rules designed to provide optimal incentives for care provide suboptimal incentives for innovation. In theory, a first best solution can be achieved in the case of patentable innovations, if patient assumption of risk is an enforceable defense. For nonpatentable innovations, assumption of risk does not guarantee an optimal rate of research. Both first-party and liability insurance markets perform poorly for permanently disabling injuries, particularly where manifestation of injury is delayed. However, in the case of vaccines, the insurance failures that have occurred are due only in part to the basic problems of nondiversifiable risk that beset medical malpractice and product liability insurance. At least as important is the mandatory nature of the vaccine programs, which involve price controls and eliminate usual contractual relations and tort duties of some participants. I conclude that there is a strong case for a special compensation program for seriously disabling vaccine injuries but not for innovative therapies in general.

Optimal Liability with Costless Insurance

ESTABLISHED THERAPIES

There is an extensive literature on the optimal assignment of liability for accidents. The starting point of any analysis must be the Coase theorem, which demonstrates that the legal assignment of liability is irrelevant if all parties are well informed about risks and can contract to allocate liability to suit their preferences. But if there is asymmetrical information or if contracting is not costless, then the liability rule does affect incentives for injury prevention. By definition, the optimal rule is that which creates incentives to minimize the sum of the utility cost of preventive measures and the cost of injuries, including nonmonetary as well as monetary loss and the overhead costs of administration and litigation.

Consider the context of a particular medical procedure, such as radiation therapy. The risk of injury depends on the frequency of performance of the procedure and on the level of care taken by the physician, the patient, and the equipment manufacturer. Standard analysis yields the intuitively obvious result: if the efficient way to prevent injuries requires effort by more than one party, the liability rule should require all parties to meet a standard of "due" care. Let us assume temporarily that adjudication and transaction costs are zero. In principle, optimal incentives for care can be obtained under three alternative liability rules: liability of physicians for negligence; strict liability of physicians; or strict liability of manufacturers. In all three cases there should be defenses of assumption of risk and contributory negligence against patients. [1]

Consider the case of physician liability for negligence. Holding physicians liable for negligence, including failure to obtain a patient's informed consent, provides appropriate incentives for physicians and patients. Eliminate the informed consent requirement and physicians might transmit too little information about risks. Consequently, patients would take too little care, and the frequency of risky treatments would be too high (assuming that uninformed patients systematically underestimate risk). In principle, it is not necessary to also hold manufacturers liable, since the Coase theorem implies that appropriate incentives could be transmitted between physicians and suppliers through contractual relations and product prices. But if contracting costs are high, manufacturer liability for negligence may also be necessary. The same incentive structure could be achieved under strict liability, provided a party held strictly liable (say the manufacturer) could sue the other (the physician) for contributory negligence. Again under the latter rule, non-negligent behavior by physicians should include obtaining a patient's informed consent, and assumption of risk by the patient should be a defense.

Let us now drop the assumption that determining cause and fault is costless. In the medical context, these costs seem to tip the balance in favor of liability only for negligence rather than strict liability. Under strict liability, more cases must be adjudicated. Litigation cost per case would be lower *only* if determining cause, under strict liability, is simpler than determining whether the due care standard has been violated, under negligence. But in the medical context, determining whether a particular adverse outcome was due to the medical treatment as opposed to the underlying condition of ill health for which treatment was sought is likely to be as costly as determining negligent performance. Since the evidence[2] suggests that non-negligent iatrogenic injuries are at least five times as numerous as those due to negligence and it is highly unlikely that adjudication cost per case could be cut to one-fifth, there is a strong presumption that strict liability for medical maloccurrences would entail even higher total costs of adjudication than the current negligence system. Indeed, only very limited no-fault proposals for medical malpractice are currently under serious consideration.[3]

INNOVATIVE THERAPIES

Let us now consider whether this conclusion of the optimality of a negligence rule for medical maloccurrences holds in the case of innovations. Innovative therapies differ in at least four ways from established therapies: the risks and benefits of innovative therapies are more uncertain; by definition there is a departure from customary practice; the physician may have a personal, research interest in using the new therapy; and there is a discrepancy between the private (expected) therapeutic benefits to the patient and the social benefits, which include the value of the information gained from experience with the new procedure. I shall argue that only the last of these—divergence between private and social benefits—undermines the conclusion that physician liability for negligence yields socially desirable incentives for care and frequency of treatment.

Uncertain Effects

By definition, the risks of adverse outcomes from innovative procedures are less well known than the risks for established procedures.[4] In principle, this alone does not undermine the conclusions of the standard analysis. The only change is that, because outcomes are less certain, the preferences of the patient for risk taking and hence the duty of the physician to inform should be more significant factors in determining the optimal course of treatment and the due standard of care.

If a negligence rule combined with a duty to inform breaks down in the context of medical innovations, it is apparently because of the reluctance of the courts to adhere to this standard in practice. Enforceability of assumption of risk is particularly problematic in cases of latent side effects, which are manifested only many years after treatment. Again by the definition of innovation, there will have been some accrual of information over the intervening years before a case is adjudicated. There is an obvious risk that the advantages of the information subsequently obtained will be used in assessing the physician's or manufacturer's performance at a prior date. Even if the courts correctly assess the manufacturer's care and the physician's duty to inform using the risks known at the time, there is obvious potential for the wisdom of hindsight in attempting to evaluate the patient's willingness to take risks *ex ante*. Consider a case where a patient has a choice between slow deterioration with loss of function and an innovative therapy that offers some chance of full recovery, together with some risk of permanent disability. *Ex ante*, the patient who values very highly an active life may be willing to take the risk, but in the event of an adverse outcome will obviously regret the choice. *Ex post*, it will be hard for the court to determine what information the physician should have had, but even harder to establish that he presented it fairly and obtained a fully informed consent.

Because the potential for the wisdom of hindsight is greater in the context of medical innovations, there is greater risk that what is a negligence rule in theory degenerates into absolute liability in practice, particularly when the manifestation of side effects is delayed. If physicians anticipate that the courts will not recognize the assumption-of-risk defense, there is a presumption that they will offer patients the choice of innovative therapies too infrequently, relative to the social optimum. Precisely the same conclusion applies if absolute liability is applied to manufacturers of innovative devices or drugs rather than to physicians. Thus uncertainty of outcome of innovative therapies undermines the optimality of the negligence rule *only* to the extent that it is unenforceable in practice, because of the difficulty of proving assumption of risk. But note that, if (1) patient incentives for care were not necessary and (2) insurance were available at actuarial rates, then the shift to absolute liability would be irrelevant. The price of the product or service would rise, to reflect the supplier's cost of liability insurance, but the patient would save the equivalent cost of first-party insurance, leaving the full cost of the product unchanged.[5]

Departure from Customary Practice

The adoption of new therapies entails by definition, a departure from customary practice, which is the norm of due care for physicians.

Although some early cases involving medical innovation seemed to hold a physician strictly liable for any deviation from standard practice, there is now considerable support for the position that liability for innovation depends on the reasonableness of the use of the innovative procedure in the circumstances of the patient.[6] The innovative departure will be reasonable if it reasonably appears the chances of providing a benefit to the patient beyond that of customary therapy outweigh the likely risk of the innovation. Thus due care is defined by weighing the risks and expected benefits to the patient, comparing the advantages of the innovative therapy to customary therapies. In principle this definition of due care protects the physician from absolute liability for innovative therapies and will yield a rate of adoption of new techniques that is optimal from the standpoint of individual patients.

Private Benefits to the Physician

It is often suggested that physicians have a personal incentive to adopt innovative therapies that may result in publication and professional advancement.[7] Again, a negligence standard that weighs the benefits and costs to the patient in principle provides an adequate safeguard against use of innovative therapies where such use violates the patient's best interests.

Divergence Between
Private and Social Benefits

The use of an innovative procedure provides not only therapeutic risks and benefits to the actual patient, but also new information that is potentially valuable to future patients. As in the case of any externality, unless the patient is given some incentive to take these social benefits into account when deciding whether or not to opt for the innovative treatment, too little innovation will be undertaken from a social standpoint. To make the point concrete, let B_p and B_s denote private and social benefits, respectively, from the treatment; let C denote the expected injury costs to the patient; and let P denote the price of the treatment to the patient (assumed equal to cost of production). Then the risk-neutral patient will opt for the treatment if

$$B_p > C + P, \tag{1}$$

whereas it is socially optimal to use the treatment if

$$B_p + B_s > C + P. \tag{2}$$

In the absence of some subsidy to the patient, private incentives for undergoing innovative therapies will be too low from a social standpoint. Under a negligence rule, if patients can expect compensation only in the event of negligent performance or failure to inform of risks, the rate of acquisition of new medical knowledge will be socially suboptimal. A rule of strict liability on physician or manufacturer, if combined with a duty to inform and an assumption-of-risk defense, results in the same set of incentives for the patient and therefore the same suboptimal rate of adoption of innovations as a negligence rule.

If the assumption-of-risk defense is eliminated, making the physician or manufacturer absolutely liable for all adverse outcomes, then the patient effectively receives a subsidy equal to the expected value of compensation. Willingness to opt for innovative therapies would presumably increase. But this solution may be nonoptimal, for two reasons. First, the optimal value of the subsidy is equal to the social benefit of the information generated by the treatment to persons other than the patient receiving the treatment. Only by chance would this equal the expected value of compensation. Since the value of additional information is likely to diminish as more experience is gained with an innovative therapy, this subsidy is likely to be too small initially, and too large as the value of additional experience falls to zero.[8] Second, if absolute liability is placed on manufacturers, the duty of physicians to inform and of patients to evaluate risks becomes moot. Physicians may have incentives to use innovative procedures when such procedures further their professional advancement. Patients may become too willing to undergo innovative procedures, particularly when their private insurance protection against adverse outcomes of established therapies is incomplete. Effectively, the manufacturer becomes an insurer who is exposed to moral hazard (reduced care) on the part of physicians and patients and to adverse selection of research-oriented physicians and high-risk patients. In principle the manufacturer could protect himself by a contract requiring indemnification if the physician failed to inform the patient of risk. But it is hard to imagine the contract that would protect the absolutely liable manufacturer against suboptimal care and adverse selection of patients.[9]

In evaluating whether simple liability rules can simultaneously provide optimal incentives for care and for innovation, it is important to distinguish patentable innovations, such as drugs or medical devices, from nonpatentable procedures or therapies. In the case of a patentable product or drug, the social benefits from gathering information are internalized to the patentee, since he can recoup the value of that information in the price charged to future patients once the product is proven safe. The price charged while the product is in the innovative stage will equal the cost of supplying it, discounted by the expected value of the information. In the above notation, the price charged to the patient would be $P - B_S$. This yields socially optimal incentives for choice of innovative products. In practice the solution may not be viable if $B_S > P$ and it is not feasible to offer a negative price, that is, a financial inducement to opt for the innovative product. In that case, an offer of indemnification to the

subject for some or all costs of an adverse outcome might be a way of circumventing an effective price control.

But the optimality of this solution, if combined with a negligence rule of
liability, depends critically on the courts' acknowledging assumption of risk.
Alternatively, if the courts engage in a cost-benefit analysis in determining
the due standard of care, it is crucial that the measure of costs include the price
paid (or financial inducement received) by the patient, which reflects the
expected social benefits. If the court defines due care as $B_p > C + P$, whereas
the patient was offered and responded to $B_p > C + P - B_s$, then, with a
negligence rule of liability, private markets cannot achieve the socially
optimal adoption of new therapies, even when patents are available to
internalize benefits.

Simple liability rules work even less well in most medical research,
which is undertaken in nonprofit university and research centers with support
from public funds. Any innovation or discovery undertaken with support from
government funds generally cannot be patented. In such cases the researchers
internalize neither the benefits nor the costs of the research. The situation is
similar in the case of physicians conducting clinical trials to gather further
information about the effects of nonexperimental but innovative uses of
established therapies.

In principle, the public subsidy to medical research could be used as a
substitute for a private patent, as a means of correcting the suboptimal
incentives for innovation that exist in private markets. The subsidy could be
used to discount the costs of treatment to the patient to reflect the social
benefits of the information gained, just as a private supplier would do in the
case of a patentable product. To the extent that physicians and hospitals use
research funds to waive fees and charges for innovative treatments, such a
crude subsidy mechanism already operates. However, given the incentives and
constraints facing agencies that fund biomedical research, there is little
presumption that the current allocation of resources and the current pattern of
subsidies mirror the social value of information.

As an alternative or supplement to waiving fees for innovative
therapies, compensation through a no-fault compensation scheme could be
used as an in-kind subsidy, particularly as a means of circumventing legal or
ethical restrictions on offering financial inducements to participate. However
the problems of absolute liability are no less, and probably greater, when the
liable party is the government rather than a private supplier. First, as argued
earlier, there is no a priori presumption that compensation for an adverse
outcome is equal to the social value of the information gained. Second, a no-
fault compensation program would be subject to the same risks of moral hazard
and adverse selection by physicians and patients, in addition to the obvious
problems of defining innovative therapies and compensable events.

An analysis of optimal incentives for medical innovation cannot ignore the impact of health insurance on the demand for medical care in general and the choice between innovative and established therapies in particular. Aside from the major public health insurance programs, Medicare and Medicaid, there are extensive subsidies to health care and health insurance in the form of the tax-exempt status of employer contributions to health insurance, the exemption of nonprofit and public hospitals from corporate income tax, and the exemption of hospital bonds from federal and state income taxes. These subsidies currently total over \$40 billion.[10] Together with other distortions in health care markets, these subsidies have led to excessive levels of insurance and inefficient forms of coverage. Because patients pay only a small fraction of the cost of health care out-of-pocket, under traditional fee-for-service coverage, utilization is pushed beyond the point where marginal benefits equal marginal social costs. This translates into excessive incentives for quality-enhancing but not for cost-reducing innovations.[11]

It cannot be determined a priori whether the stimulus from health insurance offsets the suboptimal incentives from liability rules to yield a suboptimal or excessive rate of innovation and adoption of new therapies. Cursory evidence suggests the latter. The subsidy to health insurance alone averages 31 percent at the margin.[12] On the other hand, the need for a subsidy to attract the socially optimal number of volunteers for medical trials maybe negligible or even zero if there are enough persons for whom the expected private benefits alone exceed cost ($B_p > C + P$) to reduce the social value of additional information to zero. A safe conclusion is that there is no strong presumption that incentives for innovation are suboptimal, or, if they were, that the appropriate subsidy would take the form of replacing or supplementing the current negligence rule with no-fault compensation, either through absolute liability of providers or from public funds. If rates of innovation are indeed suboptimal, achievement of the two goals—optimal levels of care and optimal rates of innovation—requires two policy tools. Given the assumption-of-risk neutrality or perfect insurance adopted so far, the liability rule should be designed to achieve optimal care, leaving to direct subsidies the role of stimulating innovation.

RISK AVERSION AND INSURANCE

The analysis so far has assumed that all parties are indifferent to risk, that is, that they are concerned only with the expected outcome (probability X expected damages). Risk neutrality is a realistic assumption only if insurance is available on actuarially fair terms to patients, physicians, and producers, in such a way that all losses can be fully compensated.[13] To the extent that first-party or liability insurance is not available at actuarially fair rates plus a reasonable loading charge for administrative expense, the costs of insurance and of residual uninsured risk cannot be ignored in determining the optimal liability rule. In the following section, I shall argue that, in practice, actuarial insurance cannot be assumed for either first-party or liability insurance.

FIRST-PARTY INSURANCE

The great majority of the U.S. population has access to subsidized, employment-based private health insurance or to the public programs, Medicare and Medicaid. Employment-based coverage has advantages in terms of economies of scale and protection against adverse selection (at least for large firms), in addition to the tax subsidy to employer contributions. However, it results in two serious gaps in coverage. First, people not in the labor force or in families without a full-time employed member and people employed in small firms face a relatively high price. Second, the fact that private insurance is tied to employment means that even the great majority of people who are covered are exposed to the risk of losing coverage, should they suffer a permanent disability that would jeopardize their employment opportunities. Athough most of the totally disabled are eligible for Medicare through Social Security Disability Insurance (SSDI), the initial waiting period, prior employment requirement, and total disability criteria for eligibility leave some of the disabled without health insurance.

For those not eligible for large employment-based private insurance plans or public programs, individual coverage is available but at premium rates at least 30 percent higher than comparable group coverage—an effective price 250 percent higher.[14] Moreover, since individual policies typically exclude preexisting conditions, they do not solve the problem of the permanently disabled or those with severe chronic conditions.

The market for first-party insurance for long-term wage loss has gaps similar to those for health insurance. Private coverage is largely employment-based. Aside from work-related injuries covered by workers' compensation, the majority of the work force relies on SSDI; but persons who have not made contributions through covered employment are not eligible. Thus, while the advocates of special funds to compensate victims of medical, products, and toxic torts may underestimate the extent of private and public insurance already in place, the gaps in the present system, especially for permanent injuries, cannot be denied. They reflect the severe risks of moral hazard and adverse selection faced by an insurer offering coverage for such events on an individual basis.

LIABILITY INSURANCE

Concern over the gaps in first-party health and disability insurance is apparently one factor underlying the move to strict liability for product-related injuries, toxic torts, and some medical maloccurrences, including adverse reactions to vaccines. However, it is a mistake to think that producer liability provides a costless means of spreading risk or a solution to the moral hazard and adverse selection risks that undermine first-party insurance. A necessary (but not sufficient) condition for actuarially fair insurance is a large pool of independent "draws" from a stable distribution whose mean can be accurately estimated from past experience.

Liability insurance violates the prerequisites of independent draws and a stable process, particularly in the case of latent injuries.[15] Liability losses depend not only on the probability of physical injury but also on the legal rules and social attitudes governing liability and damages. The longer the delay between the triggering event—the medical treatment or the sale of the product—and the manifestation of injury and adjudication of claims, the greater the potential for changes in liability rules and damage standards. This sociolegal risk introduces uncertainty as to the mean (the past cannot be used to predict the future) and destroys independence, since trends will similarly affect all policyholders. Lack of independence destroys the diversification gains from pooling large numbers of identical policyholders. The insurer may achieve some diversification through a portfolio of multiple insurance lines, a conglomerate enterprise, or ultimately through capital markets if the risk is nonsystematic. But to the extent that sociolegal risk is not costlessly diversifiable, it acts as a tax on liability insurance and hence on the insured goods and services.

Liability for medical maloccurrences may be subject to an additional "tax" because of the difficulty of distinguishing the marginal damages due to medical intervention from the underlying condition for which treatment was sought. Even if the defendant could buy actuarially fair insurance and raise the price of the product to reflect the expected liability, marginal consumers would not be willing to pay the higher price unless they accurately perceived the additional benefit and valued it at cost. Thus systematic judicial error of this type adds to the price of risky activities, thereby discouraging their use below socially optimal levels.

All these sources of liability insurance risk are even more severe in the case of innovative therapies. By definition the mean of the loss distribution cannot be estimated from past experience. Adverse side effects may affect all recipients, destroying independence. If the effects are likely to be delayed, the potential for accrual of new knowledge exacerbates the risk of retrospective application of new standards. And finally, the risk of being held liable for total rather than marginal damages is higher, to the extent that innovative therapies are more likely to be used when the patient's prognosis with established therapies is poor.

These factors tend to argue in favor of a limit on the duration of liability, under either a negligence rule or strict liability, in the form of a statute of repose running from the time of treatment or the date the product was sold, not from the time of manifestation of the injury.[16] But a curtailment of third-party liability leaves the victim dependent on first-party insurance, which has gaps. Evaluating alternative policies for filling these gaps is beyond the scope of this chapter. But since the gaps in first-party insurance for permanent disabilities and chronic conditions apply to all such cases, not just the tiny fraction that are potentially compensable through a third-party action in tort, there is a prima facie case for a comprehensive approach. One possibility would be to extend SSDI and Medicare to cover all individuals, regardless of prior employment status, for specifically defined disabling conditions that are systematically excluded from private, employment-based coverage.

Assuming the general public programs were amended to be universally available, there remains a case for establishing a special fund to treat injuries from specific causes, but only if the fund is financed from a tax on the activity generating the injuries and if there are resulting gains in market deterrence[17] that outweigh the costs of determining cause. In the case of medical innovation, the arguments against a special fund seem overwhelming. I return to this below.

"MARKET FAILURES" IN LIABILITY INSURANCE FOR MEDICAL MALOCCURRENCES

To what extent do the factors identified so far—nondiversifiable risk in general and sociolegal risk in particular—account for the apparent market failures in liability insurance for medical maloccurrences? Here, I discuss two such apparent failures: the periodic crises in medical malpractice insurance, and the unavailability of liability insurance for manufacturers of vaccines.

MEDICAL MALPRACTICE INSURANCE

Medical malpractice insurance appears to be vulnerable to periodic crises of price and availability. Most extreme was the crisis of 1975, in which malpractice insurance rates increased as much as 500 percent in a single year in some states. In other states, the stock companies that had traditionally written the business withdrew totally from the market.[18] Following several years of stable or modestly rising premiums in the late 1970s, rate increases have again exceeded 50 percent in some states, notably Florida and New York, particularly for certain specialities.

Such volatility of prices is unheard of in first-party health insurance and in other lines of liability insurance, such as automobile liability and workers' compensation, which are not subject to long delay between the pricing of the policy and the filing and ultimate disposition of claims. This delay, combined with nondiversifiable risk, leads to such uncertainty in predicting claim costs that a very safe premium (99 percent probability of premium adequacy) could be as much as three times the expected mean estimate of claim costs, plus overhead.[19] The rate actually filed within this confidence interval depends on the insurers' capital reserves and their willingness to accept risk. In 1974 a drastic upward revision in expected claim costs coincided with a serious depletion of capital. In 1975 rate increases averaging 197 percent were filed in 48 states. In 18 states, state insurance regulators denied any rate increase, and in the remaining 30 states the approved increases averaged one-third below requested rates.[20] In any competitive market, price controls result in a withdrawal of supply, and insurance is no exception. The withdrawal of malpractice insurers in 1975 and the resulting availability crisis was thus attributable most immediately to massive rate regulation. More recently, premium increases of over 50 percent in New York and Florida can be traced to prior price controls.

But more fundamentally, the problem is pricing uncertainty in the face of unlimited duration of liability and sociolegal risk. The risk is insurable—but at a price that is not politically acceptable. Moreover, state-run reinsurance mechanisms are no panacea. As the Florida experience confirms, they are vulnerable to political pressure for inadequate rates, with the attendant evils of either subsidy from other sources or delayed assessment on policyholders, or both.

LIABILITY INSURANCE FOR VACCINE MANUFACTURERS

A second area of recurrent failure of liability insurance markets is vaccines. A major cause of the collapse of the swine flu immunization program in 1975 was the apparent inability of vaccine manufacturers to obtain liability insurance. More recently, the rising costs or lack of availability of liability insurance for manufacturers of the pertussis vaccine have led to the exit of all but one manufacturer from the market. In both cases the problem of unknown risks, which is intrinsic to innovation, seems to be only a small part of the story. The swine flu vaccine was admittedly a new product, and there was some concern for unanticipated side effects. But the pertussis vaccine has been in use for many years, and the incidence of adverse outcomes can be estimated with some accuracy. Moreover, adverse outcomes are immediate, so the issue of sociolegal risk or the application of new, unanticipated liability are not major issues.

Several factors contribute to the potential for market failure in the case of vaccines. First, even if the social benefits of the vaccine exceed social costs, including costs of adverse reactions, that does not guarantee that manufacturers will be able to charge a price that will cover the cost of liability insurance for adverse outcomes. The price that any individual patient would be willing to pay for a vaccine will not internalize the social benefits from reducing the probability of infecting others. Some estimates indicate that a 75 percent rate of vaccination suffices to give herd immunity.[21] Obviously, every individual would prefer to be in the free-riding 25 percent who enjoy the benefits but suffer none of the risks and costs of vaccination.

The shortfall of private willingness to pay below social benefits is probably greater for vaccines than for medical innovations, simply because many medical innovations offer potential benefits to a relatively small number of individuals, whereas the entire population benefits from the elimination of a contagious disease. But the social benefits of vaccination cannot be captured simply by giving a patent on the vaccine to a manufacturer. In the case of therapeutic innovations, the patent enables the innovator to set a price above operating costs once the innovation has proven safe. The price future consumers will be willing to pay "internalizes" to the manufacturer the value of the information about safety that was generated by tests on the earlier individuals, thereby offsetting the costs incurred by the patentee in obtaining the information. In the case of a vaccine, the social benefits of reducing contagion are not reflected in the demand price of any consumer, which is presumably why vaccination is mandatory.

The mandatory nature of vaccination programs has contributed to the failure in the market of liability insurance. Even if patients would be willing to pay a vaccine price that would cover the costs of insurance against adverse outcomes, price controls in state-administered programs have prevented manufacturers from recovering this value. In the swine flu vaccine situation, vaccination was to be free to the public. In such circumstances, social willingness to pay for vaccination must presumably be reflected in the price at which the government contracts to buy supplies from the manufacturers. One insurer indicated a willingness to write insurance for the swine flu vaccine at a cost of a $1.76 per shot. The cost of this insurance would have amounted to 2.6 times the total congressional appropriation for the program.[22] Similarly, over half of the DPT (diphtheria-pertussis-tetanus) vaccine is purchased by state agencies. But federal funds for immunization programs were cut during the same two years that the price of the vaccine, inclusive of liability insurance, increased from 12 cents to $2.80 per dose.[23]

To the extent that these programs are funded out of tax revenues, a subsidy to offset the external benefits from vaccination is already in place, although it may be less than the full excess of social over private value of the vaccine. Moreover, to obtain the optimal demand price, the subsidy should supplement, not replace, charges to private patients. As in the case of malpractice insurance, the problem is thus not that vaccination programs are uninsurable but that the price at which private markets will bear the risk is politically unacceptable. The decisions being made through legislatures as to the social value of vaccines are inconsistent with the decisions being made through courts as to the social cost of injuries.[24]

A third problem in the vaccine context is that the mandatory nature of vaccination programs, combined with implementation through public health agencies, undermines control over the transmission of information and undermines the manufacturer's assumption-of-risk defense. All 50 states require that children be immunized before entering school. Exceptions are allowed for high-risk patients, because some of the adverse side effects are preventable with reasonable care. For example, adverse reactions to the swine flu vaccine were most likely in persons allergic to egg. Children with a prior personal or family history of susceptibility to convulsions are at high risk with the pertussis vaccine; if certain reactions occur after one dose, subsequent doses are contraindicated. If the vaccine were administered in a physician's office, the physician would presumably be held negligent if he did not screen out these high-risk cases. But the state officials and volunteers who were expected to administer the swine flu program would probably have been immune from liability.[25] Consequently, they would have less incentive to take care, thereby increasing the likelihood of liability on the manufacturers. A substantial part of the total risk faced by manufacturers was the risk of lack of due care by other participants, for example, government officials, in setting standards and verifying the safety of the vaccine; patients, in identifying their own risk of adverse outcome; and personnel, in screening patients, avoiding infections, and so on.[26] The elimination of both voluntary contractual relationships and tort liability of other parties for due care—which is inherent in a mandatory vaccination program—thus magnifies the exposure of vaccine manufacturers.[27] Moreover, even if it were feasible to obtain a meaningful informed consent to vaccination, rulings in the Sabin polio vaccine cases suggest that manufacturers may be held to a rule of absolute liability, regardless of the consent of the patient.[28]

A fourth concern in the case of pertussis is the nature of the risk—damage to the central nervous system of young infants—and the difficulty of distinguishing damage due to the vaccine from other central nervous system disorders which typically become manifest around the same age the vaccine is administered. Tort awards for severe brain damage to infants routinely run in the millions of dollars. Because there is no adequate private insurance for such events, the likelihood of the courts' bending the rules to provide some form of compensation is high. It is therefore not surprising that insurance problems are more severe for pertussis than for other vaccines, where the risk of catastrophic adverse effects is less.

Finally, the "safe" insurance premium depends in part on the insurer's capital reserves. It is no accident that apparent failures in liability insurance markets occur at times when insurer capital has been depleted. Adverse investment and underwriting experience for stock property and casualty insurers in 1973 and 1974 combined to wipe out 26 percent of insurers' capital.[29] This was one factor triggering the rate increases of 1975. Insurer capital had not yet been restored at the time of the swine flu threat and would have been significantly at risk because of the magnitude of the program. Assuming that 200 million people were vaccinated, defense costs (loss adjustment expenses) alone were estimated betwen $9.5 and $25 billion.[30] Assuming claim payments would be at least twice defense costs, this implies total costs of $30 to $75 billion. With total capital of $18.4 billion at the end of 1975, insurers were not surprisingly reluctant to assume the risk. Similarly, contraction of insurer capital has been one factor triggering the recent rise in malpractice insurance rates and withdrawal of carriers from highly risky lines, including the riskiest components of product liability, medical malpractice, and medical vaccines.

SPECIAL COMPENSATION FUNDS

VACCINES

Vaccines present distinct problems that cannot be readily resolved through existing compensation and liability mechanisms. I have argued that private markets do not internalize the social benefits of vaccination; the subsidy provided through public budget allocations is apparently too small and is used to replace rather than supplement private fees; and existing private and public programs do not adequately provide for permanently disabling injuries, particularly to children. While there is an efficiency argument for improving social insurance for all such cases, the ethical argument is perhaps even stronger in the case of mandatory vaccines. Thus a strong case can be made for providing a special fund to compensate victims of severely disabling injuries from childhood vaccines.

In principle, compensation of vaccine victims could also be achieved by holding manufacturers absolutely liable and making budget appropriations that would support a price for the vaccine sufficient to cover the cost of liability insurance. But that leaves determination of liability and of damages to the courts. If tort damage awards exceed optimal compensation,[31] then the appropriate social subsidy for vaccines and the optimal compensation to victims are more likely to be achieved if compensation is administered through a special public fund rather than through the liability system. To preserve manufacturer and provider incentives for care, the fund should be subrogated to any victim's claims for negligence, but the fund should be the sole recourse for the injured victim.[32] The fund should be financed by a tax on the vaccine, to be included in the price paid by both state and private purchasers. The correct social accounting for the cost of injuries due to vaccines would then be attained.

Of the vaccine compensation plans currently under consideration, the American Medical Association draft bill has most of these features. Its provisions include coverage of mandated pediatric vaccines only; an exclusive remedy through no-fault claims review for permanent, severely disabling injuries; payment for medical expenses, lost earnings, and pain and suffering up to $100,000; and a limit of two years on the period for filing claims. The no-fault fund would be subrogated to any victim's claim for negligence against providers. The bill's major defect is the proposal that the fund be supported by general revenues rather than a tax on vaccines.

The Hawkins-Waxman proposal calls for a generous no-fault compensation plan for a comprehensive list of vaccines and a comprehensive list of conditions, with a five-year statute of limitations running from discovery of the injury, while leaving the tort remedy as an alternative to the victim. The no-fault plan is to be funded by a vaccine surcharge and borrowed amounts from general revenues if necessary. The plan would be subrogated to all tort rights of compensated victims against manufacturers and physicians. This plan is unlikely to reduce the risk facing vaccine manufacturers. It might even increase their liability, in the likely event that the plan evolves into a general compensation fund for a variety of childhood injuries.

The Lederle proposal would establish a system of hearing panels that could award damages (subject to some limits) on a finding of vaccine relatedness, regardless of fault. A plaintiff could appeal the panel's finding, but damages in a subsequent tort action would be subject to all the same limits as those set up for the panels. By limiting the jury's freedom to set damages, this plan would go some way toward containing the defendant's risk while preserving incentives for care. Although this plan merits serious study, experience with medical malpractice screening panels suggests that the panel component could simply add another layer of cost and delay to the tort process.

MEDICAL INNOVATIONS

If a special compensation fund makes sense for vaccines, why not extend the idea to medical innovations, in recognition of the social benefits flowing from participation in such research? As argued above, a patient's incentive to participate is socially suboptimal if private benefits fall short of social benefits. In principle this could be corrected by a cash inducement. For the sake of argument, let us make the implausible assumption that the optimal subsidy is positive and equal to the actuarial cost of compensation. Then the participant would be better off with a guarantee of compensation rather than cash only if the research program could provide the compensation more cheaply than alternative insurance sources to which he might turn. If, as was argued earlier, the permanently disabled victim would in fact suffer significant increase in the cost of obtaining private insurance, and if he were not eligible for SSDI, then he would probably prefer a long-term health and disability insurance policy to the equivalent value in cash. In that case, one possibility would be to hold researchers absolutely liable for adverse outcomes. Another alternative would be to require them to provide health and disability insurance coverage as a condition of obtaining government funding for research. A third possibility would be to establish a special compensation fund.

Ignoring insurability, the second of these alternatives—that of requiring medical researchers to provide coverage as a condition of obtaining federal funding—has clear advantages. If the agency that allocates research funds is also responsible for defining levels of compensation, then both the compensation and the research funding decisions are made subject to appropriate budget constraints. An objection raised to this approach is that private insurance vendors might not be willing to write such coverage without a substantial risk markup.[33] However, if the researchers were not subject to tort liability but were simply required to furnish an injured subject with standard first-party health and disability policies, such insurance would not be subject to the sociolegal risks of tort liability. Consequently, the risk markup might be less than is now paid through liability insurance.[34] Currently, liability insurance for medical research is explicitly excluded from standard malpractice coverage and is written on a separate treaty basis through surplus lines carriers. It is possible that any increased risk due to the no-fault aspect of the coverage could be more than offset by the decreased risk obtained by codifying benefits.

While the same benefits might in principle be offered through a government program, the argument against this is largely political. The government has a very deep pocket, and the potential expansion of categories of compensable injuries is virtually unlimited, if the criterion is injury in the course of an activity that generates some socially valuable information. The line between experimental and established medical procedures is impossible to define. The fact that some innovations received federal funds and are already subject to substantial regulation does not necessarily distinguish them in terms of social benefits. Moreover, why should medical experimentation be distinguished from other forms of social experimentation, such as education, income maintenance programs, and so on? If compensability were indeed expanded in the face of such pressure, it is unlikely that costs would be internalized to the relevant activities. In that case, the market deterrence argument for a special fund, as opposed to a general social insurance program, evaporates.

CONCLUSION

Liability rules designed to induce optimal levels of care may result in suboptimal rates of innovation because research subjects have no incentive to consider the social benefits of the information generated. However, in the case of medical innovations this is probably offset by other subsidies to health care. Even if it could be shown that the current rate of medical research is suboptimal, providing stimulus in the form of no-fault compensation through either absolute tort liability or a special compensation fund is unlikely to be optimal. If compensation is the optimal form of subsidy, then requiring researchers to provide first-party coverage seems preferable. Mandatory vaccines present different problems. In this case, a special fund for severely disabled victims seems appropriate.

NOTES

1. See John P. Brown (1973), p. 323. Contrary to Brown, a comparative negligence rule could also yield optimal incentives. See David Haddock and Christopher Curran (1985), p. 49.
2. California Medical Associaton (1977).
3. For example, S. 2690.
4. This difference is only one of degree, at least on the benefits side, since the efficacy of many medical procedures is not well established.
5. This conclusion also requires that compensation through tort be equivalent to the insurance the patient would have bought voluntarily and that transactions costs be equivalent.
6. See John Robertson (1975) and J. R. Waltz and F. E. Inbau (1971), pp. 179-202.
7. Robertson (1975).
8. This assumes that the expected cost of injuries (C) is unaffected by the acquisition of knowledge. It could diminish if greater experience with a new therapy made it possible to screen out categories of patients who are at risk, or to avoid adverse drug interactions, and so on. Still, there is no presumption of equivalence between C and B_s.
9. For a similar argument—that abolition of the privity defense exposes suppliers to adverse selection and moral hazard—see Richard Epstein (1984).
10. Taylor and Wilensky (1983); Phelps (1983).
11. This distorting effect of health insurance is less true in the early phase of development of a new therapy, because health insurers typically deny coverage for procedures they classify as experimental and may also deny coverage for any adverse consequences. The decision to classify a procedure as nonexperimental is currently not based on any formal analysis of costs and benefit, but rather on such factors as how widely it is used, political pressures, pressure from physicians and patients, and so on.

12. Ginsburg (1981).
13. In principle, under a negligence rule physicians should have no incentive to buy liability insurance since it would be cheaper to prevent injuries deemed negligent than to insure against them [Shavell (1982)]. In practice, physicians consider extensive liability insurance a condition of practice, presumably insuring against erroneous imputations of negligence by the courts and settlement process [Danzon (1985b)].
14. The real price of insurance is the loading charge. If the premium for comparable coverage is 30 percent higher for an individual than for a group and the load is 20 percent of the group premium, then the real price of individual coverage is 2.5 times the real price of group coverage.
15. Danzon (1984).
16. Danzon (1984). The optimal duration of liability involves a trade-off, balancing the benefits from additional incentives for care against the higher costs of insurance and suboptimal levels of risky activities.
17. "Market deterrence" refers to the reduction in the output of a risky activity that is induced by internalizing to that activity the cost of injuries that it generates.
18. Commercial insurers were replaced by physician-owned companies (which now account for over 50 percent of malpractice insurance premium volume); mandatory joint underwriting associations, which require insurers to provide malpractice insurance as a condition of writing other insurance lines in a state; and state-operated patient compensation funds, which assume liability for losses above a specified threshold, typically $100,000 per claim per physician.
19. Danzon (1984).
20. Danzon (1985a).
21. U.S. Senate, Committee on Labor and Public Welfare (1976).
22. U.S. House of Representatives, Committee on Appropriations, Subcommittee on Labor and Health, Education, and Welfare (1976), p. 81.
23. Sun (1985).
24. This exacerbates the more general problem, that if tort awards attempt full compensation for pecuniary and nonpecuniary loss that exceeds the compensation consumers are willing to pay for, suppliers of goods and services cannot recoup in higher prices the cost of liability insurance, even without constraints due to state intervention [Danzon (1984)]. This applies a fortiori if liability is erroneously assigned for injuries not caused by the product or service. The level of activities subject to such tort liability will consequently be suboptimal.
25. The decision of the Supreme Court in *United States* v. *Orleans* (1976) established that the United States would not be liable under the Federal Tort Claims Act for the negligence of nonfederal personnel who administered the swine flu vaccine. In some jurisdictions, local governments would not be liable for the negligence of their employees [U.S. House of Representatives, Committee on Interstate and Foreign Commerce, Subcommittee on Health and the Environment (1976), pp. 30-31].

26. U.S. House of Representatives, Committee on Interstate and Foreign Commerce, Subcommittee on Health and the Environment (1976), pp. 40-41.
27. Some of these risks would not be independent, in that one error (such as in checking the safety of a batch of vaccine) could affect similarly thousands, perhaps millions of vaccine recipients. In that case, the vast numbers involved serve to multiply rather than diminish the risk.
28. *Davis v. Wyeth Laboratories* (1968); *Reyes v. Wyeth Laboratories* (1974).
29. Danzon (1985a).
30. U.S. House of Representatives, Committee on Appropriations, Subcommittee on Labor and Health, Education, and Welfare (1976), p. 86.
31. Danzon (1984).
32. This is essentially the proposal advanced by the swine flu manufacturers, who did not seek to avoid liability for negligent production.
33. National Commission for the Protection of Human Subjects of Biomedical and Behavioral Research (1978).
34. The admittedly sparse evidence suggests that the physical risks are not large. Less than 2 percent of victims of therapeutic research suffer a permanently disabling or fatal injury, and the average injury rate is less than 1 percent if nontherapeutic research subjects are included [Cardon et al. (1976)].

BIBLIOGRAPHY

Brown, J. P. 1973. "Toward an Economic Theory of Liability." *Journal of Legal Studies* 2:323.

California Medical Association and California Hospital Association. 1977. *Medical Insurance Feasibility Study.* San Francisco: Sutter Publications.

Cardon, P. V., F. W. Dommel, and R. R. Trumble. 1976. "Injuries to Research Subjects." *New England Journal of Medicine* 295:650.

Danzon, P. 1984. "Tort Reform and the Role of Government in Private Insurance Markets." *Journal of Legal Studies* 13:517

————. 1985a. *Medical Malpractice: Theory, Evidence and Public Policy.* Cambridge, MA: Harvard University Press.

————. 1985b. "Liability Insurance and the Tort System: The Case of Medical Malpractice." *Journal of Health Economics* 4.

Davis v. Wyeth Laboratories, Inc. 1968. 399 F. 3d 121 (9th Cir.).

Epstein, R. 1984. "Products Liability as an Insurance Market." Paper presented at the Conference on Critical Issues in Tort Law Reform: A Search for Principles. Yale University Law School, September 1984, New Haven, CT.

Ginsburg, P. 1981. "Altering the Tax Treatment of Employment-Based Health Plans." *Health and Society: Milbank Memorial Fund Quarterly* 59:224.

Haddock, D., and C. Curran. 1985. "An Economic Theory of Negligence." *Journal of Legal Studies* 14:49.

National Commission for the Protection of Human Subjects of Biomedical and Behavioral Research. 1978. *Ethical Principles and Guidelines for the Protection of Human Subjects of Research* (Belmont report). DHEW publ. no. (OS) 78-0012. Washington D.C.: Government Printing Office.

Phelps, C. E. 1983. "Tax Policy, Health Insurance, and Health Care." In J. A. Meyer, ed., *Market Reforms in Health Care*. Washington, D.C.: American Enterprise Institute.

Reyes v. *Wyeth Laboratories, Inc.* 1974. 498 F. 2d 1264 (5th Cir.).

Robertson, J. 1975. "Legal Implications of the Boundaries Between Biomedical Research Involving Human Subjects and the Accepted or Routine Practice of Medicine." In *Ethical Principles and Guidelines, Appendix*, vol. 2. DHEW publ. no. (OS) 78-0014, pp. 16-1—16-54.

Shavell, S. 1982. "On Liability and Insurance." *The Bell Journal of Economics* 13:120.

Sun, M. 1985. "The Vexing Problems of Vaccine Compensation." *Science* 227:1012.

Taylor, A., and G. Wilensky. 1983. "The Effect of Tax Policies on Expenditures for Private Health Insurance." In *Market Reforms*, pp. 163-84.

United States v. *Orleans*. 1976. 44 L.W. 4700 (June 1).

U.S. House of Representatives, Committee on Appropriations, Subcommittee on Labor and Health, Education, and Welfare. 1976. *Hearings on Emergency Supplemental Appropriations Poll, Swine Flu Immunization Program*. 94th Cong., 2nd sess.

U.S. House of Representatives, Committee on Interstate and Foreign Commerce, Subcommittee on Health and the Environment. 1976. *Hearings on Proposed Swine Flu Vaccination Program*. 94th Cong., 2nd sess.

Waltz, J. R., and F. E. Inbau. 1971. *Medical Jurisprudence*. New York: MacMillan.

14

Some Social Bases
of Compensation Schemes

Franklin E. Zimring

> The object of this paper is to give notice of an impending question of
> great importance; not to give an answer to the question, but to show how
> and why it arises at the present time.
> There is a movement now going on in this country for the enactment of
> legislation based upon the principle of the English Workmen's
> Compensation Act. This legislation is founded largely upon a theory
> inconsistent with the fundamental principle of the modern common law of
> torts. As to a considerable number of the accidents covered by some of the
> recent statutes, the results reached under the statute would be absolutely
> irreconcilable with results reached at common law in cases outside the
> scope of the statute. This incongruity must inevitably provoke discussion
> as to the intrinsic correctness of the modern common law of torts; and is
> likely to lead, either to a movement in favor of repealing the statutes, or
> to a movement in favor of making radical changes in the common law.
> —Jeremiah Smith
> "Sequel to Workmen's Compensation Acts,"
> *Harvard Law Review,* 1917

My object *here* is to set the discussion of compensation for medical mishaps
in a wider context than the provisions of tort law. The quotation from Smith's
classic examination of the principles of tort law and workmen's compensation
serves both as a reminder that the issues which concern us when discussing
compensation options are far from novel and as a caution against concluding
that compensation systems based on inconsistent principles cannot coexist.

The incongruity of tort and workmen's compensation principles was
evident 70 years ago and certainly did provoke discussion, but this did not lead
to the emergence of either approach as dominant in the structure of
compensation schemes for injury. Instead, American society currently
operates without comprehensive compensation programs in areas such as
income maintenance and health care. The law of torts shares sovereignty with
a wide variety of categorical benefit schemes directed at special groups or

special problems. Other activities, including medical mishaps and automobile accidents, are governed in most states by tort law.

While current circumstances may be a way station on the path toward a more coordinated and comprehensive system, a profoundly mixed set of subsystems has prevailed in the United States for at least half a century and shows no sign of imminent collapse.

For my purposes, it does not matter much whether current conditions can be characterized as a mixed system or no system at all. The fact that different areas are under very different regimes of response to losses invites an account of what determines social choice in loss distribution: what I would call a political science of compensation schemes. Of course, different disciplines would give different accounts of what constitutes the major determinants of social choice in these matters. One can imagine a lively dialogue among political scientists, economists, historians, and lawyers using different vocabularies and points of emphasis in explaining the range of societal responses to loss.

Whatever the disciplinary labels, accounting for those factors that do (rather than should) influence compensation policy is a useful exercise. Identifying a range of likely options in a political spectrum can make the use of normative criteria within the range of likely candidates a more powerful and relevant exercise.

This chapter stops well short of proposing a political science of compensation schemes. It is the sort of exercise that generates phrases such as "notes toward" or "fragments of" on title pages. I will first outline a set of societal tensions about loss spreading that characterizes modern dialogue about compensation in the United States and then speculate about the extent to which the factors associated with displacement of the tort system in other fields characterize medical innovation and experimentation.

TORT LAW AND COMPENSATION AGENDAS

The principal complaint about tort law responses to a variety of losses—the failure of these rules to achieve widespread compensation—turns out to be socially contingent in a very important way. Dissatisfaction is expressed about the tort system response to automobile accidents, for instance, because many persons injured are not paid for medical expenses or lost earnings.

This criticism is of some force only because comprehensive compensation schemes do not exist outside the tort system to perform compensation functions. If a societal decision had been made to pay for necessary medical care on a need basis, the fact that tort law did not shift losses for accident-related medical costs would not matter. Comprehensive income replacement programs would serve a similar purpose with respect to lost earnings.

The absence of broad compensation schemes, together with a social bias toward spreading losses, puts pressure on tort law doctrine and generates proposals to supplement or supplant the tort system for a variety of victim groups. The conflict between legal doctrines stressing culpability and strict standards of causation and those emphasizing the spreading of loss is obvious: once loss shifting in tort cases is institutionalized (by insurance, for example), these mechanisms can be extended to achieve broader compensation results by compromising traditional doctrine. The more important compensation becomes, the greater the number of instances where other principles will be subordinated. When tort law is viewed as an alternative to other compensation systems, then the more significant the compensation aspect of a program, the more likely the conclusion that a categorical compensation scheme is superior to the tort alternative.

There is, of course, no reason why the tort system should be regarded as the only mechanism available for loss spreading, and there may be important benefits provided by a tort system even if other loss-spreading mechanisms are in place. Even though income maintenance and medical expense schemes are frequently discussed as alternatives to tort recovery, compensation schemes and tort recovery could supplement each other without one supplanting the other. Indeed, the argument can be made that the growth of insurance and compensation programs which operate independently of the tort system could liberate tort law from compensation pressures and limit recoveries in tort to those circumstances where causation and culpability meet traditional standards for recovery.

But as long as medical care costs are not shifted from injured consumers and incomes are not maintained without tort recovery, tort doctrine will be pushed beyond moral coherence. The felt need to compensate will encompass cases that fall short of the culpability requirements which terms such as "malpractice" and "negligence" carry in ordinary language. And the parties to whom those labels are attached will not understand that they play a role in a larger compensation agenda.

Meanwhile, what I shall call categorical compensation systems spring up and operate with an ad hoc quality that bedevils political theory. Government pays over 40 percent of the medical bills in the United States and employer-paid insurance provides another major share,[1] but there is no general theory of cost spreading to be found. Instead, there are special programs for crime victims, coal miners with black lung disease, war veterans, and victims of auto accidents. The principles on which groups are selected for special compensation are elusive at best.

If tort systems can achieve compensation results only at great administrative cost and through a loss of principle, the categorical programs compensate with lower administrative cost and no theory at all. Is there a way out of this morass?

One possibility is a general compensation scheme involving medical costs and partial earnings replacement. In fact, when governmental health and disability schemes are combined wth standard employer-paid medical insurance, current expenditure patterns are not so far from this result, if not its formal theory. Among its other advantages, this development would make the special problems of compensation for losses associated with innovative medicine disappear.

Short of this solution, however, how can we locate the problems associated with losses imposed by toxic waste, violent crime, old age, and automobiles? What factors create pressure for compensation and when? Where does innovative medicine fit? That is the subject of the next section.

PRECURSORS TO COMPENSATION PROGRAMS

Can we identify some of the characteristics of loss-causing activity that generate pressure for categorical compensation systems as alternatives or supplements to the tort system? This task is necessary as a preliminary to discussing where medical experimentation stands on the spectrum of social problems which raise compensation issues. It is also a useful window into the social processes that produce compensation schemes.

Three limitations on the list of factors to follow deserve preliminary mention. First, the characteristics discussed here constitute a partial list, bordering on the fragmentary. A more complete accounting, while obviously useful, is beyond the scope of this work. Second, my discussion of factors is limited to their role in shaping compensation alternatives to tort system recovery. The same features that animate the search for alternatives to tort system recovery doubtless explain the differential pressures to bend tort law toward recovery in some areas rather than others, as well as differences in other collective resource allocations. Third, the armchair methodology that produces my short list is an effort of last resort. We really need a political science of compensation that is far more systematic than anything discussed here.

With those caveats in place, I wish, first, to distinguish between the characteristics of losses attributable to particular activities and perceptions about the loss-causing enterprise. Then I shall nominate various elements in each category that predispose the political system toward a compensation response.

The distinction between loss characteristics and enterprise characteristics is not meant to be obscure. The former concern social perceptions of the kind of harm done; the latter concern social perceptions of the nature of the enterprise associated with the harm.

LOSS FACTORS

Four loss characteristics appear to be associated with positive pressure for special compensation: the occurrence of special damages, the existence of individuals who suffer substantial loss, a social sense that the victim was not to blame and could not control events, and social identification with the victim class.

I use the phrase "special damages" as a metaphor. In the United States, there is a hierarchy of losses clearly expressed in social attitudes and in most compensation schemes. The preservation of health (at almost any cost) and the maintenance of income (but only up to working-class standards) are perceived as necessities; loss of profits, of reputation, of an earning potential far above average, and monetary compensation for pain and suffering, while parts of tort damages, do not have the same social importance.

These necessaries are usually the first—and not infrequently the only— kinds of losses to be addressed by categorical compensation systems. It thus seems likely that the frequent occurrence of these kinds of losses predisposes the political system to search for a special categorical compensation approach. The larger the proportion of all losses attributable to an activity to be found in the "necessaries" category, the higher the likelihood of a special compensation approach. And if my nomination of socially perceived necessaries is correct, the mixture of limited doses of income maintenance with unlimited doses of health maintenance biases social investment in compensation toward investing resources in health maintenance.

The occurrence of large individual losses is also an important part of the social process of isolating a particular problem for special treatment. In an important sense, you cannot have a poster without a poster child. The impetus for federal programs of disaster relief, for example, is support for the disaster victim who loses everything, even if the program compensates less drastic changes in circumstance. We would thus expect that the occurrence of catastrophic harms attributable to an activity would predispose the system toward searching for special compensatory solutions.

Two further aspects, while interrelated, deserve individual mention. American culture distinguishes, at a deep level, between the deserving and undeserving poor, and it seems likely that there is a parallel distinction between the deserving and undeserving injured. The more clearly individuals harmed lack either personal fault or personal control over the events that caused the loss, the more likely they are to appear attractive candidates for compensation. The moral judgments that condition this kind of distinction are socially determined and often problematic.

This is at least a partial explanation for the low degree of concern for compensating victims of catastrophic illness associated with cigarette smoking, alcohol, and single-car automobile accidents. This mind-set might also explain why public health approaches to automobile injury and death were retarded by the emphasis on personal fault ("the nut behind the wheel" was believed responsible) and may still explain part of the resistance to no-fault automobile compensation plans. Certainly this distinction is relevant to the palpable difference in public response to AIDS victims who contract the disease through homosexual contact or drug abuse and those who contract it through blood transfusion.

In addition to perceptions about the loser's personal control and degree of responsibility, there is a broader sense in which the social capacity to identify with victims helps select attractive candidates for compensation. I use "identify" here in a literal sense: In a situation where the average citizen can see himself as a potential victim of a loss, the particular problem giving rise to that situation will receive favorable attention as a candidate for compensation. The sense that it can happen to me, no matter how engendered, predisposes the political process toward identifying a special loss for governmental attention on a priority basis.

With respect to loss characteristics, the same features that predict investment in compensation programs should predict other collective resource allocations, such as public support for medical research and prevention programs.

ENTERPRISE FACTORS

What characteristics of the loss-causing agency predispose the political system toward compensation? Let me nominate five: a social perception of cause, a perceived ability to pay, a sense of the specialness of the loss-causing agency, an existing payment system, and the perceived failure of tort law to achieve desired results.

With respect to this list, the distinction between the political science approach I wish to take and a philosophic or economic approach must be clearly drawn: in dealing with concepts like causation and ability to pay, I am referring to social perceptions of reality, independent of any empirical truths about causation or economic ability. Two standard examples make this point.

Sparks from a New York Central Railroad locomotive ignite a wheat field next to the tracks and the fire causes the loss of 100 acres of winter wheat. The conceptual problem with attributing this loss to the enterprise of railroading is that a similar harm would not have occurred if the wheat were planted elsewhere. But if there is a social consensus that railroading is the culprit, that consensus will determine the political response to such fires.

Similarly, despite the conceptual difficulty we encounter in attributing pedestrian accidents to the enterprise of driving cars rather than to trying to cross city streets on foot, a social consensus on the matter identifies an acceptable political resolution of the difficulty. If people think cars cause the accidents, then pedestrians will be included in an auto compensation plan. Consensus of this kind on causation predisposes the system toward funding compensation programs by making assessments against drivers.

The perception of "deep pockets" is also a social construct. If people think railroads can pay, and that the enterprise of railroading rather than the railroad's customers is bearing the cost, the perception will have political consequences independent of any deeper reality.

What I call the perception of the specialness or novelty of the agency that is perceived to cause losses is one of the contributing features to a clear sense of enterprise causation. That the losses caused by a particular agency be considered special is critical in predicting legislative response. Many victim groups lobby for special legislative concern, but few are chosen for compensation. Success in focusing legislative attention depends on persuading elected representatives that a problem is both important and different from other loss-causing agencies that do not win categorical compensation treatment.

One indication of specialness is the social novelty of a particular activity. People have been raising sheep in Utah far longer than the government has been stocking nerve gas there or conducting atomic tests upwind. The perceived novelty of an enterprise seems one aspect that singles it out for special treatment, and this is at least a partial explanation of why losses caused by new technology and self-conscious experiments have special appeal with respect to compensatory treatment.

The heavy involvement of an enterprise with tort law and insurance can also encourage the shift to categorical compensation by providing an institutional precedent as well as a pool of funds available for compensation. In the evolution of no-fault automobile insurance plans, the widespread existence of car insurance and the substantial transfer payments under the tort system facilitated the identification of driving as a special compensation category and made the establishment of state-level compensation plans seem far less radical than compensation programs for areas where loss shifting was less institutionalized.

Finally, and despite problems of tautology, it seems to me that the perceived failure of the tort system to achieve equitable results with respect to particular activity probably deserves special mention. The lack of fit between the problem of industrial accidents and a tort system compete with an assumption-of-risk doctrine and the fellow-servant rule is an important part of the story of workmen's compensation. Difficulties in arbitrating between the underlying illness and innovative therapy as a cause for actions may hamper the tort system in providing compensation where many think it is needed. The problems with proof of causation in cases of radiation cancer have provoked efforts at separate compensation schemes.

Here again, one is dealing with a social perception rather than an objectively defined phenomenon. The absence of transfer payments is only a sign of failure if the public thinks that payments should be made. One would expect this to occur when loss characteristics previously discussed are present: losses that affect health maintenance and basic income, hit some individuals catastrophically, seem beyond the fault and control of the victims, and select victims who engender a sense of identification in the general public and its elected representatives.

The next step toward a general political science of compensation schemes would be to measure the settings in which compensation has been adopted or rejected against the factors outlined above. Such an exercise will not be attempted here. I suspect that reviewing case studies in compensation decisions would both add to the factors mentioned and suggest a strong role for nondeterministic factors and sheer accident in the particular history of compensation schemes.

However primitive the foregoing list may be, it may still be worthwhile to examine the case of medical innovation in light of the criteria for compensation discussed above. That is my task in the following section.

MEDICAL INNOVATION AS A COMPENSATION CANDIDATE

Is medical innovation an enterprise that is sufficiently distinct and unified to permit classification on the basis of the factors that predict compensation schemes? This, too, is a question of public perception rather than conceptual coherence. And the answer is far from easy.

Are medical innovations distinct from the larger enterprise of medical care, or are they usually regarded as a subset of the problems and losses associated with medical service? My suspicion is that the distinction between normal and experimental medicine is far more acutely felt by professionals than by the lay public and that members of the general public would be puzzled by attempts to discuss compensation for research injuries as a species apart from other medical misadventures. There is certainly no feeling currently that experimental medicine is a special problem requiring an individualized compensation solution. In such circumstances, compensation program decisions probably would concern the medical enterprise as a whole rather than its innovative aspects.

It is also not obvious that the wide array of drug experiments, introduction of new surgical techniques, and classical experiments share enough characteristics to call for common treatment. Drug innovation might better be viewed as a subset of products liability or as a separate matter altogether. The nonexperimental use of innovative therapies and techniques might best become a branch of malpractice doctrine with some special rules. Classical experiments might be viewed as unique with respect to both experimental and control subjects.

If a judgment about the likelihood of special compensation for a broad spectrum of medical innovations must be made, however, the prospects for a single compensation program limited to innovative medicine but addressing most of its aspects are not good. The barriers to compensation lie not in the loss factors discussed in the previous sections but in the enterprise factors discussed there.

The mishaps associated with innovative medicine produce large losses involving the sorts of social necessaries that provoke compensation. These injuries frequently produce the sense of social identification with victims associated with procompensation bias. But there is no clear sense that medical innovation is the culprit, no institutional precedent or pool of funds broad enough yet specific enough to spawn a compensation scheme, and no clear perceived failure of the tort system or sense that innovative medicine is a special problem.

Medical research and innovation are socially regarded as desirable rather than dangerous. I suspect that virtually nobody outside the animal rights movement would tell a public opinion polltaker that "too much medical research" is conducted in the United States. In this sense, the enterprise stands in significant contrast to many other new technologies. In the frequent case where it is not clear whether an innovative technique or the underlying illness has generated a bad effect, there may not be a social predisposition toward assuming the medical invention caused the harm.

There is also no single institutional precedent or pool of funds associated with medical innovations. Drug companies and doctors use different insurance mechanisms. Medical malpractice insurance is decentralized to the state level. Hospital liability insurance is also decentralized. All these insurance programs cover risks other than innovation and experiment and thus could not be combined to prepare a uniform system for innovation alone. Significant proprietary rights and property controls exist for drugs and for some technologies but not for many surgical procedures. The federal government, which plays a major role in underwriting medical research, takes a more limited part in stimulating new drug development.

Further, there is no strong public sense that the losses occurring as the result of medical innovation are special or distinct. The problem is either seen more broadly (medical mishaps as a whole) or as a specific crisis requiring a special, usually ad hoc solution (swine flu vaccine).

While the tort system response to medical injury is not above public reproach, there is at present no particular concern or special urgency associated with uncompensated injuries from biomedical innovation.

Of course, a sense of special urgency might be generated in the wake of a particularly catastrophic innovation. It is more likely, however, that particular branches of medical innovation will work out particular approaches to insurance or compensation, or that major shifts in social approaches to all medical mishaps will change compensation conditions for innovations.

Compensation for victims of experimental drug mishaps may be expanded as part of a loosening of the strictures on new drug development and introduction. Special insurance for clinical research subjects may be institutionalized at the behest of research institutions rather than victims, a "trickle down" compensation scenario quite unlike workmen's compensation but more similar to the campaign for crime victim programs.

More significant general changes may take place as a response to the perceived malpractice crisis and continuing efforts at containing hospital costs. If hospital medicine is more completely federalized, the institutional climate for a national solution to hospital-based medical mishaps will be far more favorable.

The most important change relating to compensation for medical mishaps may occur outside both the medical services liability field and the tort system. If we continue to build disability and medical care compensation systems into government and the employment relationship, we may solve most of the problems associated with compensating the losses from medical mishaps without ever specifically addressing them. As both a political and conceptual matter, this would not be wholly unfortunate.

The possibility that special compensation programs will emerge as part of a package of changes that will allow more risk exposure in clinical drug trials may also apply to a broader spectrum of medical innovations. Loosening the *ex ante* protections of human subjects in medical research may confer benefits that outweigh the costs. To do so, however, will create a sense of the special risk of the research subject that fits the criteria for categorical compensation more closely than my understanding of current conditions. A social compact that includes extensive compensation to subjects would then seem more appropriate.

NOTE

1.   See *Business Week*, October 15, 1984, p. 141: "Government accounts for $149 billion of the $355 billion total, with private health insurance responsible for another $110 billion. The combined share of private health insurance and all levels of government of total health care costs is 73 percent."

15

Responding to Biomedical Innovation:
A Beginning Synthesis
and Modest Proposal

Alan J. Weisbard

How are we as a society to respond to the injuries that inevitably accompany our quest for medical progress? Economists, lawyers, and public policy analysts are too often prone to see such questions as inviting a purely technical inquiry, to be solved by recourse to allegedly value-free economic theory or legal precedent. One of this book's signal contributions is to suggest an alternative form of analysis, drawing on history and philosophy, cultural analysis and sociology of professions, the history and philosophy of science and medicine, and the careful analysis of politics and political institutions, to improve our understanding of the social meaning and significance of medical innovations and the injuries that trail in their wake. The question—indeed, the challenge— is whether we can employ the fruits of this multidisciplinary inquiry to develop a better informed and more sensible public policy to govern medical innovation and the treatment of its victims.

I am not convinced that the programmatic recommendations for law and policy advanced earlier in this book have sufficiently risen to this challenge. The dominant motifs of several of the contributions—particularly those in the law and economics tradition—are such fixtures of conventional policy analysis as economic efficiency and minimization of administrative costs and burdens. There is no apparent willingness to entertain the possibility that injuries associated with medical innovations are somehow special and demand a rethinking of society's obligations to those injured. The perspective seems to differ little from that of the English court which announced in 1798 that "It is better that an individual should sustain an injury than that the public should suffer an inconvenience."[1]

I am pleased to acknowledge my indebtedness to Guido Calabresi, who introduced me to these issues and fostered a continuing fascination with tort law and its place in regulating our collective lives; to my Cardozo colleagues Paul Shupack, Steve Diamond, Arthur Jacobson, Richard Singer, David Carlson, and Chuck Yablon, for stimulating criticisms and suggestions; and to Deborah Arnowitz of the Cardozo class of 1987, for dedicated research and editorial assistance extending far beyond the call of duty. Responsibility for remaining errors is strictly my own.

This chapter proceeds from quite different premises. Taking seriously the contributions of the humanists, it attempts a beginning synthesis of the social meaning of injuries associated with medical innovation and explores the implications of that synthesis for the formulation of public policy. The analysis challenges the social values implicit in certain conventional legal and economic thinking, particularly that associated with the law and economics school of thought. The essay concludes by proposing an alternative non-fault framework for compensation for medical injuries. While only the outline of this approach can be offered here, the proposal is set forth in the hope of stimulating further debate on how social and philosophical analysis can contribute to better law and public policy.

THE SOCIAL CONTEXT OF MEDICAL INNOVATION

Stephen Toulmin aptly characterizes contemporary American society as "deliberately modernizing" and "progressive" in its pursuit of technological innovation (chapter 2). His elegant essay provides a powerful and much-needed reminder that sound analysis of potential societal responses—including legal ones—to the problem of injuries associated with technological innovation must be rooted in a careful assessment of the social and historical context in which the problem arises.

While the pace of technological progress has, if anything, markedly accelerated since World War II, recent decades have also brought increased awareness of and concern for the risks entailed in our commitment to a technological way of life. We came to see ourselves not only as the world's pioneers in technological innovation, but also as "a nation of guinea pigs."[2] Demands for action rapidly followed expressions of concern, and these demands were met in the 1960s and 1970s with new and ever-more-expansive governmental regulatory efforts to control risks and prevent technological catastrophes. The past decade has also witnessed widely publicized private litigation seeking compensation through the tort system when risks have eventuated in injuries (and sometimes even when they have not, as at Three Mile Island).

Occupational and environmental hazards in particular have been prolific sources of massive litigation in recent years. Such names as Three Mile Island, Agent Orange, asbestosis, black lung, and, most recently, Bhopal, have dominated the headlines and created powerful new images associated with our collective commitment to technology. We have become rather more skeptical in our attitudes toward the corporate—and occasionally governmental—purveyors of progress who unleased these terrors of modern life. We have sought perpetrators to blame and hold accountable for the fearsome human and economic toll imposed by several of these hazards.

The tort system, through its well-established norms of negligence and more recently evolving concepts of strict liability for abnormally dangerous activities and defective products, has provided a serviceable, if imperfect, legal means for seeking redress from the parties responsible. In so doing, it compels certain "risky technologies" to bear their costs by imposing financial liability for the injuries caused, often in the absence of clear proof of fault or negligence in any traditional legal sense.[3]

Toulmin's remarks about technological innovation in general certainly extend to and encompass medical research and, more broadly, innovative medical practices. Yet in some ways medical progress is quite special, and perhaps unique, in the responses it evokes from this society. American society is almost certainly more uniformly supportive and enthusiastic, and far less ambivalent, about technological innovations in medicine than in other spheres of economic activity. The reasons for this require fuller scholarly exploration in the directions suggested by Toulmin, but some preliminary speculations may be in order here.

The enthusiasm for medical innovation may be rooted in a subconscious quest for immortality and resistance to the inevitability of death. Perhaps it reflects a troubling symbiosis between the public relations efforts of organized medicine and the often uncritical boosterism prevalent within some sectors of the popular communications media, although the latter may simply mirror existing public attitudes. Perhaps the organization of the medical profession—the historical (but rapidly changing) lack of for-profit corporate manifestations of Modern Medicine, Inc.—helps to diffuse the anxieties generated by periodic reports of medical innovations gone awry. Indeed, the seeming exceptions—the medical cases that have most dramatically generated adverse public response, such as DES and the Dalkon Shield—may prove the rule, insofar as they represent medical products merchandised by for-profit corporations, rather than the sorts of innovative practice that arise in individual practitioner-patient encounters. If so, the increasing concentration and corporatization of what is now termed the "health care industry" may well have its impact on the climate of public support for medical innovation.

The basis for our enthusiasm about medical innovation might also be sought at quite a different, less instrumental, and perhaps more poetic level. Baruch Blumberg's evocative account of the Daedalus effect (chapter 3) captures a particular image of the scientific and technological enterprise—its insatiable quest for knowledge and understanding, as well as its sometimes unpredictable potential for increasing our power to influence, for good or ill, the natural world. Yet it also provides a moving description of certain aspects of the human spirit that we as a society have come to value most. If Blumberg has indeed succeeded in providing a plausible secular account of the ethos, and perhaps the telos, of our technological civilization, this consonance between scientific and broader secular values offers a powerful intrinsic and expressive justification for medical innovation, quite apart from the more utilitarian considerations usually adduced on its behalf. One cannot reflect on the awe inspired by organ transplants, man's creation of a functioning artificial heart, or the development of novel means of human reproduction—whatever their practical import or potentially troubling social consequences—without concluding that Blumberg has captured something very important.

These distinctive features of medical innovations, viewed in a broad social, historical, and cultural context, are critical to assessing existing legal doctrines governing liability for medical injuries and to evaluating the prospects for future legal or institutional reforms. The law's own evolution reflects changing societal perceptions, values, and mores at least as much as it is influenced by prescriptive economic theories or mechanical doctrinal analysis. Further social and conceptual analysis, both of attitudes toward technological innovation in general and of those factors which differentiate medical innovations in particular, has much to teach regarding the possibilities and limits of legal and institutional change and the shape of those political compromises likely to prove necessary in transforming social or philosophical ideals into practical realities. The value of such efforts is compellingly demonstrated by the intriguing legal, political, and institutional analysis proposed by Franklin Zimring (chapter 14). The essays by Toulmin, Blumberg, and Zimring thus begin a novel and much-needed exploration of potential approaches all too often ignored by legal, economic, and policy analysts.

THE REGULATORY AND MORAL FRAMEWORKS

If we are prepared to conclude, on both instrumental and intrinsic grounds, that medical innovation should and will go forward in American society, we must recognize the existence of the risks, and indeed the costs in human injuries and suffering, entailed in that commitment. One partial response to that inescapable fact seeks to minimize the costs of accidents by curtailing unjustifiably risky innovative activities. The imposition of various legal controls exemplifies that strategy. There is, of course, a long-running debate over which methods of control are best, pitting adherents of direct intervention through government regulations against those who favor the less direct controls and incentives associated with the potential for tort liability. That great debate cannot be resolved here, if indeed it is subject to resolution at all. Suffice it to say that neither approach seems likely to prevail exclusively, even in this era of deregulation. Nor could either approach do away with the problem of technological injuries without simultaneously closing down virtually all innovative activity. That outcome seems neither desirable nor plausible.

What remains is the painful question of how we are to look after persons unwittingly injured as an unavoidable by-product of our quest for progress. Are those persons regretfully, yet firmly, to be left by the wayside as progress marches on? Or can and should we as a society find some way to share with them, in more than a theoretical sense, the collective benefits that accrue to the rest of us from our societal commitment to innovation—the very commitment to which they were sacrificed? My approach is animated by two convictions: first, that it is right that we tax ourselves to provide for those from whose sacrifice we derive benefits;[4] and, second, that a prudent and enduring societal commitment to desirable innovative activity cannot be built on a foundation of bodies broken by our technological failures and then left in neglect.

If we are to foster an environment conducive to continuing innovation in a just and honest society, two steps seem to me to be critical: first, an enhanced commitment to acquiring the data necessary to document and clarify the social costs, as well as the benefits, of our quest for technological progress; and, second, the maintenance of public confidence in and support for the technological enterprise by treating its victims in a way that is, and is perceived as being, just and benevolent.

With respect to medical innovations specifically, the first step encompasses careful review and assessment of new medical technologies prior to their widespread and probably irreversible diffusion into routine use. Several contributors to this book have noted the very high proportion of currently accepted medical techniques that have never been adequately validated. They have stressed the difficulty, once the technology has spread into common use, of finding ethically acceptable ways to subject those techniques to proper scientific tests of safety, of efficacy, and, in the current environment, of cost-effectiveness or cost-benefit as well. My own judgment is that we would do well to adopt a much more expansive system of postmarketing surveillance and evaluation of drugs, medical devices, and innovative procedures. The adoption of such a system might, in fact, justify some adjustments to the FDA's current initial review process, with its widely decried regulatory delays, by establishing a system more capable of identifying and following up on potential side effects, including those with long latency periods, that might not be adequately recognized initially. The non-fault mechanism for compensation that I will discuss later would, as one of its important secondary effects, provide a useful vehicle for generating and keeping track of such data.

Second, I believe that continuing public support for medical innovation ultimately will (and should) depend upon the creation and fostering of a shared sense that we are, indeed, coventurers on a promising yet risky voyage of discovery and that we are mutually committed both to sharing the benefits equitably and to spreading the losses associated with injuries to individual victims. Means as well as ends are significant here: to be effective, the process should reflect a helping and communal rather than a mean and adversarial spirit. It is precisely this communal element that I find most strikingly lacking in much of the relevant law and economics literature, including some of the contributions to this book. In a society as stable and wealthy as our own, there is no compelling need to jettison the injured; we need not resort to lifeboat ethics. It is fundamentally a question of will, and of political, moral, and intellectual leadership, for our society to commit itself to realizing more fully those aspects of human sympathy, connectedness, and aspirations for community that have long been enshrined in both our religious traditions and our secular ideals. Those claiming such leadership—including scholars and intellectuals—cannot simply "leave to others the . . . difficult issues of equity and fairness" or consider questions of distribution of benefits and burdens "irrelevant" in a quest for a theoretical "optimal assignment of liability for accidents" (Danzon, chapter 13). Considerations of equity and fairness are central to the task of law in a democratic society. They should play a far greater role in shaping both our moral analysis and our public policy.

These concerns are especially compelling in the context of medical innovation and medical care more generally. Health and illness involve many fundamental human values and elicit precisely the connections of family, community, and therapeutic alliance just alluded to. Medical care thus provides a unique setting and opportunity for establishing and reinforcing these ties as a model for broader application throughout the society.

The point can be made negatively as well. We are all aware of the malignant growth of a new adversarial ethic within our system of medical care. Concerned with the rising tide of malpractice litigation, many physicians increasingly view their patients as potential adversaries. Some act accordingly, striving to minimize their potential liability, not necessarily in the fashion contemplated by proponents of improved quality of care. While the extent of the phenomenon is difficult to document or quantify, this concern with liability is believed to result in a variety of defensive practices engaged in principally "for the record" rather than for the well-being of the patient. Such practices impose unwarranted additional risks on the patient, as well as adding significantly to the cost of medical care. We would do well to reexamine any legal doctrine that encourages such practices.

In my view, we should move far more rapidly to explore alternative legal models that would reinforce, rather than undermine, those venerable medical traditions encouraging physicians to act as patient advocates rather than as potential adversaries of the patient. No legal regime will eliminate all instances of gross incompetence or recklessness, in medicine or in any other sphere of human conduct. In such cases, serious misconduct by the physician will and should continue to play some role in any plausible system of legal responsibility. But this need can be accommodated without necessarily retaining those elements of the present negligence malpractice system that are threatening the very foundations of the patient-physician relationship.

To be sure, creating an alternative to the present system will entail formidable administrative burdens and, most likely, economic costs; these must be carefully assessed and weighed in any ultimate calculus regarding significant legal reforms. Yet just as considerations of economic efficiency and administrative practicability should not be left out of that calculus, neither should the harder-to-quantify social and moral concerns. Too often such concerns *are* omitted from the analysis, perhaps because acknowledging their presence would make uncomfortably explicit the necessity for controversial value choices. Such choices cannot be escaped, although they can be obscured behind a facade of scientific objectivity.

How, then, should we approach the questions of whether and how to provide compensation to victims of our quest for medical progress? The chapters by legal scholars Richard Epstein (9) and Alexander M. Capron (10) focus primarily, indeed almost entirely, on remedies afforded by the existing tort system, with particular reference to theories of negligence and strict liability. But such theories sidestep the central issue—that the risk of injury is inherent in medical innovation, even when the innovative practice is conducted most carefully, with full attention to available knowledge, appropriate technique, and proper involvement of patients in the informed consent process. Injuries can and do occur without negligence, without apparent defect. If we nonetheless are convinced, after careful reflection, that compensation should be due when the inherent risks of the innovative enterprise miscarry, resulting, in Charles Gray's felicitous phrase, in a "failed project," then we can fairly conclude that the theories of recovery embodied in the existing law of tort fail to conform to our considered moral beliefs and thus may constitute morally as well as practically inadequate vehicles for providing such compensation. The next section of this chapter steps back a bit from the immediate debate to seek some perspective on why we and our system of tort law have come to this impasse.

THE IRRECONCILABLE CLAIMS OF COMPENSATION AND TORT DOCTRINE

THE LEGAL SETTING

Tort law, rather like classical drama, is characterized by certain fundamental unities, by confrontations in direct and relatively unmediated fashion between a victim and a tortfeasor in the setting of an isolated moral drama. Within that drama, the victim must demonstrate how the tortfeasor's actions caused his or her injury and why the costs associated with that injury should be shifted from the victim to the person who caused the injury. This particular form of drama is rooted in the early Anglo-American legal tradition, but it has correlates in many other legal systems, as Gray has so elegantly demonstrated (chapter 12).

Although the fundamental structure of this drama has remained relatively fixed, the legal principles that have been applied within it have evolved significantly over time. While historians continue to debate the particularities of given incidents, few would dispute that changes in legal doctrine have both influenced and reflected broader economic, political, and ideological tendencies, including changing social values and constructions of reality, within given societies. In England, the classic articulation of principles of strict liability arose in a dispute pitting a member of the emerging industrial sector against the entrenched interests of the landholding aristocracy. Attempts to explain the result, one favorable to the established land owners, in terms of the social and class backgrounds of the judges have proved unfounded; but the weaker claim, that the result is consonant with, and perhaps best explained by, more widespread English social values, retains its power.[5]

In the United States, the evolution of the industrial system and the rise of the railroad in the mid to late nineteenth century profoundly influenced the law's commitment to negligence principles, generally favoring the emerging capitalist class and fostering the nation's realization of its "Manifest Destiny." Once the nation's infrastructure was established and the destructive social consequences of this course became increasingly visible (in the form of industrial and other accidents), and as political alignments began to shift, significant countertrends emerged.

This development was perhaps most evident in the early part of the twentieth century, as successive state legislatures enacted statutory compensation programs for injured workers. These programs abandoned fault as the predicate for employer liability and abrogated what were termed the "unholy trinity" of tort defenses— notably, most instances of contributory negligence and assumption of risk, as well as the fellow-servant rule—which had previously posed such formidable obstacles to recoveries by injured workers.

In more recent decades, principles of strict liability have come to predominate over negligence for abnormally dangerous activities, and especially for defective products, and the defenses of contributory negligence and assumption of risk have been substantially narrowed or eliminated. Indeed, much has changed, probably far too much for those who saw in the fabric of prior tort doctrine an economically, socially, or morally optimal interweaving of certain traditional legal goals and con cerns. As that fabric has been rent by legal developments over the past century, particularly those in recent decades, it has become increasingly difficult to identify, let alone to preserve, the integrity of traditional tort doctrine.

The point is hardly a new one. As torts scholar John Fleming argued in a celebrated article a quarter century ago:

> In certain periods of the past, particularly during the nineteenth century, these apprehensions were accorded the fullest recognition in the interest of an acquisitive society bent on expansion and inclined to make light of the incidental cost to human and material assets. The subordination of the individual's security was deemed a necessary toll for achieving the more valuable goal of rapid industrial development and exploitation of the seemingly inexhaustible store of available resources. If injuries went without redress, it was but the victim's admission fee to participation in the larger benefits secured by advancing civilization. . . . But with the passage of time, these social postulates have undergone a drastic revision. The individualistic fault dogma is being eroded by the mid-twentieth century quest for social security, the welfare state replacing an outmoded order where man was expected and encouraged to fend for himself. Enhanced social consciousness has today led to the broad acceptance of the view that society can no longer afford to turn its back on the hapless victims of disaster or accident, leaving us only with the practical task of devising the economically least burdensome methods for redressing or mitigating their misfortune.[6]

THE EPSTEIN PROPOSAL

Epstein's analysis of the duty to warn of risks associated with biomedical innovations, and his urging that medical professionals and manufacturers of health care products be substantially insulated from potential liability so long as they recite government-approved warnings to patients and product users, must be evaluated against this background.

As I understand Epstein's proposal, seemingly concurred in by Patricia Danzon but questioned by Capron, formal disclosure of risk statements would be reviewed and approved (or perhaps drafted in the first instance) by the government and recited to all potential patients, with appropriate written documentation. This process would create a legal safe harbor for medical innovations in the event of bad outcomes for particular patients. The responsibilities of the medical team would apparently be satisfied, virtually in their entirety, by compliance with this duty to warn. Expressed somewhat differently, the patient would be considered to have assumed the risk of the medical innovation and would therefore be disqualified, as a matter of law, from pursuing compensation through the legal system.

The proposal is certainly a logical and coherent one, and it may seem particularly compelling to those not acquainted with the infamous history of the assumption-of-risk defense and the evolution of objections to it over the decades. As already noted, this defense played a prominent—perhaps preeminent—role in defeating the tort claims of injured workers against their employers (including employers who negligently maintained unsafe working conditions) in the nineteenth century. The revulsion it aroused helped to stimulate successful efforts to oust common-law tort principles from the work-place in favor of a non-fault-based system of workers' compensation. In other settings as well, the scope of the assumption-of-risk doctrine has been steadily eroded over succeeding decades. In recent years, most courts have discarded the doctrine almost entirely. What remains viable as a defense—at least in the negligence setting—are those unreasonable volitional decisions properly regarded as contributory or comparative negligence. Those decisions bear little resemblance to decisions by patients to follow their doctor's advice regarding innovative therapies. The legal system has thus moved firmly and consistently over many decades to reject precisely that doctrine which Epstein and Danzon seek to rehabilitate in modern guise. The rejection rests on a widely shared and well-founded perception that the assumption-of-risk defense is readily susceptible to being—and often has been—unfairly and unrealistically invoked to deny the socially mandated compensatory goals of the tort system. Any broad reassertion of the defense must bear the heavy burden of responding to these arguments from history and policy.

The role of the duty to warn, and correspondingly of a narrower conception of express assumption of risk following adequate warnings, has evolved somewhat differently in the context of product-related injuries, in which strict liability principles rather than negligence have come to predominate. In limited circumstances, primarily those in which product defects cannot reasonably be prevented without destroying the utility of the product, courts have permitted manufacturers to satisfy their legal duties by providing adequate warnings to consumers. It would, however, be a consid-erable oversimplification to suggest—as Epstein's proposal seems to do—that risk disclosure does or should serve in all instances as a full and complete substitute for making products safe in the first instance. The implicit suggestion that medical innovators should be insulated from tort liability for defective innovations (and perhaps even for negligence in choosing to go forward with unduly risky innovations) solely on the basis of a government-certified warning simply cannot be reconciled with the thrust of recent developments in tort law, developments amply supported by legal and policy justifications set forth in detail in numerous judicial opinions and scholarly treatises. And one cannot help noting in passing the endearing trust in gov-ernmental omnipotence inherent in the proposal's reliance on government-authored or -approved disclosure statements, a trust not always associated with either the law and economics movement or with lawyers or economists making their intellectual home at the University of Chicago. Even unreconstructed New Dealers might have some difficulty mustering such enthusiasm following the swine flu experience.

Finally, it is worth drawing an explicit comparison between the conceptions of risk disclosure and assumption of risk set forth by Epstein and Danzon and the evolving doctrine of informed consent as applied to medical treatment and research. The legal doctrine of informed consent has developed in response to powerful social and judicial perceptions of unequal knowledge and power in the physician-patient and investigator-subject relationships. The doctrine is intended as a source of enhanced protection for the patient-subject's well-being and autonomy and is properly understood as a necessary, but not sufficient, condition for therapeutic or research interventions. The informed consent of the patient will not necessarily excuse a negligent treatment recommendation by the physician; nor, in the research setting, will the subject's informed consent legally justify the conduct of research properly rejected by an institutional review board on scientific or risk-benefit grounds. Respect for autonomy is indeed an important value, but it is not the only value in medical or research settings. Further, there are numerous reasons, many of them usefully canvassed by Capron, for concern about the adequacy of existing informed consent processes, particularly in the context of medical innovations. Epstein's proposal would do little to allay these general concerns and would transform informed consent from an added layer of protection for patients' interests into a weapon to be used against them in the event of injury.[7] To justify this step on the ground that the patient, rather than the physician or researcher or manufacturer, is somehow better situated to make the scientific risk-benefit calculation regarding use of the product or innovation is to turn the behavioral assumptions underlying informed consent on their heads with no logical or empirical support whatever.[8]

This theoretical analysis is perhaps best illustrated by discussion of an actual case, and the particular case mentioned by Epstein provides as good an example as any. *Reyes* v. *Wyeth Laboratories, Inc.*[9] involved a lawsuit on behalf of a young girl who developed polio after having been given the oral polio vaccine. While a good deal of expert testimony suggested that the girl had contracted a wild strain of polio, not one related to the vaccine, the girl's physician testified otherwise. The physician's testimony apparently was convincing to the jury, which found for the plaintiff and awarded substantial damages against the manufacturer of the vaccine. The verdict was predicated on a failure to warn theory, not on allegations that the vaccine was negligently manufactured. The verdict favoring recovery was then upheld by the appellate court in an opinion by John Minor Wisdom.

Judge Wisdom's decision has been the subject of much scholarly commentary, and I am not surprised that Epstein, as the editor of a renowned torts casebook, takes the legal doctrine of the case seriously indeed. That is entirely appropriate: the *Reyes* case and others that have followed it have transformed the legal environment in which vaccines are manufactured and distributed. The doctrine deserves to be taken seriously, and I agree with

Epstein's conclusion that, for better or worse, the legal principles enunciated in Judge Wisdom's opinion mark a departure from prior tort law. What I find more remarkable, however, is what is left out of Epstein's discussion: namely, some account of our societal response, as reflected through the legal system, to the plight of a young girl afflicted with polio. Perhaps—and here I am speculating—Judge Wisdom's novel legal analysis was prompted by his own human response to the failure of conventional legal doctrine to provide an adequate remedy. On this view of the case, the central issue was not the theoretical "economics of information transfer," but the very real plight of the individual in need and the lack of other mechanisms to help her. Two passages in the opinion support this reading. First, there is an explicit judicial recognition that other, arguably more appropriate responses are unavailable:

> It can also be argued, of course, that since all society benefits from universal immunization against infectious disease, the loss should be borne by the local, state or federal government. Unless the doctrine of sovereign immunity is signifcantly altered, however, such a loss distribution scheme does not appear to be likely.[10]

Second, Judge Wisdom sets forth an explicit, although hardly uncontroversial, view of the appropriate role of courts and judge-made common law in such circumstances:

> Until Americans have a comprehensive scheme of social insurance, courts must resolve by a balancing process the head-on collision between the need for adequate recovery and viable enterprises. . . . [A] strong argument can be advanced that the loss ought not to lie where it falls (on the victim), but should be borne by the manufacturer as a foreseeable cost of doing business, and passed on to the public in the form of price increases to his customers.[11]

To be sure, some may argue that Judge Wisdom's humanity got the better of his intellect, or invoke the familiar nostrum that hard cases make bad law. But that, I believe, would miss the point. Whatever academic commentators think of Judge Wisdom's modification of prior tort doctrine, other judges have followed and, indeed, extended his lead. The entire episode exemplifies the transformation of modern tort law from a system that often seemed designed to manufacture obstacles to recovery by injured victims toward a system increasingly determined to provide compensation to the injured and to spread the losses associated with the risks of our technological way of life. The modern system represents, at the least, a different balancing of the multiple objectives of a system of tort law. This new primacy of the compensation objective and the downgrading in salience of traditional concepts of fault reflects changing perceptions by both the legal profession and the society at large. In the modern period, "public convenience does *not* outweigh individual compensation [emphasis added]."[12]

IMPLICATIONS

If this analysis is correct, then repeated calls for a return to the true faith, to the integrity of traditional tort doctrine, are simply out of step with evolving social norms favoring more expansive compensation. Efforts to yoke the two together within the tort framework are doomed to incoherence.

That is not to say that tort law should be abandoned in favor of an all-purpose non-fault compensation system, or even to assert that Judge Wisdom's resolution of the *Reyes* case represents the socially ideal resolution of the problem of vaccine injuries. I do not believe that Judge Wisdom's imposition of liability on the vaccine manufacturer for failure to meet a nearly impossible to satisfy duty to warn achieves any such ideal, either with respect to vaccine injuries or to injuries associated with medical innovations more generally. (Nor, I suspect, does Judge Wisdom.) At a doctrinal level, I consider this legal innovation to be questionable, at least as a permanent fixture. But I am also inclined to see additional layers of meaning in Judge Wisdom's approach. His decision gives powerful voice to evolving societal attitudes toward the compensation objective, and, still more significantly, it prods other potential actors in this drama (health officials, legislators, pharmaceutical companies, and representatives of the insurance industry) to take the problem of vaccine injuries more seriously, thereby spurring development of alternative, and probably preferable, means of providing compensation.[13] Indeed, many commentators with diverse ideological perspectives, including those represented in this book, seem now to agree on the desirability and practicality of a non-fault mechanism for compensating vaccine injuries, and the legislative enactment of such a proposal has become a distinct possibility. One may doubt whether this congruence could or would have been achieved in the absence of Judge Wisdom's departure from conventional wisdom in *Reyes*. Similarly, other recent doctrinal innovations in tort law may perhaps best be understood as temporary but nonetheless necessary prods to rethink conventional modes of dealing with compensation for accidental injuries, particularly those associated with technological innovations.[14]

Contrast with this analysis an alternative approach based on the theory of "*ex ante* consent and assumption of risk" or of "the optimal economics of information transfer." Does it not strain credulity to believe that an educational informed consent campaign would, or should, discourage large numbers of children, or their parents, from participating in immunization programs— particularly when participation is publicly mandated or legally required for entry into schools? In such cases, to deny compensation for known risks of immunization on grounds of assumption of risk is to push beyond legal fiction into the realm of collective fantasy. The relevant question is whether we are prepared to assume and spread the costs of socially desirable activities—public health immunization programs or medical innovations more generally—or prefer instead to visit their financial consequences, as well as the unavoidable physical injuries, on random victims who have done nothing worse than follow the advice of their physicians and their government—and then to add insult to injury by blaming them for doing so. That is, I fear, what the alternative approach comes down to. It is an approach we must reject, even if that course is not economically "optimal."

TOWARD A MODEST PROPOSAL

Most analysts of the tort system believe that it does and should serve important social purposes in addition to providing compensation to injured victims; some argue that these other goals should predominate. The system should provide, *inter alia*, appropriate incentives for safety (what Calabresi has called the "maximum reduction of the sum of accident costs and the costs of avoiding accidents that can be accomplished in a just way"[15]), a means for social expression of the priority of safety goals, and a vehicle for holding morally and financially accountable those who engage in unacceptably risky and antisocial conduct. These goals are important ones, but under modern conditions they are increasingly at war with emerging social attitudes favoring compensation. Any single system aimed at pursuing all these goals simultaneously is likely to become intolerably complex, convoluted, and chaotic. In the view of many, that is an apt characterization of the current state of tort law.

Perhaps the time has come to ask some fundamental questions and to contemplate proposals for systemic reform.[16] I believe that such proposals offer the only hope of simultaneously meeting our felt obligations to provide compensation to injured victims in accordance with current social values and of providing a context in which the other important purposes of tort law can be pursued effectively and with intellectual and practical coherence. I am also convinced that such proposals offer greater promise of successfully addressing the special characteristics of maloccurrences associated with medical innovations than the more traditional tort theories discussed by Epstein and Capron. While (for reasons explored with great insight by Zimring and discussed further near the end of this chapter) I do not expect ready adoption of these proposals, particularly in the limited context of biomedical innovations, I consider it imperative to expand the range of discourse beyond that assumed by several of the other contributors to this book.

What I want to suggest is that the integrity of tort doctrine will remain endangered as long as we fail to provide some adequate alternative means, consistent with evolving norms of basic decency and human dignity, for meeting the needs of people suffering serious injuries. If we remain wedded to the classical unities of tort litigation, particularly to the nexus by which the victim's ability to recover compensation is directly tied to the court's ability and willingness to assess the tortfeasor for those costs, then the felt imperative for providing for victims is unlikely to be adequately reconciled with the other goals of the tort system. If there is to be a reconciliation, it must be founded on a new and different mix of compensatory and regulatory policies, a mix not governed by the fundamental unities of traditional tort litigation.

The framework I propose as a basis for further exploration and debate would entail the creation of a special compensation fund which would utilize separate processes to achieve the compensatory and regulatory objectives of the program. The fund might be private, quasi-public, or governmental in character and might be limited to narrow categories of risks or integrated into a more comprehensive, societywide program of social insurance. Compensation awards would be provided to individual victims, in the first instance, according to non-fault principles. Recoveries would be less than those provided to successful litigants in tort actions, perhaps approximating those now provided by the federal and more generous state workers' compensation plans. Claims would be processed within an administrative structure similar to those that handle first-person health and disability insurance or governmental social insurance claims. Ideally, this relatively efficient and inexpensive administrative structure would permit claims to be handled expeditiously and benefits to be paid out speedily, maximizing the rehabilitative potential of the claimant and returning that individual to customary activities quickly and without the need for lengthy litigation prior to receipt of basic compensation. In its broad outline, the compensatory aspect of this approach bears a close relationship to the Accident Compensation Act now in effect in New Zealand.

How would the compensation fund be financed? That is a critical matter for social choice. Most simply, the system could be funded entirely out of general revenues. That approach would not, however, best promote the regulatory objectives of the system, and it is not the course I would endorse. A second possibility, which would retain many aspects of current tort law, would be to subrogate the compensation fund to the tort claims of the accident victim, thus permitting the fund, rather than the victim, to proceed against the tortfeasor. The fact that the victim had already been compensated would be known to both court and jury, thus ameliorating any problems of excessive jury sympathy for the plight of the victim in the trial of the case. This approach would substantially reduce or eliminate the system's dependence on contingent fee arrangements and would do much to promote the orderly trial or settlement of most claims. The system could thus promote many of the worthy goals of the tort system in a far more coherent fashion than is currently possible, and it might even serve to restore something of the integrity of traditional tort doctrine. To be sure, the compensation fund would most likely not recover its full costs, in which event additional methods would be required to cover the shortfall.

To this end, or as an alternative approach to financing the entire system, a mechanism could be devised to secure complete or partial funding on a class, rather than an individual case basis. A mandatory surcharge might be imposed on designated innovative procedures, perhaps in the form of required first-party private insurance, perhaps as a required contribution to a governmental fund. The surcharge would fall initially on the patient but might be covered through other health insurance mechanisms or subsidized with public funds in those instances in which the government wishes to promote the particular innovation. Alternatively, to reduce administrative costs and burdens, taxes might be levied directly on those conducting innovative activities, to be recovered through higher prices for medical products and services. Still another possibility would be for the compensation fund to pursue a new form of quasi-tort actions against classes of activities that create risks of injury.

At least in theory, such approaches to financing the system could be calibrated to provide suitable incentives for safety. There would be no need to show a close causal nexus to injuries in particular cases. What is fundamental is that the system would disengage the provision of compensation to injured persons from the mechanisms for charging the costs of those injuries to those whom society decides to hold financially responsible.

In addition to providing compensation on a more just basis, such a system could provide an important institutional mechanism for accumulating data on risks associated with medical and other technological innovations. It would permit issues of causation to be treated in ways that are more consistent with the epidemiological and philosophical perspectives presented so compellingly by Kenneth Schaffner (chapter 6). Finally, the system could be structured to permit additional (punitive or quasi-punitive) damages to be collected, either through the compensation fund or perhaps by individual plaintiffs, in cases in which society wishes to say something special about faulty or grossly improper behavior on the part of the tortfeasor.

In moving to this sort of system, society would have to face a number of fundamental questions that are largely finessed in a tort system characterized by the classical unities. To illustrate, one might compare the status of claims for compensation, none involving allegations of unprofessional conduct, that might be advanced by three young women with adenocarcinoma: the first, a DES (diethylstilbestrol) daughter whose claim is advanced following publication of studies documenting the relationship of DES exposure to that disease; the second, a DES daughter whose claim is being considered prior to proof of the connection; and the third, a woman whose mother did *not* take DES and whose disease cannot be explained by any known or suspected linkage to any human agency. Is it clear that any one of these women should have a greater claim to assistance, judged on its intrinsic nature? Should the fact of injury as opposed to illness, or of known human agency as opposed to fate, justify differential treatment? Or might we ultimately believe that the fact of adenocarcinoma (and the need it generates) should be the only, or at least the principal, test of eligibility for assistance? That is, do we ultimately wish to compensate for harms, or only for wrongs? I cannot fully address these questions here, but I do wish to suggest that adoption of the proposed approach would make it more difficult to avoid them and other questions growing out of this book's themes of causation, liability, and responsibility. We would do well to begin to consider these questions.

First, with respect to causation, it seems most unlikely that the world is so organized as to assist us in identifying single, deterministic "causes" of many of the injuries and illnesses with which we are concerned. Existing science—and perhaps the very nature of reality—may correspond poorly with the law's traditional requirements for proof of causation in such situations. But that realization may well foster a fruitful if unaccustomed inquiry: Why need we be concerned with causation in that narrow sense? To the degree that our concern is to identify those products and activities (and those combinations of them) that increase the probability of future injury to the population at large or to specified subpopulations, statistical methodologies that do not focus on causation in an individual case may be perfectly appropriate to our needs. The backward-looking tasks of assessing liability and providing compensation require individualized causal determinations in the traditional tort system, but they need not do so in the proposed alternative. We could simply decide to provide compensation from a central fund based on the fact of injury and to assess liability in relation to overall statistical patterns of contribution to increased risk over a *class* of cases, without the need for complex and expensive individualized determinations. This capacity might be especially relevant for classes of injury associated with multifactorial causation or synergistic effects. While the results would likely be rough-and-ready rather than finely honed, they would be no more imprecise than many traditional or emerging techniques in the law, which have rarely functioned at the level of conventional norms of scientific certainty. (Thus, the law is more inclined to utilize formulas such as "more likely than not" than to test hypotheses for significance at the 5 percent level!) The traditional focus on individualized cause in tort law is, in many current contexts, expensive, uncertain, and unnecessary to our larger objectives. It has become dysfunctional and should be changed or abandoned.

Second, with respect to legal liability, the tort system has already abandoned, in a great many contexts, even the pretense that ultimate liability rests on the outcome of a close moral inquiry into the fault of the actor. In such fields as product liability and abnormally dangerous activities, strict liability is imposed in accordance with a variety of social objectives that may bear little or no relationship to fault as traditionally conceived. Even in those areas in which negligence principles continue to hold sway, it is increasingly clear that the real party in interest in much tort litigation is the insurance company, not the named defendant. The moral relevance of the connection between the insured's fault and the insurance company's obligation to pay is obscure at best. While experience-rated policies and the emergence of self-insurance may limit the scope of this conclusion in some settings, the costs of liability only rarely reflect the degree of moral culpability.

What is perhaps most troubling about this phenomenon is that, as the law has moved away from traditional conceptions of fault as the true basis for tort liability, lawyers have not always made clear to the broader public the growing distinction between legal liability and moral responsibility. The public may be too quick to conclude that persons found legally liable are necessarily also morally blameworthy. This observation may be especially relevant to the current medical malpractice situation, in which juries seem often to stretch norms of professional conduct in order to facilitate compensation of needy plaintiffs. While humanly understandable, such decisions are likely to be accompanied by unjustified stigmatization of the professional reputation and competence of the defendant and to reinforce the adversarial aspects of the physician-patient relationship. Perhaps an alternative approach, one that enlisted the physician as patient advocate and did not, even nominally, require assertions of malpractice as a predicate for recovery, would promote a healthier relationship.

With respect to responsibility, it is undoubtedly true that tort litigation, despite its increasing attention to compensation and incentive objectives, retains a dimension of primitive justice or vengeance. As so vividly documented by Gray, this punitive element has a powerful hold, transcending our own culture, time, and place. I suspect that efforts to divest the system of this residual moral element would be unavailing, as well, perhaps, as ill-advised. That said, it does not follow that its current scope is necessarily optimal. I would be inclined to retain a place for fault— more properly, for some concept of aggravated fault—but only with respect to clear deviations from socially mandated standards of behavior, not for what are today close jury questions on whether basic compensation is to be provided.[17] While such an approach is not plausible today, it might become so if basic compensation were provided in an assured, alternative fashion.

On Idealism and Practical Politics

Assuming the merits of my modest proposal, is there any reason to believe that such an approach might be susceptible to legislative adoption? If so, in what form? I have argued that a number of considerations, some of them unique to the domain of medical innovations, justify the exploration, and perhaps the creation, of an alternative system of compensation for victims of medical innovation, what has sometimes been termed a "tailored" or "categorical" compensation system. Detailed efforts to structure an analogous scheme for the narrower domain of research injuries are documented in a three-volume report by the President's Commission for the Study of Ethical Problems in Medicine and Biomedical and Behavioral Research.[18] Similar proposals have been developed to provide compensation for injuries associated with immunizations and vaccines, particularly in the context of mandated public health measures. Commentators representing diverse ideological starting points have coalesced in finding moral and economic policy justifications for non-fault compensation programs for vaccine injuries and, to perhaps a lesser degree, injuries associated with so-called nontherapeutic research. The rationales for such positions are reviewed by Capron.

While the constellation of forces favoring the substitution of a tailored compensation system for tort liability in the vaccine field may yet prove sufficient to win enactment, I am dubious, for reasons substantially similar to those adduced by Zimring, that medical research and nonvaccine medical innovations more generally are politically promising candidates for legislative action. The magnitude of the problem is not sufficient, the intellectual and practical problems of implementation too formidable, the community of supporters too fragmented, and the political and budgetary environments too hostile to entertain even a flicker of optimism.

The problem of injuries associated with medical innovations bears a close relationship, however, to two other areas of current social concern in which the likelihood of systemic reform appears considerably more promising. First, as the medical malpractice system continues its steady descent toward intellectual incoherence and practical collapse and as Band-Aid modifications are demonstrated to be inefficacious in curing the system's underlying ills, the antagonists may come to see the wisdom of a basic rethinking of the system's needs and objectives and possess the political strength to prompt legislative action. On a second front—the emerging field of technological torts associated with the multifarious hazards of workplace and environment—the size, cost, and complexity of existing tort litigation, in conjunction with efforts by corporate defendants to seek shelter under provisions of the bankruptcy laws, may yet lead to scandalous breakdowns and public demands for major institutional reforms. If systemic reform should occur in either of these contexts, injuries associated with medical innovations might well be brought along as stepchildren into a new legal structure. A tailored compensation plan addressed generally to medical injuries or technological torts is perhaps less likely to resolve ideally the niceties unique to medical innovations, but it is considerably more likely to win legislative enactment.

As the political pendulum swings back, one might also contemplate a broader set of changes in social welfare legislation. Such changes would provide more adequately for income substitution and health care and rehabilitative costs for those wholly or partially disabled, without regard to the occasions creating such need. This system could supplement the system of tort or compensation law—or, indeed, substitute for it, at least in its compensatory function. New Zealand's decision to limit its innovative non-fault-based compensation system to injuries caused by accident and to exclude from coverage certain other misfortunes of life (specifically including illness) can only be understood in the context of that nation's social welfare system. That system provides far more comprehensive and generous coverage for illness than the patchwork of social insurance provisions now applicable in the United States. Were such extensive coverage currently in place in the United States, I doubt that the debate in these pages would be so heated or so necessary.[19]

While I would applaud movement toward a more comprehensive system of social entitlements in this country, both on its intrinsic merit and as a preferable substitute for or supplement to the compensatory function of the tort system, this more comprehensive system would do little, in itself, to promote other important goals of tort law—either in providing appropriate incentives for safety or in meting out justice to blameworthy tortfeasors. While there is ample room for skepticism as to how well existing tort law satisfies these goals, they remain appropriate goals for some instrument of social policy. A fully articulated non-fault model—one developed with far greater specificity than possible within the compass of this essay, or, indeed, this book—would necessarily have to address those difficult issues in some detail.

Tort law has a long and venerable history. It has served the needs of our society, for better or worse, for many generations. But tort principles arose in a world very different from our own in material circumstances, scientific understanding, pace of change, and social ideals. Tort law is a tool of human society, not its master. If we are to face the moral, social, and economic demands presented by biomedical innovation, as well as other innovative and risky activities, we should not allow our imaginations to be bound by past solutions. Law, like medicine, is capable of innovation. To be sure, legal innovations, like scientific ones, may be subject to their own Daedalus effect. The suggestions set forth here carry their own risks of unintended consequences. Yet they do so in the service of a moral vision that, for me at least, offers greater inspiration than the competing vision of the law and economics scholars. If this vision is not yet capable of being realized, it is perhaps still useful as a reminder of, and stimulus to, our higher aspirations as compassionate individuals and as a caring community. Intellectual leaders might well consider the enduring social costs of abandoning those aspirations.

NOTES

1. *Russell* v. *Men of Devon*, 100 Eng. Rep. 359, 362 (1798).
2. Marshall Shapo, *A Nation of Guinea Pigs: The Unknown Risks of Chemical Technology* (New York: Free Press, 1979)

3. These costs may be reflected industrywide in higher charges for insurance or self-insurance and then passed on as some combination of lower returns to investors, lower wages for workers, and higher prices for consumers.

4. I do not mean to suggest that our obligations can necessarily be satisfied exclusively through the payment of money. But in a society like our own, money is the measure of most, if not all, things, including redress for physical injury. Those who would deny the provision of financial compensation to the injured should bear the burden of justifying an alternative approach.

5. *Rylands* v. *Fletcher*, L.R. 3 H.L. 330 (1868). See Francis H. Bohlen, "The Rule in *Rylands* v. *Fletcher*," *University of Pennsylvania Law Review* 59(1911):298-326, 373-93, 423-53; Robert Thomas Molloy, "*Fletcher* v. *Rylands*: A Reexamination of Juristic Origins," *University of Chicago Law Review* 9(February 1942):266-92; Clarence Morris and C. Robert Morris, Jr., *Morris on Torts*, 2nd ed. (Mineola: Foundation Press, 1980), pp. 232-33.

6. John G. Fleming, "The Passing of *Polemis*," *Canadian Bar Review* 39(December 1961):489-529, pp. 505-6.

7. It must, of course, be recognized that, under some extraordinary conditions, recourse even to dangerous and relatively untried innovations may be urgently desired by both physician and fully informed patient. The requirement of compensation for known risks may impose unsustainable costs on the process and perhaps go beyond any social consensus favoring its provision. The implantation of artificial hearts in desperately ill, imminently dying patients may provide an example, although hardly one free of controversy in its own right. In such highly unusual circumstances, there may be a more persuasive, although still troubling, case for relying on concepts of risk disclosure, informed consent, and the assumption of certain risks of uncompensated bad outcomes. That case, however, must be balanced against the serious concern that this approach would unduly promote the premature application of untested technologies to desperate patients.

   Even then, one would need to engage in a far more searching process of disclosure and consent than has characterized even some of the most highly publicized innovations in recent medical history. One might usefully contrast the distressingly limited nature of the informed consent processes in Christiaan Barnard's early heart transplants or in Denton Cooley's implantation of an artificial heart in Haskell Karp with the far more extensive, although still imperfect, educational process developed for Barney Clark at the University of Utah. [For documentation and masterful analyses of the failings of informed consent in the early heart cases, see Renée C. Fox and Judith Swazey, "The Case of the Artificial Heart," in *The Courage to Fail: A Social View of Organ Transplants and Dialysis*, 2nd ed., rev. (Chicago: University of Chicago Press, 1978), pp. 135-97, and Jay Katz, *The Silent World of Doctor and Patient* (New York: Free Press, 1984).]

   Whether such extraordinary cases are sufficiently frequent or compelling to justify the elaboration of a different set of compensation rules and procedures, or to incur the administrative costs and burdens of resolving problematic issues of classification, is a difficult problem, defying armchair empiricism. Perhaps within this quite limited sphere, Epstein's proclivity for contractual solutions might find its most persuasive application.

8. Richard Epstein defends his reliance on the assumption-of-risk defense by asserting that "the defense is required by the principle of individual autonomy" and that what he identifies as "the weakness of the defense," namely, the risk of imperfect information, can be corrected by government-approved warnings (chapter 11, note 7). I disagree on both counts.

To be sure, the assumption-of-risk defense bears some relationship to powerful principles of individual autonomy and personal responsibility for one's actions. But it does not follow that the defense is "required" by these principles. As a society, we have long distinguished our legal responses to some exercises of autonomy, for example, decisions by explorers and adventurers to scale mountain peaks, parachute from tall structures, or encounter obvious risks of amusement park rides, from certain other important life choices, most notably decisions by workers to encounter known risks of hazardous lines of employment. We have also marked an important distinction in permitting individuals to embark upon dangerous courses of action while constraining their ability to relinquish certain protections provided by law. The workplace example is again instructive: we respect the freedom of individuals to choose a hazardous line of work (and to contract for "risk premiums" increasing their remuneration) but do not generally permit employers and employees to "contract out" of socially mandated compensation programs in the event these risks eventuate in injuries. Thus, even when we believe fairness *ex ante* has been approximated, we retain a social interest in the fairness of outcomes *ex post.*

Further, there is little reason to believe that this felt social commitment would be abrogated by improved warnings. One may fairly doubt whether the erection of large signs reading, "Abandon hope all ye who enter here," over the entrance gates of factories—or hospitals and clinics—would or should serve to immunize those who cause injuries from potential liability. The argument that informed participation in contemporary civilization necessarily constitutes an assumption of all the risks inherent in modern life simply does not extend so far.

Thus, contrary to Epstein's suggestion, the risk of imperfect information has not been the sole, or necessarily even the primary, weakness of the assumption-of-risk defense. The troubling issues have not concerned whether the isolated (even if fully informed) individual autonomously accepts the terms of a proffered bargain; they have involved the substantive terms of that bargain, how those terms are set, and the context in which the decision is made. While the multifarious settings in which these questions have arisen have proved recalcitrant to any overarching theoretical formulation, the courts have been alert to disparities in power and bargaining position, the possibilities of overreaching and abuse by the stronger party, the dependency of the weaker party, and the nature and importance of the interests at stake. Here, as elsewhere, the law has proceeded case by case, reflecting societal perceptions and values; the question for us is where to place the situation of endangered patients along these several spectrums.

The persons we are talking about here—patients confronting difficult choices about innovative therapies—often face limited, unpleasant, and sometimes dismal alternatives and must make choices under constraints imposed by their disease and the limits of available knowledge and technology. It does not follow that their decisions are necessarily involuntary or coerced or lacking in autonomy, or that these individuals should not be able to choose; but one may well ask how their exercises of autonomy compare to the idealized image of adventurers deciding whether to assault a dangerous mountain, and consider how the choices put to them are most justly framed. In such circumstances society may well wish to say, "The decision whether to accept the risks of physical injury is and must be yours, but the decision whether any injury must go uncompensated need not be implicated in your decision and is properly a matter for *social* choice."

The National Aeronautics and Space Administration might well have been able to recruit astronauts interested in a one-way trip to the moon, or willing, as a condition of employment, to sign away any claims for injury or death in the event of an accident. Such a practice may well save the government money, and it would respect the autonomy of the participants. I suspect most of us would not endorse such an arrangement, viewing it as unnecessary and incompatible with our social ideals. Just as we would be reluctant to ask such an unnecessary sacrifice from an astronaut, so we might conclude, for the reasons discussed here and elsewhere in this book, that it would be a poor idea to demand such a sacrifice from participants in innovative medical activities. Or we might not. But that is the question for decision. Ritual incantations of individual autonomy and the principle of assumption of risk beg that question, they do not answer it.

9. 498 F. 2d 1264 (5th Cir. 1974), *cert. denied*, 419 U.S. 1096.
10. 498 F. 2d, p. 1294, note 57.
11. 498 F. 2d, p. 1294.
12. *Muskopf* v. *Corning Hospital District*, 55 Cal. 2d 211, 359 P. 2d 457, p. 459 (1961) (Traynor, J.).
13. Some pharmaceutical companies have responded to the expanded potential for tort liability by withdrawing from the manufacture of one or more vaccines. The resulting threat to the availability of vaccines has served to place the compensation issue high on the agenda of public health and other government officials and may ultimately contribute to the adoption of an alternative compensation scheme. While the path is perhaps more circuitous than might have been anticipated at the time of Judge Wisdom's decision, the destination is the same.
14. Richard Epstein (chapter 11, note 18) appears to misapprehend the point of my argument here, and some response may help to clarify the nature, and limits, of our disagreement.

My point is expressly *not* that the substantive rule of law announced by Judge Wisdom in *Reyes* and followed in subsequent cases constitutes the ideal permanent resolution to the problem of vaccine injuries. Indeed, I am inclined to agree with Epstein's observation that, under this approach, "the theory of improper warnings becomes an elaborate, expensive, and erratic pretext for compensation for bad outcomes alone." My difference with Epstein concerns what should flow from that observation. Epstein bemoans the bias of the "modern common law . . . intensified by the discretion left to juries, toward finding all warnings inadequate when judged by the standard of hindsight," but he never seems to consider just why judges, juries, and indeed the "modern common law" might be drawn to this result or whether they might be trying to tell us something. In particular, they may be reflecting a social judgment that in such circumstances "bad outcomes alone" *ought* to be compensated, although perhaps not at exorbitant levels. In the absence of a simple, honest, and straightforward program designed to provide such compensation outside the tort system, the use of "pretexts" within that system may be about the best the common law can provide.

The genius of Judge Wisdom's resolution is that it does more than that; it shifts the burden of seeking a sensible legislative resolution away from isolated and largely powerless injured plaintiffs (and trial lawyers who may have their own reasons for resisting an administrative compensation program) to potential defendants—pharmaceutical companies and the insurance industry—who are far better situated to place the matter high on the legislative agenda. My defense of Judge Wisdom's approach thus rests not only on its provision of an imperfect, second-best remedy for individual plaintiffs, but on an appreciation of its dynamic potential to stimulate additional desirable changes in the law. I quite agree with Epstein that if Epstein's separate arguments against the creation of a non-fault compensation system for injuries associated with medical innovations are heeded (and applied to the vaccine context), and if pharmaceutical companies respond to a continuation of the existing legal regime by withdrawing from the vaccine market, injurious social consequences will follow. That, for me, is an argument in favor of a non-fault compensation system (which I believe will eventually be adopted, at least in the limited context of vaccine injuries) and not an argument against Judge Wisdom's attempt to prod government policymakers toward resolving these issues.

[It is perhaps worth noting in passing, with respect to the withdrawal of some pharmaceutical manufacturers and insurers from the vaccine market, that Epstein's interesting analysis of the economic basis for this phenomenon is no less speculative than an alternative hypothesis. That hypothesis would view these highly publicized actions as carefully considered elements of a longer-term political strategy designed to frighten and intimidate policymakers, physicians, and the public into reshaping the governing legal regime into a configuration limiting potential liability and precluding injured victims from seeking even such redress as is now erratically available. Recent events suggest that such a strategy, if it exists, has found a receptive environment in the current political climate.]

Finally, Epstein's comments regarding the so-called we-they dimension of the vaccine injury problem once again obscure the distinction between *ex ante* and *ex post* analysis. Judged *after the fact*, it is simply not true that, in the absence of compensation, "reducing the overall level of illness leaves *everyone* better off." Those few who would not have developed the disease and who take the vaccine, suffer a vaccine-related injury, and are not compensated are *not* better off after the fact. The critical issue is *not*, as Epstein suggests, the *individual's* choice "between a 10 percent chance of the natural disease and a 0.1 percent chance of vaccine injury"; rather, it is the *social* choice with respect to our responsibilities toward that unfortunate 0.1 percent: Should we as a society, who benefit after the fact from this and other medical innovations, share some small portion of the value of our real benefits with those who *might* have benefited, but who *in fact* suffered real injuries? Further, if the test is minimization of avoidable injuries and illness, as Epstein seems to suggest, I am inclined to think that a public health program coupled with an adequate, non-fault compensation mechanism would secure greater public participation and accompanying public health benefits (although probably at greater budgetary cost) than the legal regime advocated by Epstein, which rests on the asserted desirability of putting worried parents to an unnecessary choice between foregoing an apparently beneficial vaccine and accepting the risks not only of serious possible injury to their children, but of social abandonment in the name of respecting their "autonomy."

15. Guido Calabresi, *The Costs of Accidents: A Legal and Economic Analysis* (New Haven: Yale University Press, 1970), p. 31.

16. Important earlier studies raising such questions and advancing proposals for reform include Calabresi, *The Costs of Accidents*; Marc A. Franklin, "Replacing the Negligence Lottery: Compensation and Selective Reimbursement," *Virginia Law Review* 53(May 1967):774-814; Richard J. Pierce, Jr., "Encouraging Safety: The Limits of Tort Law and Government Regulation," *Vanderbilt Law Review* 33(November 1980):1281-1331; and the extensive writings of Robert Keeton and Jeffrey O'Connell on no-fault plans. More recently, a number of intriguing critiques of the tort law system and proposals for alternatives have been set forth in "Symposium: Alternative Compensation Schemes and Tort Theory," *California Law Review* 73(May 1985):548-1042. See especially Stephen D. Sugarman, "Doing Away With Tort Law," pp. 555-664. See also the symposium on "Catastrophic Personal Injuries," *Journal of Legal Studies* 13(August 1984): 415-622. Unfortunately, these stimulating collections arrived too late for consideration in the preparation of this chapter.

17. Compare John G. Fleming, " The Collateral Source Rule and Loss Allocation in Tort Law," *California Law Review* 54(1966):1478-1549; p. 1548:

If deterrence . . . has any continuing appeal as a justification for tort liability, it will be confined to situations where it can realistically perform an admonitory function, namely, only against defendants guilty of serious misconduct. Somewhat paradoxically, tort law would shrink, at least in this respect, to its original starting-point as an adjunct of the criminal law in sanctioning immoral conduct.

18. President's Commission for the Study of Ethical Problems in Medicine and Biomedical and Behavioral Research, *Compensating for Research Injuries*

(Washington, D.C.: Government Printing Office, 1982).
19. I am less hopeful than Zimring that the patchwork of public and private provisions in the United States will eventually mesh into an effective social safety net, and I despair at the manifest inconsistencies and irrationalities inherent in such a tattered fabric.

Index

About the Editors

MARK SIEGLER, M.D., a practicing physician, is Professor of Medicine and Director of the Center for Clinical Medical Ethics at the University of Chicago. He is a coauthor with A. R. Jonsen and W. J. Winslade of *Clinical Ethics: A Practical Approach to Ethical Decisions in Clinical Medicine* and a coeditor with E. J. Cassell of *Changing Values in Medicine.*

STEPHEN E. TOULMIN is Avalon Foundation Professor of the Humanities at Northwestern University and Assistant Director of the Center for Clinical Medical Ethics in the University of Chicago Department of Medicine. He was a staff member of the National Commission for the Protection of Human Research Subjects (1975-78) and has written extensively on ethics, philosophy of science, and history of ideas.

FRANKLIN E. ZIMRING is Professor of Law and Director of the Earl Warren Legal Institute at the University of California at Berkeley. Prior to 1985, he was Karl N. Llewellyn Professor of Jurisprudence and Director of the Center for Studies in Criminal Justice at the University of Chicago. He is a coauthor with Gordon Hawkins of *Capital Punishment and the American Agenda* and *The Citizen's Guide to Gun Control.*

KENNETH F. SCHAFFNER, M.D., is Professor of History and Philosophy of Science, Professor of Philosophy, and Adjunct Professor of Medicine at the University of Pittsburgh. He is currently Codirector of the University of Pittsburgh's Center for Medical Ethics and has been Chairman of its Department of History and Philosophy of Science. He served as Editor-in-Chief of *Philosophy of Science* from 1975 to 1980. He has written a number of papers on computer-assisted medical diagnosis and on causation in science and the law and is the editor of *Logic of Discovery and Diagnosis in Medicine.* With Siegler, he developed the initial research agenda for the Chicago EVIST project.